Lung Function In Health And Disease: Basic Concepts of Respiratory Physiology and Pathophysiology

Authored By

Camillo Peracchia & Nasr H. Anaizi

Department of Pharmacology and Physiology
University of Rochester, School of Medicine and Dentistry
601 Elmwood Ave.
Rochester, NY 14642-8711
USA

DEDICATION

To our wives Lillian Mae Leverone Peracchia and Fawzia Alsharif Anaizi

CONTENT

Foreword *i*

Preface *ii*

Introduction *iv*

CHAPTERS

1. **Historical Background** **3**
   Camillo Peracchia

2. **Basic Lung Structure** **35**
   Camillo Peracchia

3. **Respiratory Mechanics** **47**
   Camillo Peracchia

4. **Gas Exchange** **80**
   Camillo Peracchia

5. **Gas Transport** **100**
   Nasr H. Anaizi

6. **Acid-Base Balance** **122**
   Nasr H. Anaizi

7. **Ventilation-Perfusion Distribution, Blood Shunts and Alveolar Dead Space** **150**
   Camillo Peracchia

8. **Control of Breathing** **197**
   Nasr H. Anaizi

9. **Respiration at Rest and During Exercise at Sea Level and High Altitude** 215
Camillo Peracchia

10. **Functional Consequences of Respiratory Diseases** 233
Camillo Peracchia

Clinical Cases 270

Tests 354

Problem Based Learning 373

Problem Based Learning 381

Problem Based Learning 390

Appendix 1 391

Appendix 2 399

Appendix 3 403

Appendix 4 415

Further Reading 420

Index 423

FOREWORD

We now have an unprecedented understanding of the cellular and molecular basis of lung function in health and disease. The lung is made of dozens of different cell types, which integrate signals from other body systems to maintain homeostasis. Although the lung has the remarkable ability to rapidly adapt to environmental stressors, compensatory mechanisms can be overwhelmed leading to disease states. Despite recent advances in the cellular and molecular analysis of lung structure and function, an integrated understanding of lung physiology is the cornerstone upon which all other knowledge rests. This new book fulfills this vital role and provides a step-by-step explanation of key aspects of pulmonary physiology.

Written by a team of experts with decades of teaching experience, the authors' passion for their subject is apparent from the first page. Chapter 1 provides an illuminating yet concise review of how the lung was viewed through history, and culminates in the "golden decades" of 1940-1970 when key theoretical and practical aspects of pulmonary physiology were established by pioneers in the field. Subsequent chapters cover basic principles of lung structure, respiratory mechanics, gas exchange, gas transport, acid-base balance, ventilation-perfusion distribution, control of breathing and respiration during exercise at sea level and high altitude. Although the concepts covered are not new, the authors' experience in teaching complex concepts shines through in the numerous practical examples and detailed illustrations.

This ebook will be a useful resource for medical students, residents and trainees specializing in pulmonary medicine. Whether encountering dyspneic patients in the outpatient clinic, or managing intubated patients with respiratory failure, a solid understanding of the concepts contained in this ebook will provide the practitioner the insights and confidence needed to provide effective medical care.

Steve N. Georas
University of Rochester
School of Medicine and Dentistry
Rochester, NY
USA

PREFACE

The goal of this ebook is to present mechanistically basic concepts of respiratory function in normal and diseased states. While the book stresses the quantitative approach, more importantly it attempts to explain in detail the basic elements of respiratory mechanisms and to train students to become "clinical detectives" - a physician in the process of analyzing data from a patient's history and lab reports should reason based on the data by determining whether abnormal values are primary abnormalities or compensatory changes, by relating each lab value to other relevant values, and by making an educated interpretation of the major abnormalities in terms of ventilation, pulmonary blood perfusion, venous admixture, wasted alveolar ventilation, tissue oxygenation, acid-base balance, respiratory mechanics, control of breathing, and so on.

The present ebook is intended for first and second year medical students, as well as for residents and fellows, especially in disciplines such as anesthesiology and pulmonary medicine. In addition, this book attempts to provide a useful reference to teachers of respiratory physiology who are not directly involved in pulmonary research and/or have not been specifically trained in organ-system physiology. It is common knowledge that present faculty of physiology/biophysics departments are most often composed of cell physiologists, biophysicists and molecular biologists, many of whom have limited knowledge of organ-system physiology, while the basic needs of medical education in organ-system physiology have not changed. This book tries to fill this gap by offering to modern physiology faculty some basic tools for understanding the "nuts-and-bolts" of this major field of basic medical education.

In short, the key features of the ebook are: 1. Mechanistic and quantitative presentation of most important elements of respiratory physiology and pathophysiology. 2. In-depth analysis and detailed explanation of the most relevant aspects of respiratory functions. 3. Detailed analysis of functional consequences of respiratory diseases and differences from healthy pulmonary maintenance. 4. Thorough derivation of equations used for evaluating respiratory functions in health and disease.

Following the preface and a brief introduction, ten chapters cover the major subjects of respiratory structure and function, including: historical background, basic lung structure, respiratory mechanics, gas exchange, oxygen and carbon dioxide transport, respiratory regulation of acid-base, ventilation-perfusion distribution, right-to-left blood shunt (venous admixture) and alveolar dead space ventilation, chemical and neurological controls of breathing, respiratory adaptation to high altitude, both at rest and during exercise, and functional consequences of major respiratory diseases. These chapters are followed by the quantitative presentation of ten clinical cases, two tests and a case study structured for problem-based-learning. Finally, there are four appendices, which provide normal values, equations and examples of methods used for quantitatively evaluating pulmonary disorders, a list of books for further reading, and a index.

ACKNOWLEDGEMENT

Declared none.

CONFLICT OF INTEREST

The author confirms that this eBook content has no conflict of interest.

Camillo Peracchia

Department of Pharmacology and Physiology

University of Rochester, School of Medicine and Dentistry

601 Elmwood Ave.

Rochester, NY 14642-8711

USA

E-mail: camillo_peracchia@urmc.rochester.edu

INTRODUCTION

To define "amazing" the structure and function of the lungs is quite an understatement. Just think of the incredible surface area available for the exchange of oxygen and carbon dioxide between blood and environmental air. If we were able to dissect from the lungs each one of the roughly three hundred million alveoli - the microscopic gas-filled polyhedral sacs specialized for gas exchange - flatten and paste them side by side on the floor, we would easily cover the surface of half a tennis court. Just as astonishing is the efficiency of the alveolar respiratory membrane - the air-blood partition where gas exchange takes place; its width, as thin as a ten-thousandth of a millimeter, enables in a quarter of a second the complete equilibration of gas partial-pressures between alveoli and blood vessels, represented by the astronomic number of approximately one hundred billion capillaries. This allows the diffusion of large volumes of gases - in heavy exercise, for example, the diffusion of oxygen and carbon dioxide can increase from a few hundreds of milliliters to several liters per minute. The extensive airway tree, with its efficient cilia-dependent garbage-disposal apparatus, effectively cleans, warms and humidifies the inspired air so efficiently that even in dusty, cold and dry environments the gas that enters the alveoli is clean, warmed to body temperature and saturated with water vapor.

The major function of the lungs is obviously to exchange respiratory gases between blood and environment, a function of fundamental importance for the normal operation of the cellular metabolism. But, the lungs have other important tasks as well. Most relevant is their function in regulating the organism's acid-base balance. While the kidneys play a major role in regulating acid-base, their compensatory mechanism is relatively slow, as it can alter the blood's bicarbonate concentration by only a couple of milliequivalents (mEq) per liter plasma per day. In contrast, the lungs can alter the partial pressure of carbon dioxide in blood very rapidly, dramatically increasing or decreasing the blood's pH in seconds by increasing or decreasing the ventilation rate, respectively. Another important function of the lungs is their ability to generate appropriate pressures and gas-flows for speaking, singing, playing wind instruments, coughing and sneezing; in addition, the pressure exerted on abdominal organs by expiratory muscles complements the work of abdominal muscles in defecation and parturition. Finally, a very useful byproduct of having lungs is the buoyancy they provide the body with for floating and swimming - just think how hard it would be to swim without the help of such a large gas reservoir.

Camillo Peracchia

Department of Pharmacology and Physiology

University of Rochester, School of Medicine and Dentistry

601 Elmwood Ave.

Rochester, NY 14642-8711

USA

CHAPTER 1

Historical Background

Camillo Peracchia

Abstract: This chapter reviews major steps in the history of respiratory physiology, without laying claims to completeness. Throughout the centuries, the growth to present knowledge of pulmonary physiology and pathophysiology has not been a smooth steady climb, but rather a slow, often clumsy, walk punctuated by clever inventions, startling discoveries and amazing insights, but also by backward steps, misunderstandings, mistakes, controversies, rediscoveries, conflicts, prejudices and superstitions. In this brief review, we will travel in time from centuries before common-era to present, witnessing the progress of knowledge through periods such as the Greco-Roman era, the Middle Ages, the Renaissance, the 17th, 18th, 19th and early 20th centuries, the three golden decades of the 20th century (1940-1970) and beyond.

Keywords: Acid-Base Balance, Alveoli, Animal Heat, Bohr Effect, Capillaries, Carbon Dioxide, Dead Space, 2,3-Diphosphoglycerate (2,3-DPG), Gas Diffusion, Haldane Effect, Hemoglobin, Inert-Gas-Elimination Technique, Lung-Chest Compliance, Lung Diffusion, O_2-CO_2 Diagram, Oxygen, Respiratory Centers, Surfactant, Three-Compartment-Model, Tissue Metabolism, Ventilation-Perfusion Distribution.

SYMBOLS, ACRONYMS AND NORMAL VALUES: See Appendix 3

In spite of many centuries of scientific curiosity on the meaning of breathing, the properties of gas and blood, the function of lungs, heart and vessels, the source of body heat, and so on, only recently detailed knowledge of the mechanisms that drive lung and heart functions has been acquired. Undoubtedly, technological advances have played a major role in the exponential growth of knowledge in this and other fields of biological science that has taken place in the past two centuries, but much of the unprecedented growth in scientific discoveries has also resulted from greater freedom of experimentation from cultural restrictions, religious intolerance and bigotry, often based on superstition, prejudice and taboos.

RESPIRATORY CONCEPTS "BEFORE COMMON ERA (BCE)"

In distant past, a major obstacle to progress in biomedical knowledge was the misunderstanding of what arteries actually contain. The belief that arteries carry air rather than blood was perpetuated for at least seventeen centuries from Egyptian times to the work of the Greek physician Galen in the 2nd century of the Common Era (CE). This mistake was based on the observation that after death arteries are totally empty - it wasn't known then that blood pools into veins after death; therefore, only veins were believed to contain blood in living animals. This led ancient scientists to assume that arteries are filled with air and, consequently, arteries were thought to be conduits of inspired air.

Perhaps the earliest interpretation of the meaning of breathing is found in a Chinese document of 2000 BCE, in which respiration is understood as a process by which air is transformed into "soul substance", a life needed "essence". Evidence from the Ebers Papyrus, a document that dates to the 16th century BCE, indicates that Egyptians believed that air travels from the mouth to the lungs, and then *via* arteries to the heart and the rest of the body. This is perhaps the earliest scientific attempt to understand the mechanism of respiration.

In the 4th century BCE, the Greek physician Erasistratus of Ceos (born ca. 304 BCE) made a crucial observation that should have enabled him to understand what arteries actually contain, but he missed the chance because the conviction that arteries contain air was still too ingrained. Erasistratus correctly noted that arteries bleed when cut in a living animal, but assumed that air had first escaped from the arteries and subsequently venous blood had flooded into them from unknown structures connecting veins to arteries.

A clear distinction between veins and arteries was made by Herophilus, a contemporary of Erasistratus, who also proposed the existence of connections between veins and arteries, for which he is credited of being the first to suggest the existence of capillaries; it took many centuries, however, for convincing evidence of the existence of capillaries to emerge – the 17th century's Italian physician Marcello Malpighi deserves credit for it (see below). Erasistratus is also recognized to be the first to propound the "pneumatic" theory of respiration.

GRECO-ROMAN TIMES

In the 2nd century CE, the Greek physician Galen (Pergamum, Asia Minor, 130-199 CE) finally proved that arteries contain blood rather than air, and made a clear distinction between venous and arterial blood. Galen believed that components of inspired air were carried from the lungs to the left ventricle through the mitral valve, and waste products were regurgitated through the same valve into the pulmonary vein and delivered to the lungs, but was puzzled on how the mitral valve could separate inspired components from waste products. However, Galen correctly understood that blood "also" reaches the lungs *via* the pulmonary artery (vena arteriosis).

Galen mistakenly believed that some blood made its way from right to left ventricle *via* postulated pores in the inter-ventricular septum, a passageway whose existence was still accepted as late as in the 11th century by the Persian physician Avicenna - this hypothesis was finally put to rest by Ibn-al-Nafis in the early 13th century (see below). In spite of this mistake, Galen deserves credit for having correctly represented for the first time in history the topographic anatomy of the major arteries, and for having demonstrated that arteries carry blood; he also correctly believed that arteries and veins must be connected.

Galen also understood the fundamental mechanism of breathing, as he recognized that air enters the lungs by "active" expansion of the chest, which results in "passive" lung expansion. Amazingly, this concept was disputed for the following fifteen centuries, as most physiologists continued to believe that inspiration involves lung activity. Galen is believed to have written over five hundred books, but only eighty have survived a fire that destroyed his Roman house.

Over the centuries, fire has been responsible for many other major losses; in 391 CE, Christian fanatics caused a very serious setback to scientific progress by burning the library of Alexandria, which contained priceless manuscripts from the Greco-Roman era. The damage that resulted, however, would have been much greater if it hadn't been for the meticulous work of Persian, Syrian and Spanish physicians who had translated into Arabic many Greek manuscripts. Additional books also survived due to the zealous work of Byzantine scholars such as the Greek physician Oribasios (325-403), who succeeded in preserving many classic documents of anatomy and physiology.

MIDDLE AGES

A significant step forward occurred in the 11th century CE through the work of the Persian physician Avicenna (ca. 980-1037). Although he still accepted Galen 's mistaken belief of the existence of inter-ventricular pores, Avicenna deserves credit for having correctly described the cardiac cycle and the function of cardiac valves.

The first accurate description of circulation, however, was only documented two centuries later by the Arab physician Ibn-al-Nafis (1213-1288), and later independently reported by Servetus (see below). Ibn-al-Nafis clearly understood that the inter-ventricular septum is not perforated, and that blood from the right ventricle flows to the lungs *via* the pulmonary artery, where it comes in contact with air, and eventually makes its way back to the heart *via* the pulmonary veins. Additionally, Ibn-al-Nafis, as Galen, had a clear hint that there must be tiny channels or pores connecting arteries to veins.

RENAISSANCE

The great intellectual ferment that characterized the Renaissance significantly advanced knowledge of anatomy and physiology mainly through the work of three scientists: Leonardo da Vinci (1452-1519), Michael Servetus (1511-1553) and Andreas Vesalius (1514-1564). Leonardo made careful studies of the human body, describing in detail the anatomy of the heart and large blood vessels. Servetus is credited for having rediscovered the pulmonary circulation, originally described by Ibn-al-Nafis. Correctly, he recognized that the blood reaches the left heart from the right heart not through the septum but through the lungs, by flowing from the pulmonary artery to the pulmonary veins. Servetus' book, titled: "*Christianismi Restitutio*" was thought by the clergy to be heretical; therefore, tragically in 1553 both Servetus and his book were burned at stake in Geneva. Vesalius is rightfully recognized as the founder of modern anatomy - in his publication *De Humani Corporis Fabrica Libri Septem* (1543) he accurately described for the first time with superb anatomical illustrations the detailed topography of the pulmonary circulation. Vesalius' studies also convinced him that contrary to previous beliefs arteries do not actively pulsate, the arterial pulse resulting entirely from cardiac contraction. He also made the important observation that the lungs collapse following chest opening but, in spite of this finding and the work of Galen (see above), physiologists of the 16th century continued to believe that inspiration involves independent lung activity.

17th CENTURY

Circulation

Our understanding of blood circulation took a major leap forward in the early 17th century through the work of the English physician William Harvey (1578-1657). Harvey's publication *De Motu Cordis* (Frankfurt, 1628) accurately described for the first time the systemic circulation and the pumping function of the heart. He clearly understood that blood pumped by the heart eventually returns to the heart following the same route over and over - a concept that seems so obvious to us now, but was not so in the 17th century.

In spite of significant progress in the understanding of the anatomy and physiology of circulation, in the early 17th century knowledge of respiratory physiology was not much greater than at Greco-Roman times. The major reason for this lag in knowledge was the absence of technology for observing structure at microscopic level. This technological gap was soon to be filled by the invention of the compound microscope.

Structure

A rudimentary compound microscope was invented in 1590 by the Dutch spectacle makers Hans Lippershey (1570-1619) and Zacharias Janssen (c1580-c1632). This instrument, later perfected and named "compound microscope" (1625) by Italian physicist, mathematician, astronomer and philosopher Galileo Galilei (1564-1642), enabled the Italian physician Marcello Malpighi (1628-1694) and the Dutch microbiologist Antoine van Leeuwenhoek (1632-1723) to view structure at the cellular level.

Malpighi made two crucial discoveries: he succeeded in viewing the lungs' alveoli, which he described as flask-shaped structures, and provided convincing evidence that arteries and veins are connected by tiny vessels. Van Leeuwenhoek described for the first time similar microscopic vessels in the tail of tadpoles as well as in fish and mammals. These structures were later named "capillary vessels" by the English clergyman Stephen Hales (1677-1761), who is also credited for having developed the "pneumatic trough", a clever instrument for collecting gases.

Chemistry and Physics of Gases

The 17th century also witnessed significant advances in physics and chemistry. The Flemish chemist, physiologist, and physician Jan Baptiste van Helmont (Brussels, 1580-1644) discovered the gas carbonic acid, which he named "gas silvestre", and realized that this gas extinguishes flames and asphyxiates animals. He invented the word "gas", deriving it from the Greek word "chaos" to depict its wild nature.

A few years later, the Neapolitan physiologist, physicist and mathematician Giovanni Alfonso Borelli (1608-1679) realized that air is essential for animal life. More importantly, Borelli was the first to describe the basic processes of gas diffusion, as he demonstrated that gases dissolve in liquids and pass through membranes without the need of pores. In spite of this important discovery, two centuries will pass for the concept of gas diffusion across membranes to be accepted - gas diffusion was finally demonstrated by the work of Edward F.W. Pflüger (1829-1910; see below).

The Italian physicist and mathematician Evangelista Torricelli (1608-1647), a contemporary of Borelli, was the first to realize that air has weight. For measuring its weigh he invented the mercury barometer, a clever instrument that was later perfected by the Anglo-Irish chemist and physicist Robert Boyle (1627-1691) into the U-shaped column still used today.

Both Boyle and the English natural philosopher, architect and mathematician Robert Hooke (1635-1703) found that vacuum kills both flames and animals. They also realized for the first time that respiration and combustion are similar processes, and performed experiments on combustion and respiration by means of an ingenious machine invented by Hooke: the "New Pneumatic Engine". In collaboration with the English physician Richard Lower (1631-1691), Hooke demonstrated that the change in blood color from dark bluish-red to bright red, as blood passes through the lungs, is due to its interaction with air. Lower went a step further, as he demonstrated that tracheal occlusion darkens arterial blood, turning it into venous.

Respiratory Mechanics

In the 17th century, some progress in respiratory mechanics took place as well. Borelli was the first to measure the inspiratory volume and to recognize the existence of the residual volume. Lung volumes were later measured by other scientists, including Lavoisier and Hales.

A significant advance in the understanding of respiration resulted from the work of the English chemist and physiologist John Mayow (1643-1679), who was the first to recognize the nature of oxygen. Through experiments in which he placed candles or animals inside a glass bell immersed in water, he proved that both combustion and respiration absorb something from the air that causes a decrease in volume. He named the lost substance "nitro-aereal" - by a fortunate accident, the carbon dioxide generated by combustion, that would have replaced oxygen by a similar volume, had dissolved into water.

In 1660, the Dutch physician, physiologist and chemist Francisco Sylvius de le Boë (1614-1672) laid to rest the mistaken understanding that inspiration involves lung activity. His view was shared by most scientists of the time, including Boyle, Lower, Mayow and Borelli, but alternative hypotheses still surfaced and were not fully discarded until a century later through the careful work of the Swiss anatomist and physiologist Albrecht von Haller (1708-1777).

18th CENTURY

The 18th century became pervaded by a theory of combustion known as "phlogiston". According to this theory, first proposed by the German chemist and physician Johan Joachim Becher (1635-1682) and widely propounded by his student Georg Ernest Stahl (1659-1734), any combustible material contains a fire-element, phlogiston, which is released by combustion. Once burned, the "dephlogisticated" material leaves ashes, acquiring its true state: the so called "calx". The phlogiston theory, which was believed to apply to the body as well, survived for many decades and was finally put to rest eighty years later primarily by the work of Antoine Lavoisier.

The 18th century also witnessed the revival of van Helmont's "gas silvestre" concept, renamed "fixed air" (non-respirable gas) by French-Scottish physician and chemist Joseph Black (1728-1799), who correctly mentioned van Helmont's work. Black understood that material becomes lighter when it is heated because it loses fixed air. He believed that fixed air represented all of the non-respirable gas in air, not yet recognizing the existence of nitrogen, which was discovered in 1772 by Daniel Rutherford (1749-1819) and named "noxious air" or "phlogisticated air".

Oxygen

One of the most important advances of the 18th century was the independent discovery of oxygen by the English theologian and chemist Joseph Priestley (1733-1804) and the German-Swedish chemist Carl Wilhelm Scheele (1742-1786). Priestley noticed that the addition of a sprig of mint to a sealed bell in which a candle had burned out allowed another candle to burn very well. Rightly, he concluded that plants reverse the effect of combustion (or respiration) by preventing its noxious effect on animals. By means of Hales "pneumatic trough", which he perfected, Priestley determined that the fraction of "respirable air" (oxygen) in air is ~20%. Unaware of Priestley's work, in 1777 Scheele reported a different method for generating "fire-air" (oxygen); he also reported important new data on combustion, and succeeded in isolating new gases.

Their contemporary Henry Cavendish (1731-1810), an English chemist and physicist, determined the density and solubility of different gases and succeeded in producing hydrogen, "inflammable air", by applying acid to either zinc, copper or tin. By burning a mixture of hydrogen and air Cavendish produced pure water. The discovery that water is made of oxygen and hydrogen is attributed to four scientists: Henry Cavendish (1784), Antoine Lavoisier (1781), Gaspar Monge (1783) and James Watt (1784).

The 18th century also witnessed the birth of chemistry as quantitative science, mostly through the work of the French chemist Antoine Lavoisier (1743-1794). Most relevant for respiratory physiology is Lavoisier's work on combustion and respiration. With the help of his wife and laboratory assistant Marie Paulze, Lavoisier demonstrated that these two processes are similar in nature, as both involve absorption of "oxygine" (oxygen) from the air and production of "carbonic acid gas". The similarity of the two processes was proven through experiments that Lavoisier performed in 1782-4 in collaboration with the French mathematician Pierre Simon Laplace (1749-1827) by means of an ice calorimeter ideated by Joseph Black in 1761; these studies enabled them to determine for the first time the value of the respiratory quotient (RQ = 0.82 - the fraction of CO_2-production over O_2-consumption per unit time).

Animal Heat

In spite of significant progress in the understanding of respiratory and combustion processes, the source of animal heat was still unclear. Most of the 18th century's scientists, including Lavoisier, believed that combustion takes place in the lungs, and that heat is transported by blood to the other organs. This misunderstanding was based on the general belief that gases cannot diffuse through pulmonary membranes; therefore, oxygen conversion to carbon dioxide was believed to take place in the lungs. Curiously, this view was generally accepted in spite of Borelli's work that clearly demonstrated gas diffusion a century earlier (see above).

A serious blow to the lung-combustion theory was given by the Italian biologist Lazzaro Spallanzani (1729-1799). Spallanzani, working on a large number of cold-blooded animals as well as birds and mammals, found that tissue samples taken from recently killed animals continue to absorb oxygen and release carbon dioxide for quite some time. This finally proved that metabolism takes place in all tissues. Still mysterious, however, was the mechanism by which oxygen and carbon dioxide are transported to and from the various organs, because Spallanzani as well as others continued to believe that venous blood does not contain carbon dioxide.

Control of Breathing

The French physiologist Julien Jean César Legallois (1770-1814) demonstrated that the removal of brain and cerebellum in rabbits does not stop respiratory movements, but removal of the entire medulla oblongata does. This determined for the first time the general location of the respiratory centers.

19th CENTURY

Oxygen, Carbon Dioxide and Metabolism

Proof of the presence of carbon dioxide in venous blood finally came in the 19th century through the work of Heinrich Gustav Magnus (1802-1870), a German chemist and physicist. Magnus proved it by demonstrating that bubbling hydrogen into venous blood releases carbon dioxide. Working with his improved gas analyzer, Magnus also showed that arterial blood contains more oxygen that venous blood, which provided convincing evidence that oxygen is consumed at the periphery rather than in the lungs.

Additional important evidence for tissue metabolism soon came through the work of the French physiologist Claude Bernard (1813-1878). Bernard demonstrated that heat production occurs in tissues because thermoelectric measurements showed that temperatures are higher in the organs than in the arterial blood they receive. Further evidence came from the work of the German physiologist Edward F.W. Pflüger (1829-1910), who demonstrated that tissues have a lower oxygen partial pressure than their capillary blood, indicating that tissue oxygen-consumption is the cause of oxygen diffusion from blood.

Surprisingly, the first clear evidence of the relationship between tissue metabolism and heat was produced by a German country doctor, Julius Robert von Mayer (1814-1878), who happened to work as ship physician on a voyage to the East Indies. Von Mayer noticed that the color of the sailors' venous blood was brighter-red in the tropics than in Europe. Correctly, he attributed it to the fact that in the tropics the metabolic rate needed for maintaining the body warm is lower than in Europe. This simple observation convinced him that heat and work are interchangeable. Thus, for the first time the law of energy conservation was found to apply to the body as well. This was soon to be unequivocally proven by the German physiologist and physicist Herman von Helmoltz (1821-1894), who fathered the first law of thermodynamics.

Mechanics of Breathing

Knowledge of pulmonary mechanics progressed in the 19th century through the work of the Dutch physiologist and ophthalmologist Franciscus Cornelis Donders (1818-1889) and the English physiologist John Hutchinson (1811-1861). Donders recognized that the lungs collapse because of their elastic properties; he proved it by monitoring the positive intra-tracheal pressure in cadavers following chest opening, and comparing it to the negative intra-pleural pressure before chest opening. Hutchinson was the first to draw rudimentary versions of lungs' and chest-wall's compliance curves. He also named the subdivisions of lung volumes and described methods for measuring them by an early spirometer.

Additional progress took place late in the 19th century through the work of the Danish physiologist Christian Bohr (1855-1911). In collaboration with the German physiologists Nathan Zuntz (1847-1920) and Adolf Löwy (1862-1937), Bohr developed the concept of conductive (anatomical) dead space. In 1890 Bohr introduced the famous equation for measuring dead space, which takes advantage of partial pressure differences between average-alveolar ($\bar{A}$; end-tidal) and mixed-expired (E) gases.

Control of Breathing

The 19th century also witnessed significant advances in the understanding of the chemical and neural control of breathing. Donders reported that carbon dioxide regulates breathing *via* a vagal reflex, and the English physician and physiologist Marshall Hall (1790-1857) suggested that both breathing rhythmicity and exercise-dependent hyperpnea depend on carbon dioxide partial pressure. In 1868 Pflüger was the first to demonstrate the independent role of oxygen in breathing regulation.

The quantitative role of carbon dioxide in the control of breathing was first reported by the Scottish physiologist John Scott Haldane (1860-1936). By means of his famous gas analyzer, Haldane showed that dyspnea develops when carbon dioxide increases in inspired air by fractions as low as 3%, and that in the absence of carbon dioxide a 14% drop in inspired oxygen stimulates breathing. Haldane and Priestley developed a reliable method for sampling alveolar gas, which enabled them to determine that the alveolar pressure of carbon dioxide remains relatively constant at different barometric pressures, while the oxygen pressure dramatically drops. In addition, they found that alveolar ventilation doubles with an increase in alveolar carbon dioxide by only 0.2%, while hypoxia stimulates ventilation only when inspired oxygen drops to 13% or lower.

Haldane and Priestley originally believed that breathing depends entirely on the direct action of carbon dioxide on the respiratory centers. However, in view of data from subsequent experiments performed by Haldane in collaboration with C.G. Douglas, which showed that hyperventilation in vigorous exercise is caused by an increase in blood lactic acid rather than carbon dioxide partial pressure, they concluded that the respiratory centers are stimulated by "total acid, including that due to free CO_2".

In late 19th century, the German physiologist Karl Ewald Konstantin Hering (1834-1918) and his pupil Joseph Breuer (1842-1925) described the famous "Hering-Breuer" reflex. This reflex is a neurological feedback mechanism which regulates breathing by inhibiting over-inflation *via* vagal activity.

Hemoglobin

What carries oxygen in blood was much of a mystery up to the middle of the 19th century. This mystery was solved in 1842 when the German chemist Justus von Liebig (1803-1873) made the pivotal observation that "red globules" (red blood cells) contain iron and are capable of binding gases. Seventeen years later, the German physiologist and chemist Felix Hoppe-Seyler (1825-1895) made a comprehensive study on hemoglobin, firmly establishing its function as oxygen carrier. His extensive work determined the absorption spectra of both oxygenated and reduced hemoglobin, provided the formulas of hemin, hematin and hematoporphyrin, and described methemoglobin and hemochromogens.

In 1872, the first hemoglobin dissociation curves of oxygen and carbon dioxide were constructed by the French zoologist and physiologist Paul Bert (1833-1886) - the S-shape of the oxygen dissociation curve, however, was first reported by Bohr fourteen years later. Bert was also the first to recognize the physiological role of oxygen and carbon dioxide partial pressures, and to make it very clear that barometric pressure is irrelevant as long as partial pressure of oxygen is maintained. He proved it by showing that a bird survives well at barometric pressures as low as 100 mmHg if the oxygen fraction is increased to 90%.

EARLY 20th CENTURY

Hemoglobin's Curve-Shifts

In 1904 Bohr, Hasselbalch and the Danish physiologist Schack August Steenberg Krogh (1874-1949) published important data on the effect of carbon dioxide on the hemoglobin's oxygen carrying capacity, which demonstrated that an increase in carbon dioxide partial pressure induces a right shift in the O_2 dissociation curve - this phenomenon is still referred today to as the "Bohr effect". This phenomenon was first thought to depend entirely on carbon dioxide partial pressure, but soon after it was found to result primarily from pH changes – a small independent effect of carbon dioxide on the dissociation curve, however, was reported in 1933 by the Italian physiologist Rodolfo Margaria (1901-1983), in collaboration with the American chemist Arda Alden Green (1899-1958). In 1909, Bohr also developed a clever method for estimating the mean value of PO_2 in the alveolar capillary blood. This method is now known as the "Bohr integration method"; in the same study Bohr also succeeded in calculating the O_2 diffusion capacity.

Temperature was also found to affect the O_2 dissociation curve. For over a decade (1914-1928) the effect of temperature on the oxygen dissociation curve was studied in detail by the English physiologists Joseph Barcroft (1872-1947) and W.O.R. King (a travelling student of Sidney Sussex College, Cambridge), who demonstrated that a temperature rise causes a right-shift as well. In 1967 two groups: A. Chautin and R.R. Curnish, and R. Benesh and R.E. Benesh, independently discovered that the O_2 dissociation curve is also right-shifted by an increase in 2,3-diphosphoglycerate (2,3-DPG) concentration.

The effect of hemoglobin's O_2 saturation in reducing the CO_2's blood content - the reverse of the Bohr-effect - was described in 1914 by Johanne Christiansen, C. Gordon Douglas and J.S. Haldane. This phenomenon was named the "Haldane effect".

In 1933, the role of carbonic anhydrase in accelerating carbon dioxide's hydration-dehydration processes was first reported by N.U. Meldrum and H.W.

Rougton, and in 1925 G.S. Adair was the first to recognize that hemoglobin combines sequentially with four oxygen molecules.

Oxygen Diffusion *Versus* Secretion

In 1906 Krogh found that nitrogen does not participate in respiration and in collaboration with his wife, the renowned physician Birthe Marie Jørgense Krogh (1874-1943), proved that O_2 and CO_2 are transferred across the lungs by diffusion alone. In spite of this, however, they didn't completely abandon the stubbornly ingrained belief that lungs secrete oxygen, as they thought that diffusion alone would be insufficient to account for oxygen transfer during exercise and at high altitude.

Most famous among the contributions of the Krogh's couple is the invention of the single-breath carbon monoxide method for measuring the lung's diffusing capacity. This method was first published in Marie's doctorate-degree thesis (1914) and a year later in the Journal of Physiology. In spite of Marie's clear demonstration that oxygen diffusing capacity increases in exercise due to increased cardiac output, Haldane still remained convinced that oxygen secretion plays a role in exercise, in carbon monoxide poisoning and at high altitude's hypoxic conditions.

What was believed to be the final "kiss-of-death" for the thirty year old "oxygen secretion hypothesis" came through Barcroft's work. In a brave experiment, for which he remained in a closed chamber for six days resting and exercising under hypoxic conditions, Barcroft's blood measurements showed that his arterial oxygen saturation was always lower than that of blood simultaneously exposed to a sample of his alveolar gas - this was obviously expected if there were an oxygen diffusion gradient. Note, however, that in those years they were not aware of the fact that the alveolar-arterial oxygen gradient, (Ai-a)PO_2, even under hypoxic conditions is mostly due to the normal anatomical (conductive) right-to-left blood shunt (venous admixture, 2-4% of cardiac output), complemented by a small amount of shunt-like effect due to the gravity-dependent ventilation-perfusion ($\dot{V}/\dot{Q}$) maldistribution (see Chapter 7).

Respiratory Dead Space and Alveolar Ventilation-Perfusion Distribution

Following the original studies of Bohr and coworkers, further work on dead space measurement, as well as additional controversy, took place in the first half of the

20th century. Careful dead space measurements were performed in 1925 by the Swiss physiologist Fritz Rohrer (1888-1926), who also clarified the relationship between lung volume and static alveolar pressure, estimated airway resistance, and determined the optimal respiratory frequency for minimizing respiratory work load. Remarkably, in the span of ten years Rohrer developed the first thorough treatment of respiratory mechanics.

Dead space measurements were also performed by Krogh and Lindhard, and independently by Douglas and Haldane. In collaboration with the Danish physician Johannes Lindhard (1870-1947), Krogh used 20-30% hydrogen as gas indicator and collected samples from expired volumes as low as 0.5 liters, while Haldane and coworkers made measurements using carbon dioxide. Data from the two groups agreed on values of approximately 150 ml when samples were taken at rest, but not when gases were collected during exercise. Douglas and Haldane measured dead space volumes of 0.5-0.6 liters during exercise, whereas Krogh and Lindhard reported only minimal increases from resting values. One of the reasons for this controversy, that lasted several decades, was the lack of knowledge of the difference between conductive and physiological dead space. More reliable data were published in 1938 by Henrik Enghoff, who used arterial rather than alveolar carbon dioxide values for the calculations - this allows one to distinguish between physiological and conductive (anatomical) dead space ventilations (see Chapter 4). The dead space controversy was finally settled in 1948 when the American physiologist Ward S. Fowler developed the single-breath-nitrogen-washout method, which accurately measures the conductive (anatomical) dead space volume.

Significantly, the dead space controversy brought to light a more important aspect of respiratory physiology, namely the non-homogeneity of alveolar gas composition. Indeed, up to the early 20th century it was generally believed that all of the alveoli behave identically in terms of ventilation and perfusion. The first indication that there might be differences among lung regions came from the anatomical work of Arthur Keith (1909), who divided the lungs into three zones: a radical, containing bronchi and vessels, an intermediate, containing bronchial and vascular branches as well as lung tissue, and an outer one, only about 3 cm thick, entirely composed of alveoli and capable of expansion – thus, better ventilated than the intermediate zone.

Early evidence for regional differences in ventilation-perfusion distribution came through the work of Krogh and Lindhard (1913-1917). By sampling expiratory gases following inspiration of a hydrogen mixture they determined that end-expiratory gases contain less hydrogen. This finding created a controversy with the Haldane group, which in 1919 reported of having sampled pure air at the end of deep expiration, leading them to believe that there is no gas exchange in the air sacs. In 1938 the Danish physiologists Carl Sonne and his collaborator Ejnar Roeslen (1938) confirmed the work of Krogh and Lindhard, and the controversy was finally settled in the 1940s when faster methods of gas analysis became available.

In 1913 W.H.F. Addison and H.W How were the first to observe that the lungs of fetal mammals are filled with fluid, and in 1930 C.M. van Allen and coworkers were the first to report evidence for inter-lobular communication, enabling gas exchange between adjacent lobules.

Respiratory Mechanics

The 19th century work of Donders and Hutchinson on lung elasticity was expanded in 1929 by the Swedish-Swiss physiologist Kurt von Neergaard (1887-1947), who demonstrated the crucial role of surface tension in lung elasticity, and in 1934 by the studies of the English physiologist Ronald V. Christie, who demonstrated that lung recoil - the lung's tendency to collapse due to its elastic properties (see Chapter 3) - is reduced in emphysematous lungs, and understood that this is the cause of airway collapse in expiration. Ten years later, C.L. Bayliss and G.W. Robertson provided the first detailed description of the viscoelastic characteristics of normal lungs.

Blood Gas Measurement

Important methodological advances in blood gas measurement took place in the early 20th century. Arterial oxygen and carbon dioxide were first measured in 1912 by the German physician Heinrich von Hürter, who sampled arterial blood from a number of normal subjects and found it to be 93-100% saturated with oxygen. Seven years later, measurements of oxygen saturation in pneumonia patients were performed by the American physician William Christopher Stadie (1886-1959) and in 1924 careful measurements of arterial oxygen saturation were made by the American biochemists Donald Dexter Van Slyke (1883-1971) and James M. Neill, who vacuum-extracted blood gases and analyzed them by manometry. Thanks to the work of the German physician Werner Theodor Otto Forssmann (1904-1974), who in 1929 reached his own right heart *via* a catheter that he had introduced into his arm's vein, in 1945 the French physician André F. Cournand (1859-1988) and coworkers, using the Forssmann's cardiac catheterization method, succeeded for the first time in analyzing mixed-venous blood sampled in the right atrium. In recognition of their pioneering work, Forssmann and Cournand were awarded the 1956 Nobel Prize in Medicine.

Control of Breathing

In the early 20th century, the American physiologist Lawrence Joseph Henderson (1878-1942) noticed that the blood's acid-base balance depends on three factors: respiration, red blood cells and kidney function. He expressed their relationship into an equation, converted into logarithmic form in 1916 by the Danish physician and chemist Karl Albert Hasselbalch (1874-1962), which is known today as the "Henderson-Hasselbalch equation" - this equation inter-relates partial pressure of carbon dioxide, total carbon dioxide, plasma bicarbonate and blood pH. However, the effect of blood acidity on respiratory centers wasn't fully understood until 1921, when the German physiologist Hans Winterstein (1879-1963), the developer of the "reaction (acidity) theory", demonstrated that it isn't blood acidity that stimulates the respiratory centers, but rather the acidity of center neurons.

The early 20th century also witnessed significant progress in the understanding of the roles of CNS, carotid body and carotid sinus in regulating respiration. In 1905, Haldane and Priestley demonstrated that respiration at rest is regulated by CO_2 rather than O_2. By witnessing the consequences of brain-stem sectioning, Thomas Lumsden in 1923-4 succeeded in locating in the caudal pons, the center responsible for sustained inspiratory drive, which he named "apneustic center". Lumsden also identified the "pneumotaxic center" in the rostral and lateral regions of the pons, and believed that this center inhibited the apneustic drive. Although subsequent studies questioned the existence of the apneustic center, as different interpretations of the transection experiments were reported, Lumsden is rightfully recognized as the founder of the rhythmic-breathing-regulation field.

In 1925-8, the Spanish anatomist Fernando De Castro determined through careful microscopic studies the function of the carotid body as a sensory organ stimulated by changes in blood composition. A couple of years later, the Belgian physiologist and pharmacologist Corneille Heyman demonstrated that hypercapnia, acidosis (↑[H^+]) and hypoxemia stimulate ventilation by acting on the carotid body and carotid sinuses – for this work, Heyman was awarded the 1938 Nobel prize in Physiology and Medicine.

In 1933 the English physiologist Edgar Douglas Adrian (1889-1977) discovered the role of the afferent fibers of the vagus in the respiratory cycle. Adrian is credited as being the first to succeed in recording nerve impulses from single fibers. For his work on the function of neurons Adrian was awarded the 1932 Nobel Prize in Physiology and Medicine.

THE THREE GOLDEN DECADES OF THE 20th CENTURY – 1940-1970

While there is little doubt that war is one of the worst expressions of human behavior, it is also undeniable that a byproduct of wars has often been the spurt of innovations and discoveries. To mention just a few examples, the World War II years have witnessed the rapid development of radars and sonars, the invention of synthetic rubber and multi-track recording systems, the fast growth of computer technology, the creation of jet engines, and so on. Similarly, the war years have seen unprecedented advances in respiratory physiology research.

Much of the rapid growth in our understanding of gas exchange and respiratory mechanics had to do with the American Air Force. In the early forties, airplanes did not have pressurized cabins. This was a problem because air supremacy in combat could only be achieved if fighter pilots were able to reach the highest altitudes possible - flying above the enemy is a major advantage. Due to low barometric pressure at high altitudes, pilots were losing consciousness due to hypoxia. The need for research on pressure breathing became obvious, but scientists at that time were concerned that pressurizing airplanes could be dangerous; some even felt that the lungs may rupture or circulation may stop.

Gas Exchange and Ventilation-Perfusion Distribution

In 1941, soon after the attack on Pearl Harbor, Wallace O. Fenn (1893-1971) - the first Chair of Physiology at the University of Rochester, School of Medicine -

driven by the desire to contribute to the war effort began studying the physiological effects of pressure breathing at high altitude. This was a daring decision because Fenn, who had received a Ph.D. in "plant physiology" at Harvard in 1919 and was working at that time on muscle contraction and membrane transport of potassium ions, seemed an unlikely candidate for work on respiratory physiology. Nonetheless, surprising all experts in the field, in a few years Fenn and a number of equally unprepared collaborators, foremost among them Herman Rahn (1912-1990), who was working on pituitary hormones in frogs and Arthur Otis (1913-2008), who was studying tyrosinase activation in grass hopper eggs, succeeded in clarifying fundamental concepts of pulmonary gas exchange and mechanics of breathing.

Originally supported by the Office of Scientific Research and Development (OSRD) with a sum of $500, and later by a grant from the U.S. Air Force, Fenn and coworkers assembled some rudimentary equipment, which included their masterpiece, "the high-altitude chamber" (fruit of Fenn's ingenuity), which in fact was nothing more than a steel tank originally designed for processing and transporting beer. Nonetheless, this chamber was capable of simulating altitudes as high as 5,000 meters achievable at a rate of 5,000 feet/min. Fenn always volunteered to be the first to test new procedures in his "beer" chamber until a day in which, due to a mask leak, he passed out. That was going to be his last time in the chamber because by chance the Dean of the Medical School, the 1934 Nobel Laureate George H. Whipple (1878-1976), happened to walk by. Instantly and categorically, Whipple forbade Fenn to experiment on himself.

At first, Fenn and coworkers focused on the effect of pressure breathing on gas exchange at different altitudes. This led to the development of the alveolar-gas-equation and its graphic representation, the famous O_2-CO_2 diagram (often referred to as the "Fenn-Rahn diagram"). This equation and its graphic form represent a cornerstone of pulmonary gas exchange as they contain all of the parameters of ventilation and alveolar gas composition, and enable one to graphically predict changes in alveolar and arterial blood gases under various conditions such as hyper- or hypo-ventilation, hypoxia, hypercarbia, high altitude breathing, hyperbaric pressure, and so on - in 1951, the O_2-CO_2 diagram was modified by R.L. Riley and A. Cournand, who extended it into a four-quadrant diagram, where the complex gas-blood relationship is more easily visualized. Unquestionably, the Fenn's team was the first to demonstrate that respiratory physiology can be studied mathematically in detail.

In 1949, the role of ventilation-perfusion ($\dot{V}/\dot{Q}$) distribution in hypoxemia was studied in detail by Herman Rahn; in this study, Rahn also further developed the concept of average alveolar ventilation, extending the early-century's work of Bohr (1909, see above). Two years later, the effect of $\dot{V}/\dot{Q}$ maldistribution on arterial PO_2 was further analyzed by Richard L. Riley (1911-2001) and coworkers, and the role of mechanics in $\dot{V}/\dot{Q}$-distribution were clarified by Otis and coworkers (1956).

In 1951, further understanding of alveolar O_2-diffusion came through the studies of R. Austrian and coworkers, who described a new syndrome of impaired alveolar-capillary diffusion, known as "alveolar-capillary-block". This syndrome is caused by a variety of diseases such as pneumonia by Pneumocystis carnii, lupus, rheumatoid arthritis, scleroderma, sarcoidosis, idiopathic fibrosis, obstructive bronchiolitis with organizing pneumonia, granulomatous lung disease, alveolar cell carcinoma, multiple micro-embolism, hemosiderosis, and pulmonary alveolar proteinosis. A decade later, J. Piper and coworkers further advanced the concept of uneven pulmonary gas exchange by demonstrating that diffusion capacity is unequally distributed among lung regions, and in 1966 the uneven distribution of inspired air was demonstrated by the Italian-Canadian physiologist Joseph Milic-Emili and coworkers.

The relationship among alveolar surface area, oxygen consumption and body weight was demonstrated by S.M. Renney and J.E. Remmers in 1963. Their studies reported that lung-volume is a constant fraction of body weight among animal species, although the number of alveoli per kilogram of body weight is greater in small mammals.

One of the very first studies on pulmonary hypoxic vasoconstriction was performed by the American physiologist Thomas C. Lloyd Jr. in 1968. In this study, Lloyd reported that perivascular tissues play a role in triggering hypoxic vasoconstriction by releasing vasoactive chemical factors.

Respiratory Mechanics

The gas exchange studies of Fenn and coworkers, presented in an OSRD Report in 1944, were followed a year later by a report on respiratory mechanics, which is the second masterpiece of this team. The mechanics studies focused on the work of breathing, which was analyzed during intermittent *versus* continuous pressure-breathing and classified by Otis and coworkers in 1950 as elastic, viscous and resistive. This work, aimed at estimating lung and chest wall compliances, led to the creation of the famous "pressure-volume diagram", which enables one to individually analyze the elastic properties of lungs, chest wall and the combined lung-chest-wall system. In this diagram one can define the limiting values of muscle force and the effects on pulmonary mechanics of postural changes, pressure breathing, artificial ventilation, and so on. Furthermore, areas on the diagram allow one to quantify the mechanical work, the effect of different maneuvers such as singing, diving and playing wind-instruments, and the mechanical consequences of devices and procedures employed in anesthesiology and respiratory therapy.

In 1948, Arthur Otis and the American physiologist Donald F. Proctor (1914-2006) succeeded in calculating airway resistance by measuring alveolar pressure with the "interrupter method", and eight years later the Canadian physiologists Peter T. Macklem (1931-2011) and Jere Mead (1920-2009) developed a method for distinguishing central *versus* peripheral airway resistance, which demonstrated that changes in small airway resistance present in chronic diseases may be undetected by conventional pulmonary function tests - appropriately, this lung region was called "silent zone". The mechanism of airway collapse in expiration was further addressed by Robert E. Hyatt and coworkers (1958), who determined that the maximum expiratory flow-rates decrease as lung volume drops, and drew iso-volume pressure-volume flow curves. Much progress in understanding the mechanism of airway collapse in expiration took place in the following decade through the studies of Solbert Permutt, Richard L. Riley, Donald F. Proctor, John B. L. Howell, and coworkers.

In 1961, Howell and coworkers focused on the effect of pressure on lung vessel. Their study demonstrated that the effect of Positive End Expiratory Pressure (PEEP) depends on vessel location - with an increase in alveolar pressure, alveolar capillaries are compressed but large extra-alveolar vessels tend to be dilated, as PEEP expands the lungs to larger volumes. In 1956 Arthur B. DuBois and coworkers developed a fast method for measuring thoracic gas volumes with a body plethysmograph, and years later the elastic properties of the respiratory system were described in detail by Jere Mead and coworkers (1972), who propounded the so called "interdependence theory of the lung parenchyma" which explains how the elastic properties of lung parenchyma affect airways mechanics.

Starting in late forties, great interest in the fifties and sixties was devoted to alveolar surface tension and surfactant [1]. In 1947, the findings of the American pathologist Peter Gruenwald on alveolar surface tension were truly ahead of time, as he stated that "*Surface active substances reduce pressure necessary for aeration. This suggests the administration of surface active substances to the air or oxygen which is being spontaneously breathed in or introduced by a respirator might aid in relieving the initial atelectasis of newborn infants*". In the same study, Gruenwald also addressed the concept of "opening pressure", the pressure necessary to reopen collapsed alveoli.

In 1952, Frank N. Low (1911-1998), who was one of the first cell biologists to study lung structure by electron microscopy, finally provided convincing evidence for a continuous cellular layer in alveoli, putting to rest a long standing controversy on the nature of the alveolar air-blood interface. This finding was soon confirmed by Chris C. Macklin (1954), who also reported evidence for the presence of a liquid layer coating the alveolar surface, a finding later confirmed by E.R. Weibel and J. Gil (1968). Macklin correctly recognized that the alveolar liquid is secreted by the alveolar epithelial cells type 2 (EP2), but believed surface tension to be constant. A year later, evidence for a surface active substance in alveoli came from a keen observation of Richard E. Pattle, who noticed that air bubbles embedded in the fluid of lung edema were stable. Correctly, Pattle concluded that the surface tension at the air-fluid bubble interface was zero – this provided the first convincing evidence for the presence of surface active substances in alveoli.

Further progress on surface tension and surfactant took place in 1956 by the independent studies of Elwyn S. Brown and John A. Clements. In calculating lung compliance, Brown noticed that the alveolar surface tension drops to very low values as lung volume decreases, and Clements demonstrated that the characteristics of lung compliance depend on the presence of a surface active agent in the alveoli. A year later, Clements made a major breakthrough in surfactant research by reporting that lung extracts prevent alveolar collapse by lowering surface tension to less than 10 dynes/cm. Indeed, Clements pioneered the clinical use of exogenous surfactants in the treatment of the Infant Respiratory Distress Syndrome (IRDS).

In 1959, E.S. Brown, Rudolph P. Johnson and J.A. Clements reported for the first time the presence of hysteresis in the pressure-volume curve recorded during lung's inflation and deflation, which demonstrated that the surfactant's surface tension is area dependent. In the same year, Mary Ellen Avery and Jere Mead found that lung-extracts from infants weighing over 1.0-1.2 kg, as well as from children and adults, greatly lowered surface tension, whereas lung-extracts from premature babies who died from hyaline membrane disease had minimal effects on surface tension. This important observation, together with the fundamental work of Clements and coworkers, sparked great interest in the surfactant field, but it took an additional three decades for exogenous surfactants to be employed routinely in neonatology wards – as a result of this treatment, in the past two decades the mortality rate of premature infants has dramatically dropped.

The survival of premature infants was also improved by infusion of corticosteroids, a treatment suggested in 1969 by the New Zealander gynecologist Graham Collingwood Liggins (1926-2010) which proved that corticosteroids activate the maturation of surfactant metabolism. In 1968, definitive microscopic evidence for the presence of surfactant in the alveolar lining layer came from the study of Ewald R. Weibel and Joan Gil, who observed the presence of tubular myelin-like structures, later postulated to be precursors of the monolayer surfactant film. Weibel is also credited for having pioneered modern morphometric and stereological methods, as in 1963 he published a superb book in which lung anatomy and pathology are quantified by precise morphometric methods.

Knowledge of fetal lung physiology improved in late forties through the work of P. Alfred Jost and Albert Policard, who in 1948 discovered that trachea ligation in fetal rabbits causes the lungs to become distended with fluid - this indicated that the lungs are the source of the fluid. This work was expanded in 1963 by Forrest H. Adams and coworkers, who confirmed the pulmonary origin of the lung fluid by showing that its composition differs from that of fetal plasma. In 1968, T.M. Adamson and coworkers further strengthen these findings by demonstrating that the electrolyte composition of alveolar liquid differs from that of lymph and plasma - alveolar fluid must be a special fluid secreted by the fetal lung. Indeed, both flow and composition of lung's lymph had been reported in 1942 by M.F. Warren and C.K. Drinker, who were the first to develop methods for cannulating lymphatic vessels draining from heart and lungs. Three decades later, N.C. Staub and coworkers (1975) further advanced the field by developing methods for measuring lymph flow through chronic lung-lymph-fistulas in anesthetized sheep.

The understanding of how pulmonary edema develops improved in 1959 through a study of Arthur C. Guyton (1919-2003) and coworkers, who determined the role of plasma proteins in edema formation. Eight years later, the sequence of edema formation was carefully described by N.C. Staub and coworkers.

The Three-Compartment-Model

While the Fenn's team was focusing mostly on the gas side of pulmonary physiology, at the U.S. Naval School of Aviation Medicine (NSAM) another team led by Richard L. Riley (1911-2001) was focusing on the blood side of the blood-gas barrier.

In the early forties, several aviation cadets had died during flight for unknown reason. Surprisingly, no one suspected high altitude hypoxia as the cause; rather, the general belief was that the casualties had resulted from carbon monoxide poisoning. This prompted the NSAM to order Lt. Joseph L. Lilienthal, Jr. to determine the carbon monoxide level in cockpit's air and pilots' blood. For this task, Lilienthal used a novel syringe analyzer, invented by P.F. Sholander and J.W. Roughton (1943), which consisted of a tuberculin syringe connected to a calibrated capillary.

By lucky coincidence, Riley was working near Lilienthal's lab. As he became progressively more interested in Lilienthal's work, Riley had the brilliant idea that the syringe analyzer could also be used for measuring oxygen and carbon dioxide in blood if one were to add a small bubble of gas to a milliliter of blood in the syringe. Correctly, he reasoned that the partial pressures of the gases in the bubble, after equilibration with blood, would correspond to those in the blood sample. The success of the "bubble method" for measuring arterial blood gases induced Riley to devote all efforts to the complicated field of pulmonary ventilation-perfusion distribution.

In the mid-forties, the existence of inequalities in ventilation/perfusion ratio among lung regions was well known, but no one knew how to quantify them and what would be the functional consequences of their alteration. An unfortunate accident in Riley's life – his 1948 contraction of a mild case of tuberculosis – ended up being beneficial to the field. With plenty of time to think during his forced rest at home, Riley succeeded in developing the "three-compartment-model" of the real lung, which he published in 1951 in collaboration with A. Cournand and K.W. Donald. This was a major step forward, because it provided a powerful method for quantifying the extent of maldistribution between ventilation and perfusion in pulmonary patients. This model, still widely used today, simplifies the complexity of the lungs' gas exchange into three compartments: "ideal", where gas exchange is perfect, "alveolar dead space", where alveoli are ventilated but unperfused, and "shunt", where alveoli are perfused but unventilated (see Chapter 7).

In 1953, a significant advance in the technology for measuring oxygen partial pressure in blood resulted from the development of the platinum electrode, invented by L.C. Clark and coworkers. This was complemented in 1956 by J.W. Severinghaus and A.F. Bradley's invention of an electrode for measuring carbon dioxide partial pressure. Soon after, both electrodes were successfully incorporated into a single probe that allowed the measurements of arterial PO_2 and PCO_2 to be routinely performed in hospitals.

LATE 20th CENTURY

A major breakthrough in the field of ventilation-perfusion distribution occurred in the early seventies through the work of John B. West and coworkers. This was prompted by the independent contributions of G.R. Kelman, and A.J. Olszowka and L.E. Farhi, in developing early computer procedures for describing oxygen and carbon dioxide dissociation curves. John West, recognizing the great power of the computer application, successfully developed a technique for determining regional patterns of ventilation-perfusion inequalities which involves a series of gases with different solubilities. This technique, invented by West in 1974 in collaboration with P. Wagner, J. Evans and H.A. Saltzman, and named the "inert-gas-elimination technique", is undoubtedly the most reliable method for determining regional ventilation-perfusion mismatch.

The last four decades of the 20th century also witnessed great progress in the understanding of mechanisms of expiratory airflow limitation and of the contribution of alveolar and intra-pleural pressures in pulmonary circulation - the American Physiologist Solbert Permutt (1926-2012) and his team deserve most of the credit for having advanced knowledge in these fields. Their major contribution was the Pride-Permutt's model of expiratory flow-limitation [2], which helped understanding the mechanism of the obstructive Sleep Apnea-Hypopnea Syndrome (SAHS) and the effect of cardio-pulmonary resuscitation (CPR) on pulmonary blood flow. Permutt was also the first to define the three major zones in the lung, which are determined by the pressure gradients among alveolar, arterial and venous pressures. The three-zone model is generally attributed to John West [3], but actually West published it two year after Permutt's original report [4]. In addition, Permutt demonstrated the potential lung-protective effects of Positive End Expiratory Pressure (PEEP). He also suggested the employment of spirometry for diagnosing pulmonary diseases, and helped understanding the pathophysiology of asthma.

The last three decades of the 20th century also witnessed a wealth of additional discoveries on alveolar surfactant and surface tension properties (reviewed in [5]). In 1973, a J.A. Clements' team (R.K. King, D.J. Klass, E.G. Gikas and J.A. Clements) succeeded in identifying the lung-specific apoproteins of canine surfactant, and in the same year F.M. La Force, W.J. Kelly and G.L. Huber recognized the bacteriostatic properties of surfactant proteins. Three years later a Clements' team (S. Schürch, J. Goerke and J.A. Clements) performed a direct determination of alveolar surface tension and demonstrated its changes to very low values caused by lung deflation.

The first clear evidence that instillation of cow surfactant in the airways of premature infants dramatically improves survival was reported in 1980 by the Japanese pediatrician Tetsuro Fujiwara and coworkers. This study prompted a large scale clinical trial of exogenous surfactant instillation in premature infants suffering from hyaline membrane syndrome. These trials led R.H. Phibbs and coworkers to definitively state in 1991 that the intra-tracheal instillation of natural surfactant, or a protein-free synthetic surfactant named "exosurf", is lifesaving in the prevention and treatment of the hyaline membrane disease.

Progress also took place in the understanding of mechanisms involved in lung remodeling. In 1981, H. Sahebjami and J.A. Wirman reported that the reduced oxygen consumption resulting from caloric-restrictive diets reversibly induces alveolar remodeling. This demonstrated for the first time the alveoli's plasticity properties, suggesting that alveolar size and formation can change to adapt for changes in the organism's oxygen requirements.

Work on the function of airway's smooth-muscles in asthma led R.C. Levitt and W. Mitzner (1989) to succeed in demonstrating the autosomal-recessive inheritance of airway hyperactivity to serotonin (5-hydroxytryptamine). Airway studies of K.T. Takema and coworkers (1999) discovered the role of the epidermal growth factor in regulating mucin production *via* increased expression of MUC5AC – selective EGF-R tyrosine kinase inhibitors blocked its induction. A 1993 study by C. Youngson and coworkers improved knowledge on the oxygen-sensing mechanism of airway chemoreceptors, by reporting that cells of neuro-epithelial bodies express an O_2-sensitive K-channel coupled to an O_2-sensor protein.

MORE RECENT DEVELOPMENTS

In the past few years, much of the progress in our knowledge of pulmonology has resulted from the applications of modern technology to respiration research, diagnostic and treatment of respiratory disorders, and from major advances in the biochemistry, molecular biology and pharmacology of processes operating in the alveolar epithelium. New technologies have been successfully applied to the assessment and treatment of the Sleep Apnea-Hypopnea Syndrome (SAHS) and the Chronic Obstructive Pulmonary Disease (COPD), to a more precise monitoring of pulmonary circulation, and to methods for evaluating, as well as potentiating, the activity of respiratory muscles. At the cellular level, significant progress has been made in understanding the pathophysiological processes that cause COPD and asthma, and in defining the biochemistry and molecular biology of alveolar proteins involved in the surfactant system.

For monitoring SAHS, non-invasive sensors of air flow have generally replaced the classic pneumotachograph (reviewed in [6-8]). Modern devices used for monitoring flow include thermistors/thermocouples and nasal prongs. The former monitors flow by measuring changes in the electrical properties of the thermo-sensors. The latter measures flow by recording pressure at the nostrils, as pressure generated by flow-turbulence at the nostrils is directly related to flow rate. Another method for monitoring pulmonary ventilation capitalizes on changes in the cross-sectional area of chest and abdomen, which are monitored by thoraco-abdominal bands. Other methods for assessing airflow obstruction involve measurement of airway resistance by the so-called Forced Oscillation Technique (FOT), or the evaluation of both the upstream resistance and the critical pressure of the upper airways. The FOT method records changes in nasal pressures and flows during the application of low-amplitude, high frequency, pressure oscillations.

New methods have also been developed for assessing dynamic hyperinflation in COPD patients (reviewed in [9]). The Negative Expiratory Pressure (NEP) method involves the rapid application of negative pressure by a Venturi device attached to a mouthpiece. While in normal subjects the sudden increase in pressure gradient between alveoli and airway opening results in rapid increase in flow rate, there is minimal or no increase in flow rate in COPD patients. The data indicate that in COPD patients the NEP technique is a significantly better predictor of chronic dyspnea than the traditional Forced Expiratory Volume in 1-second (FEV1) method.

Recently, our understanding of COPD's pathogenesis has been enhanced by evidence for the involvement of oxidative stress and proteases - anti-protease imbalance plays a role in COPD development (reviewed in [10]). Neutrophil and macrophage invasion of inflamed airways have been shown to add internally generated oxidants to external oxidants caused by cigarette's smoke, and new data indicate that the expression of anti-oxidants, such as components of the hemoxygenase (HO)-1 pathway in lung macrophages of COPD patients, is significantly reduced. Lung proteases mainly produced by phagocytes are normally regulated by anti-proteases such as α1-antitrypsin, but cigarette smoke inhibits anti-proteases, adding to COPD's progression. Indeed, proteases have been known to play a major role in COPD, as inherited α1-antitrypsin deficiency is the cause of COPD in non-smokers. Evidence for an increase in neutrophils and macrophages in COPD lungs explains the increase in oxidants and proteases.

Novel techniques have also been developed for the non-invasive monitoring of changes in pulmonary hemodynamics. They include: Magnetic Resonance Imaging (MRI) and Computed Technology (CT), by which the perfusion of small lung vessels is viewed in real time, measurement of electrical impedance during the cardiac cycle, estimation of capillary flow by acetylene absorption, which capitalizes on the perfusion limitation of this gas, and monitoring of endothelin-factors production, in particular that of nitric oxide (NO) in expired gas (rev. in [11]).

Recently, the mechanisms involved in pulmonary edema have been studied in greater detail by a team [12] that has succeeded in developing a microfluid device called "Lung-on-a-Chip Microdevice" which simulates the alveolar-capillary interface and enables one to study the mechanical forces involved in edema formation. This clever device is capable of reproducing *in vitro* the intimate mechanisms of fluid leakage from capillaries into alveoli.

Progress has been made in analyzing more precisely the function of respiratory muscles, by quantifying strength, endurance and fatigue (reviewed in [13]). This field has been helped by the development of the magnetic method for stimulating respiratory nerves. This method, originally used mainly for respiratory research, has found useful applications in the diagnosis and treatment of neuromuscular diseases and COPD, and is being frequently used in intensive care and pediatric wards. Magnetic stimulation generates rapidly changing intense magnetic fields, which induce currents at sufficient depth for depolarizing neural tissue. Magnetic stimulation can be used for stimulating both inspiratory and expiratory muscles. For diaphragm contraction, the phrenic nerve can be activated by Cervical Magnetic Stimulation (CMS), anterior pre-sternal Magnetic Stimulation (aMS) or unilateral/bilateral anterolateral stimulation (UMS/BAMPS).

Significant progress has also been made in our understanding of the function of alveolar proteins and their role in the surfactant system (reviewed in [14]). While in the past the function of surfactant has been thought to involve just its surface-tension regulatory activity, recent studies have greatly amplified its importance to include a major role in lung protection, which involves the inhibition and inactivation of a large spectrum of pathogens. This is accomplished by the presence in surfactant of two groups of proteins: the large hydrophobic SPs (SP-B and SP-C), which regulate the interfacial lipid adsorption, and the large hydrophilic SPs (SP-A and SP-D), which are surfactant collectins able to inhibit foreign pathogens. In addition, the alveolar defense against foreign pathogens has been found to be enhanced by anti-microbial peptides such as defensins and cathelicidins.

Significant advances have also been made in the use of Hyperbaric Oxygen (HBO) in various syndromes associated with trauma [15, 16]. HBO has been shown to be particularly beneficial to patients with femoral head necrosis (FHN), as significant pain improvement and increased range of motion was observed with 20-30 treatments. All patients remained substantially pain-free seven years later, and none required hip arthroplasty. Substantial radiographic healing of the osteonecrosis was observed in almost 80% of their cases.

It should be understood that this review of recent findings only touches a few aspects of the active research presently carried out in the field of respiration. Much progress in many other areas is taking place as we write, but due to space limitation it will not be presented here. Great advances in the field are expected in the future, as modern technologies, advanced computer applications, and more detailed analyses of diseases continue being developed. Modern techniques of molecular biology, biochemistry and biophysics, applied to genetics, pathology and physiology of pulmonary science will continue enhancing our knowledge of respiratory mechanisms down to the cellular and molecular levels, providing a clearer understanding of the etiopathogenesis and pathology of lung diseases, and allowing us to develop more selective and better targeted therapeutic procedures. For a review of present trends in respiratory research see [17].

REFERENCES

[1] Halliday HL. Sufactants: past, present and future. J Perinatol 2008;28:S47-56.

[2] Pride NB, Permutt S, Riley RL, Bromberger-Barnea B. Determinants of maximal expiratory flow from the lungs. J App Physiol 1967;646-662.

[3] West JB, Dollery C, Naimark A. Distribution of blood flow in isolated lung; relation to vascular and alveolar pressures. J App Physiol 1964;713-724.

[4] Permutt S, Bromberger-Barnea B, Bane HN. Alveolar pressure, pulmonary pressure, and vascular waterfall. Med Thorac 1962;19:239-269.

[5] Parmigiani S, Solari E. The era of pulmonary surfactant from Laplace to nowadays. Acta Bio Medica 2003;74:69-75.

[6] Farré R, Montserrat JM, Navajas D. Noninvasive monitoring of respiratory mechanics during sleep. In: Polkey MI, Farré R, Dinh AT, Eds. Series "Respiratory monitoring: revisiting classical principles with new tools". Eur Respir J 2004; 24:1052-1060.

[7] Scano G, Stendardi L, Grazzini M. Understanding dyspnea by its language. In: Polkey MI, Farré R, Dinh AT. Eds. Series "Respiratory monitoring: revisiting classical principles with new tools". Eur Respir J 2005;25:380-385.

[8] Polkey MI, Farré, R, Dink-Xuan AT. Respiratory monitoring: revisiting classical physiological principles with new tools. Eur Respir J 2004;24:718-719.

[9] Calverley PMA, Koulouris NG. Flow limitation and dynamic hyperinflation: key concepts in modern respiratory physiology. In: Polkey MI, Farré R, Dinh AT. Eds. Series "Respiratory monitoring: revisiting classical principles with new tools". Eur Respir J 2005;25:186-199.

[10] Bourdin A, Burgel P-R, Chanez P, Garcia G, Perez T, Roche N. Recent advances in COPD: pathophysiology, respiratory physiology and clinical aspect, including comorbidities. Eur Resp Rev 2009;18:198-212.

[11] Vonk-Noordegraaf, A., van Wolferen, S.A., Marcus, J.T., Boonstra, A., Postmus, P.E., Peeters, J.W.L. and Peacock, A.J. Noninvasive assessment and monitoring of the pulmonary circulation. In: Polkey MI, Farré R, Dinh AT. Eds. Series "Respiratory monitoring: revisiting classical principles with new tools". Eur Respir J 2005;25:758-766.

[12] Huh D *et al.* A Human Disease Model of Drug Toxicity–Induced Pulmonary Edema in a Lung-on-a-Chip Microdevice. Sci Transl Med. 2012;4:159ra147.

[13] Man WD-C, Moxam J, Polkey MI. Magnetic stimulation for the measurement of respiratory and skeletal muscle function. In: Polkey MI, Farré R, Dinh-Xuan AT. Eds.

Series "Respiratory monitoring: revisiting classical principles with new tools". Eur Respir J 2004;24:846-860.

[14] Orgeiga S, *et al.* Recent advances in alveolar biology: evolution and function of alveolar proteins. Respir Physiol Neurobiol 2010;173S:S43-S54.

[15] Camporesi EM, Moon RE, Grande CM. Hyperbaric medicine: an integral part of trauma care. Crit Care Clin. 1990;6:203-19.

[16] Camporesi EM, Vezzani G, Bosco G, Mangar D, Bernasek TL. Hyperbaric oxygen therapy in femoral head necrosis. J Arthroplasty. 2011;25(6 Suppl):118-23.

[17] Kiley JP. Advancing respiratory research. Chest 2011;140:497-501.

CHAPTER 2

Basic Lung Structure

Camillo Peracchia

Abstract: This chapter briefly reviews major elements of pulmonary anatomy and histology. In particular, it describes the anatomy of lungs, airways, respiratory muscles and nerves, and both vascular and lymphatic circulation. It reviews the histology of airways: nose, pharynx, larynx, trachea, bronchi, bronchioles, alveolar ducts, alveolar sacs and alveoli. The histology of the pleura and neuroreceptors is also briefly described.

Keywords: Alveoli, Bronchi, Bronchioles, Clara Cells, Diaphragm, Epithelial-Cells Type-1, Epithelial- Cells Type-2, Feyrter's cells, Intercostal Muscles, J-receptors, Kohn's pores, Lungs, Lymphatic Circulation, Macrophages, Mucous-Secreting Cells, Neuro-Receptors, Pleura, Pulmonary Circulation, Pulmonary Innervation, Respiratory Muscles.

SYMBOLS, ACRONYMS AND NORMAL VALUES: See Appendix 3

Anatomy

Lungs

Right and left lungs occupy the thorax separated by the mediastinum. The lungs are shaped as smooth truncated cones pointing upward. Their upper end, the apex, extends just above the first rib and their concave base rests on the diaphragm. The lungs are composed of lobes: three in the right lung: superior, middle and inferior, and two in the left: superior and inferior. In turn, the lobes are composed of lobules, bordered by connective-tissue partitions known as trabeculae which contain branches of airways, pulmonary artery and veins.

Both lungs and chest wall are lined with a serous membrane known as pleura. The pleural membrane that coats the lungs is the visceral pleura, while the one that lines the internal surface of the chest wall is the parietal pleura. The gap between visceral and parietal pleural membranes is the pleural space, which is actually a virtual space rather than an open space because the two membranes are practically in contact with each other, being separated by only a very thin liquid layer whose function is to enable the pleural membranes to slide on each other during the breathing cycle.

Airways

The respiratory airways include: nose and sinus cavities, pharynx, larynx, trachea, bronchi, bronchioles, alveolar ducts, alveolar sacs and alveoli. The trachea branches at the carina into right and left primary bronchi - the right one is slightly larger and departs from the trachea at a steeper angle, making it easier for inhaled contaminant to find their way into the right lung. Below the carina, the bronchi subdivide into twenty three sequential airway generations (bifurcations), of which the first sixteen are purely conductive, those from the seventeenth to the nineteenth are partly conductive and partly gas-exchanging, and those from the twentieth to the twenty third are entirely gas-exchanging (Fig. **1**).

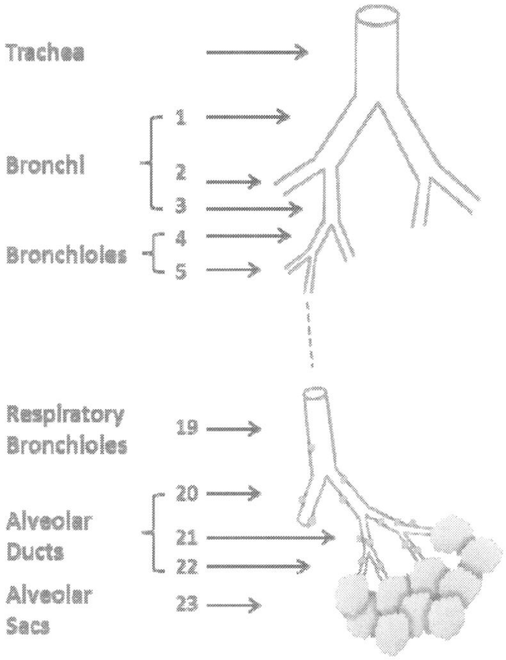

Figure 1: The trachea branches into 23 sequential generations of airways. The first 16 are conductive, those between 17 and 19 are partly conductive and partly gas-exchanging, and those beyond 20 are progressively more gas-exchanging.

The trachea is a cylindrical tube approximately 11 cm in length and 2.5 cm in diameter. Its lumen is kept open by the stiffening architecture of 15-20 cartilaginous half-rings open to the rear. Both the trachea and the two principal bronchi are extra-pulmonary. As the two bronchi branch into intrapulmonary bronchi, lobar bronchi, and tertiary (segmental) bronchi, the wall cartilage progressively decreases in size, being completely absent in terminal bronchioles.

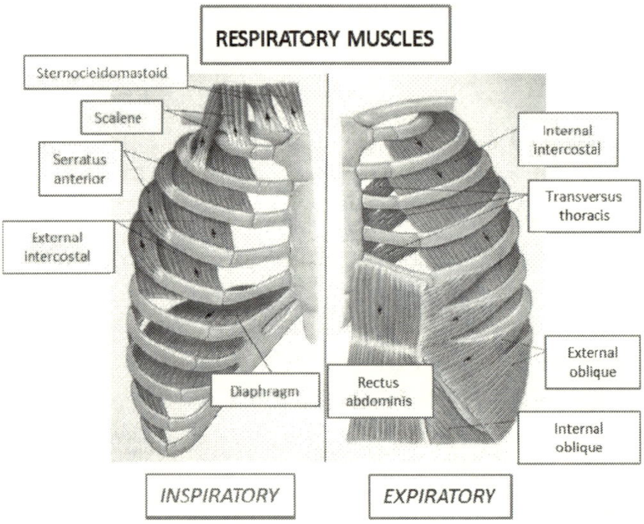

Figure 2: Inspiratory and expiratory respiratory muscles. In normal, quiet, breathing inspiration results from contraction of diaphragm and external intercostal muscles, while expiration is passive. The additional respiratory muscles shown here are only used in heavy breathing (vigorous exercise) or in certain diseased states. Adapted from: Martini FH and Timmons MJ, Human Anatomy, 1st Edition, © 1995. Reprinted by permission of Pearson Education, Inc., Upper Saddle River, NJ. Englewood Cliff, NJ, 1995.

The terminal bronchioles (16th generation) are as small as 0.3 mm in diameter and number over six thousand. Each of them branches into several generations of respiratory bronchioles, where some gas exchange with blood begins to take place. Distal bronchioles are interconnected by microscopic collateral airways known as "canals of Lambert" (first described by the American histologist Avery Eldorus Lambert, 1873-1950).

Respiratory bronchioles branch into alveolar ducts and alveolar sacs, all of which are gas-exchanging units. Multiple polyhedral-shaped alveoli, about 300 μm in diameter, line the alveolar sacs. The alveolar diameter progressively increases for lung base to apex due to gravity (see Chapter 7). Small passageways (10-15 μm in diameter), known as "Kohn's pores" (first described by the German physician Hans Kohn, 1866-1935), connect neighboring alveoli, allowing for gas exchange among them.

Respiratory Muscles

Diaphragm and inter-costal muscles are the principal muscles operating during the breathing cycle (Fig. **2**). With normal breathing (at rest), muscular activity is only involved in inspiration. Most of the inspiratory function is provided by the diaphragm, a dome-shaped muscle that creates a partition between abdominal and thoracic cavities. The contraction of the diaphragm increases the lung volume by lengthening the vertical diameter of the chest. In addition, by compressing the abdominal organs it causes the lower ribs to be displaced outwardly, which increases both the antero-posterior and lateral dimensions of the chest as well. Partially involved in inspiration at rest are also the external intercostal muscles (Fig. **2**), which span from the inferior border of a rib to the superior border of the next (more caudal) rib. The contraction of these muscles elevates the rib cage and expands the chest by increasing its antero-posterior and lateral dimensions.

Additional respiratory muscles are only involved in heavy breathing (vigorous exercise) and in illnesses such as asthma, emphysema, fibrosis, or extra-thoracic airway obstruction. In forced inspiration, accessory muscles such as scalene, sternocleidomastoid and serratus anterior (Fig. **2**) cooperate with external intercostal muscles in lifting the chest wall. In forced expiration, the contraction of internal intercostal muscles, which span from the superior border of a rib to the inferior border of the adjacent (more cranial) rib, reduces the chest volume by lowering the ribs. In addition, the transverus thoracis and both external and internal oblique muscles (Fig. **2**), cooperate with internal intercostal muscles in lowering the ribs. The contraction of the rectus abdominis (Fig. **2**) also contributes to expiration efforts by adding pressure to abdominal organs - this raises the diaphragm and reduces the vertical chest dimension. Expiratory muscles are also essential for coughing and sneezing.

Pulmonary Circulation

Two vascular networks perfuse the lungs: pulmonary and bronchial. The pulmonary artery carries venous (deoxygenated) blood, whereas bronchial arteries carry arterial (oxygenated) blood. The pulmonary artery, which originates from the right ventricle, whose thickness is just 4-5 mm (approximately a third of the thickness of the left ventricle) first divides into two smaller arteries that perfuse right and left lungs (Fig. **3**) and then progressively into smaller arteries, arterioles and capillaries. The wall of the pulmonary artery is mostly made of elastic fibers (eight layers) interspaced by a thin layer of smooth muscle fibers which only represents ~2% of the wall thickness. As the pulmonary artery branch into smaller arteries the elastic layer diminishes, being replaced by smooth muscle fibers that represent the major component of the wall thickness down to arterioles ~100 μm in diameter. As the arterioles become smaller, the smooth muscle layer progressively diminishes, such arterioles smaller than ~30 μm in diameter are virtually muscle-free. The smallest arterioles (~13 μm in diameter) branch into ~100 billion capillaries (10-12 μm in diameter), which perfuse the 300-500 million alveoli forming a vascular network within the alveolar wall.

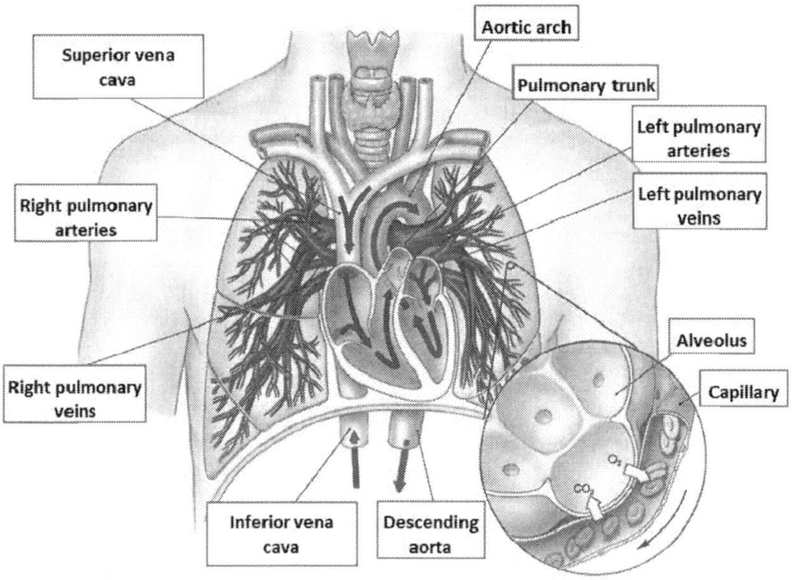

Figure 3: Representation of pulmonary vascular system. Venous blood entering the heart's right atrium from the venae cavae is injected into the pulmonary artery by the right ventricle. Oxygenated blood exiting from the lungs *via* pulmonary veins enters the left atrium and is injected into the aorta by the left ventricle. The inset shows the alveolar-capillary barrier. Adapted from: Martini, F.H. and Timmons, M.J., Human Anatomy, 1st Edition, © 1995. Reprinted by permission of Pearson Education, Inc., Upper Saddle River, NJ. Englewood Cliff, NJ, 1995.

Oxygenated blood from alveolar capillaries flows into progressively larger branches of pulmonary veins, eventually emptying into the left atrium *via* four pulmonary veins, two from each lung (Fig. **3**). The wall of the pulmonary veins is much thinner than that of the arteries, as it is mostly composed of collagen and a thin smooth muscle layer. While the branches of the pulmonary artery run next to airway branches, pulmonary veins are located within interlobular septa, and come near arteries and airways only at the lungs' hilum.

In addition to the pulmonary artery tree, the lungs are perfused by minor arteries known as "supernumerary" arteries. These vessels arise at right angles from pulmonary vessels ~1 mm in diameter, and provide a source of blood which may be very important for maintaining alveolar perfusion if the main blood supply were blocked.

The trachea is vascularized by branches of the inferior thyroid artery; the bronchial tree, instead, receives blood from different arteries. The left bronchial arteries (superior and inferior) usually originate directly from the thoracic aorta, whereas the right bronchial artery may originate from the thoracic aorta, the left (superior) bronchial artery, or several right intercostal arteries. Bronchial arteries follow the bronchial tree all the way down to terminal bronchioles. The smallest bronchial vessels form extensive anastomoses with the smallest branches of the pulmonary artery, resulting in some mixing of venous and arterial bloods. Venous blood from capillaries of the larger (extra-pulmonary) bronchi empties into the azygos vein, eventually flowing into the right atrium. In contrast, blood coming from smaller (intra-pulmonary) airways drains into pulmonary veins after mixing with oxygenated blood at the anastomoses. This bronchial (deoxygenated) blood adds an additional small source of venous admixture to the right-to-left conductive (anatomical) blood shunt (see Chapter 7).

Lymphatic Circulation

A network of lymphatic vessels located within the interstitial spaces of alveolar sacs and pleural surfaces provides the means for conveying the lymph to the systemic circulation. Lymph flows at a rate of ~0.5 ml/min *via* the right lymphatic duct and the left thoracic duct, eventually reaching the innominate vein.

Innervation

Lungs and pleura are innervated by branches of parasympathetic (vagal) and sympathetic fibers, which originate from the anterior and posterior pulmonary plexuses at the lung's hilum. The vagus contains both efferent and afferent fibers. The former innervate bronchial smooth muscles, pulmonary vessels, and secretory glands; their activation causes bronchoconstriction, vasodilation and mucous secretion, respectively. The latter are sensory fibers activated by stimuli to the airway epithelia, such as touch, pain and stretch.

Sympathetic innervation involves efferent fibers which, upon stimulation, exert an inhibitory effect on bronchial smooth muscles and glands, causing bronchodilation and reduced mucous secretion, and a stimulatory effect on pulmonary vessels, causing vasoconstriction. The parietal pleural membrane is innervated by branches of phrenic and intercostal nerves, and the visceral membrane by branches of vagus and sympathetic nerves.

In addition, there are non-adrenergic, non-cholinergic (NANC) nerve fibers. NANC fibers create inhibitory pathways to airway smooth muscles that regulate muscle tone *via* secretion of peptide neurotransmitters (reviewed in [1]). There is evidence that defects of this system may play a role in airway hyperactivity in asthma and Chronic Obstructive Pulmonary Disease (COPD).

For further reading on lung anatomy see reference [2].

Histology

Airways

Nose

The anterior nasal cavity is lined with a stratified squamous epithelium containing stiff hairs, which protect the air passages from dust particles and other macroscopic environmental contaminants. The posterior nasal cavity is lined with a mucous-secreting ciliated epithelium interspaced with receptors of the olfactory organ. Beneath the epithelium there are mucous glands, connective tissue and an extensive venous plexus, which helps maintaining warm the nasal passages and adds humidity to inspired air.

The paranasal sinuses are lined with a ciliated epithelium similar to that of nasal cavities. The cilia help clearing mucous from the sinuses by flowing it into the nasal cavity.

Larynx

From the anterior surface of the epiglottis down to the vocal cords the larynx is lined with a stratified squamous epithelium containing 3-5 µm long cilia. Below the vocal cords the epithelial lining changes into a pseudo-stratified columnar epithelium that contains numerous mucous-secreting goblet cells. The laryngeal wall includes a layer of cartilage, which provides a framework for laryngeal shape and stiffness, and two muscle layers: intrinsic and extrinsic. The activity of intrinsic muscles provides the larynx with different shapes needed for phonation. The extrinsic muscles link the larynx to adjacent muscles and ligaments, and participate in the deglutition mechanism. Laryngeal blood is supplied by branches of the superior and inferior thyroid arteries and empties into the thyroid veins. An extensive lymphatic plexus leads to upper cervical and tracheal lymph nodes.

Trachea and Bronchi

Trachea and bronchi are lined with a ciliated columnar epithelium rich in goblet cells, which produce and secrete mucous into the lumen of the airways (Fig. **4** (**A**). A network of tight junctions (zonulae occludentes) seals the extracellular space between luminal and basolateral sides of epithelial cells, preventing diffusion of inhaled contaminants. The structure of columnar cells' cilia is the same as that seen in other tissues. In cross-section the cilia display two central microtubules and nine radially arranged sets of double microtubules (doublets). Two small processes called "dynein arms" project from each doublet.

Slightly below and intermixed with ciliated cells there are basal cells in the process of differentiating into either ciliated or goblet cells. Scattered among basal cells are Feyrter's cells - also known with various names such as: Kulchitsky's cells (K-cells), Amine Precursor Uptake Decarboxylation cells (APUD), and small-granule cells. Feyrter's cells appear to have a neuroendocrine function because they contain vasoactive substances such as 5-hydroxytryptamine (serotonin), bombesin and calcitonin. They extend narrow cytoplasmic processes into the bronchial lumen. These processes are believed to sense the gas composition of inspired air, suggesting that Feyrter's cells might be involved in fine tuning ventilation-perfusion distribution. These cells are aggregated in groups called neuroepithelial bodies. A type of lung cancer known as small-cell carcinoma (common in smokers) is believed to result from malignant transformation of Feyrter's cells.

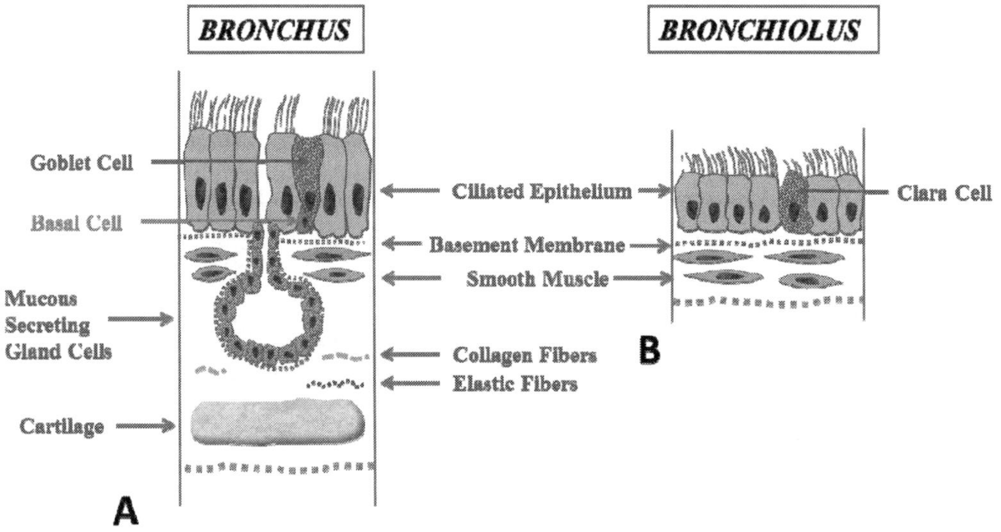

Figure 4: The pseudo-stratified epithelium lining trachea and bronchi (A) consists of ciliated columnar cells interspaced with mucous-secreting goblet cells and basal cells. A basement membrane separates the epithelium from the sub-mucosa, which contains mucous secreting glands, smooth muscle, collagen, elastic fibers and cartilage. Glands and cartilage are absent in bronchioles (B). Bronchioles also contain a few Clara cells (glycosaminoglycan-secreting cells; B).

The epithelium rests on a thick basement membrane which separates it from the sub-mucosa, a layer that contains numerous mucous secreting glands - the major mucous producers (Fig. **4A**). A loose connective tissue known as lamina propria separates the epithelium from the twenty or so C-shaped cartilaginous segments, which are linked to each other by elastic annular ligaments. Cartilage is absent at the posterior tracheal wall, where it is replaced by a layer of smooth muscle fibers oriented perpendicularly to the long axis of trachea and bronchi (Fig. **4A**). As the bronchi enter the lungs, their cartilaginous rings disappear, being replaced by irregularly shaped cartilaginous plates (Fig. **4A**) that encircle the bronchial circumference.

The sub-mucosa contains an extensive lymphatic network that leads to lymph nodes scattered along the length of the trachea. Innervation is supplied by the recurrent branch of the vagus and by sympathetic nerves.

Bronchioles

As we follow the airways down to smaller and smaller bronchi, eventually to reach the level of bronchioles, we notice that the cartilage progressively decreases, being completely absent where the bronchioles' diameter is reduced to 1 mm or less. At this level, the cartilage is replaced by smooth muscle fibers that completely surround the bronchiole (Fig. **4B**). Bronchioles are lined with a mucous epithelium similar to that of the trachea. Scattered among the epithelial ciliated cells are the Clara cells (Fig. **4B**), which are dome-shaped cells with short microvilli. Clara cells (first described by the German physician Max Clara, 1899-1966) are believed to secrete glycosaminoglycans, which protect the luminal surface of the bronchioles. The basement membrane separates the epithelial cells from the lamina propria mucosae, which is a thin layer of connective tissue containing some lymphoid cells as well as collagen and elastic fibers.

Mucous secreting glands, deeply nested below the muscle layer, are found as far down as the smallest cartilage-containing bronchioles. A diffuse lymphatic network penetrates the mucosa and the collagenous layer. As bronchioles decrease in diameter, their wall becomes progressively thinner and loses much of the fibrous layer, but maintains smooth muscle fibers as far down as to alveolar ducts.

Respiratory Bronchioles and Alveolar Ducts

As airways narrow down to ~ 0.5 mm in diameter, the bronchioles are called "respiratory" because through their wall some gas exchange with blood begins to occur. Some of their surface is lined with a cuboidal cilia-free epithelium, which coats a thin layer of connective tissue containing collagen, elastic fibers and smooth muscle cells. Some areas begin to display a few alveoli, where cuboidal cells are gradually replaced by alveolar epithelial cells.

Respiratory bronchioles branch into several alveolar ducts, which further branch into a tree-like arrangement of tortuous and thin-walled tubes. As in respiratory bronchioles, the wall of alveolar ducts contains smooth muscle as well as collagen and elastic fibers.

Alveolar Sacs and Alveoli

Alveolar sacs and individual alveoli originate from alveolar ducts at openings known as "atria". The alveoli are polyhedral sacs lined with a continuous layer of very thin and delicate squamous cells known as Epithelial Cells Type 1 (EP1, Fig. **5**). Intermixed with the squamous cells are few larger cells known as Epithelial Cells Type 2 (EP2, Fig. **5**) - these cells are filled with dense bodies, 0.2-1.0 μm in diameter, consisting of multiple parallel lamellae of phospholipid secretion known as "surfactant". The surfactant coats the entire alveolar surface and drastically reduces surface tension at the interface between the alveolar gas and the thin liquid layer that coats the epithelium. The epithelial surface is maintained clean by macrophages (Fig. **5**), also known as alveolar phagocytes or dust cells, which capture small contaminant particles that had not been trapped by the mucous of upper airways.

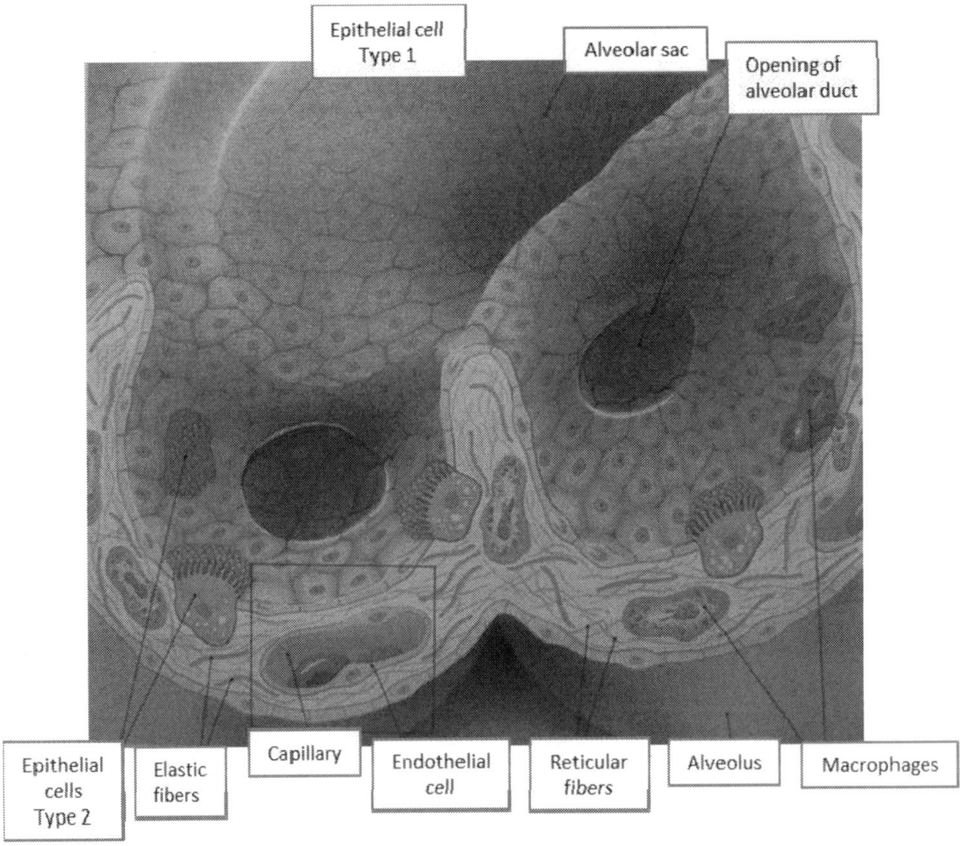

Figure 5: Structure of alveolar sacs. The alveoli are lined with squamous cell Type 1 (EP1) and a few epithelial cells Type 2 (EP2). EP2 cells contain dense bodies (0.2-1.0 μm) composed of multiple parallel lamellae of a phospholipid secretion (surfactant). Adapted from: Martini, F.H. and Timmons, M.J., Human Anatomy, 1st Edition, © 1995. Reprinted by permission of Pearson Education, Inc., Upper Saddle River, NJ. Englewood Cliff, NJ, 1995.

The alveoli are completely surrounded by an extensive network of capillaries filled with blood coming from the pulmonary artery. The alveolar epithelium is only separated from the capillary endothelium by the basement membrane, such that the total thickness of the blood-gas barrier only ranges from 0.1 to 0.5 μm.

Pleura

Visceral and parietal pleural membranes are composed of a thin layer of connective tissue containing collagen, elastic fibers, fibroblasts, macrophages, and a network of capillaries, lymphatic vessels and nerves. Both membranes are coated by a single layer of mesothelial cells somewhat similar to peritoneal cells. Branches of phrenic and intercostal nerves innervate the parietal membrane, while the visceral membrane is innervated by vagal and sympathetic branches.

Neuro-Receptors

A number of stretch- and irritant-sensitive neuro-receptors are found in airway walls. Stretch receptors respond to changes in lung volume and are located within the smooth muscle layer. Irritant receptors respond to inhaled chemicals and dust particles and are located superficially just below the epithelium. When activated by irritants, these receptors induce fast and shallow breathing (tachypnea). Juxta-capillary receptors (J-receptors) are located near capillary walls and respond to interstitial edema and/or inflammation; their activation also induces tachypnea. Additional neuro-receptors are found in chest-wall's intercostal muscles. These receptors are believed to function as modulators of breathing. For further reading on lung histology see reference [2].

REFERENCES

[1] Barnes PJ. The third nervous system in the lung: physiology and clinical perspectives. Thorax 1984;39:561-567.

[2] Martini FH, Timmons MJ, Tallitsch RB. Human anatomy. 7th Ed. San Francisco: Pearson - Benjamin Cummings; 2011.

CHAPTER 3

Respiratory Mechanics

Camillo Peracchia

Abstract: This chapter focuses on the elastic properties of the respiratory system and on the mechanisms by which gases are flown in and out of the lungs during the breathing cycle. It begins by defining the lung volumes (capacities) and describing methods used for measuring them. Then, it describes the mechanisms of inspiration and expiration and the relationship between respiratory muscles and elastic characteristics of the respiratory system. The properties of respiratory mechanics are then divided into two sections: static and dynamic. Static mechanics deals with elastic characteristics of lungs, chest wall and the combined lungs + chest wall system, and with methods used for quantifying them. The relevance of surface tension and surfactant in modulating lung compliance and in maintaining the alveoli dry is discussed in detail. Dynamic mechanics discusses how gases flow through airways during the breathing cycle. Alveolar and intra-pleural pressures changes during normal breathing and while breathing through narrowed airways are described, as well as mechanism causing airway collapse in patients with loss of lung elasticity (emphysema), or suffering from extra-thoracic airway obstruction. The last two sections deal with the work of breathing and the most common pulmonary function tests.

Keywords: Airway Collapse, Airway Resistance, Bernoulli Principle, Breathing Cycle, Chest-Wall Compliance, Diaphragm, Elastance, Expiratory Muscles, Inspiratory Muscles, Intercostal Muscles, Laminar Flow, Lung Compliance, Lung Volumes, Plethysmography, Pulmonary Function-Tests, Respiratory Work, Spirometry, Surface Tension, Surfactant, Trans-Pulmonary Pressure, Turbulent Flow.

SYMBOLS, ACRONYMS AND NORMAL VALUES: See Appendix 3

Lung Volumes

The amount of gas present in the lungs obviously depends on the stage of the breathing cycle at which one is, as well as on different respiratory maneuvers such as maximal inspiration or expiration. By convention, the amount of gas present in the lungs at different stages of breathing is referred to as "volume" or "capacity". Lung volumes are classified as follows (Fig. **1A**):

- Functional Residual Capacity (FRC): gas volume that remains in the lungs at the end of a normal expiration.
- Tidal Volume (VT): gas volume that flows in and out of the lungs during the breathing cycle.

- Inspiratory Reserve Volume (IRV): largest gas volume that can be inspired from the end of a normal inspiration.

- Inspiratory Capacity (IC): largest gas volume that can be inspired from FRC (VT + IRV).

- Expiratory Reserve Volume (ERV): largest gas volume that can be expired from FRC (FRC - RV).

- Residual Volume (RV): gas volume that remains in lungs after maximal expiration (FRC - ERV).

- Vital Capacity (VC): largest gas volume that can be expired after maximal inspiration (TLC - RV).

- Total Lung Capacity (TLC): gas volume in the lungs at end of maximal inspiration (VC + RV).

Lung volumes can be measured by the inert gas dilution method. This method consists of filling the chamber of a spirometer with a known volume (V_1) of an inert gas (He or N_2) of known concentration (C_1) and asking the subject to breathe in and out of the spirometer several times, starting the breathing experiment at the lung volume (V_2) that needs to be measured. At the end of the experiment the final gas concentration (C_2) is measured and V_2 is calculated as follows (Eqs. 1 and 2):

$$V_1 \times C_1 = (V_1 + V_2) \times C_2 \; ... \qquad \textbf{(1)}$$

$$V_2 = \frac{V_1 \times C_1 - V_1 \times C_2}{C_2} \; ... \qquad \textbf{(2)}$$

The residual volume (RV) can only be measured by the inert gas method, while the other lung volumes can also be measured by spirometry. The old-fashion spirometer is an instrument composed of an inverted cylinder inserted into an upright cylinder filled with water. As respiratory gases enter or exit the spirometer, the inverted cylinder is displaced upward or downward, respectively. The inverted cylinder is connected to a pen that records the displacements of the inverted cylinder on the paper of a rotating cylinder (a record of volume changes is shown in Fig. **1B**).

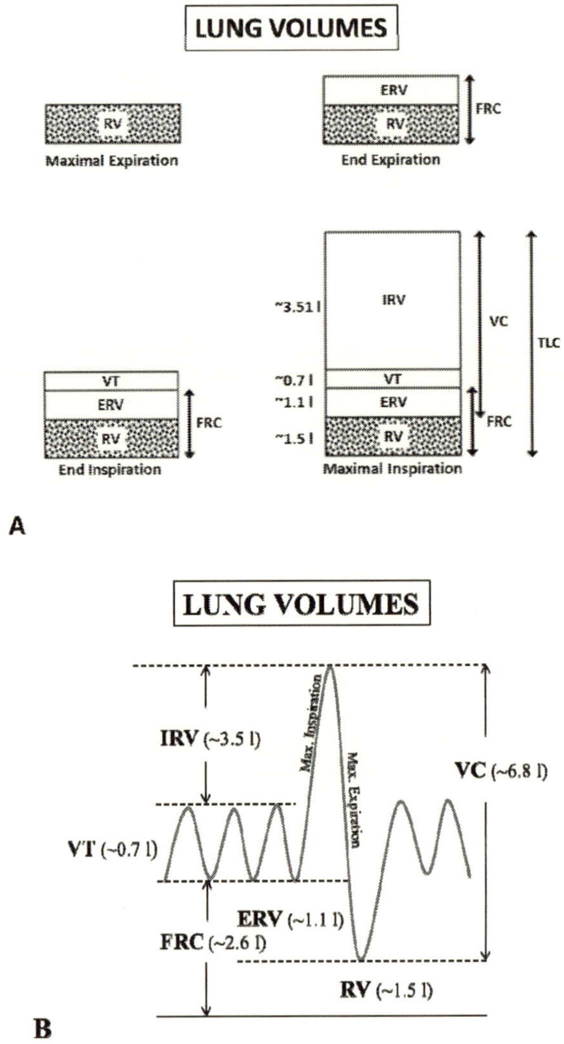

Figure 1: A). Classification of lung volumes. B). Tracing of changes in lung volume recorded from an old-fashioned spirometer during the normal breathing cycle, and at maximal inspiration and expiration.

While the old-fashion water spirometer provides a very demonstrative illustration of lung volume measurements, nowadays newer instruments and methodologies are more commonly used. One is the whole-body plethysmography, a technique first developed in 1956 by DuBois and coworkers [1, 2]. The body plethysmograph is a rigid box in which the subject sits; small changes in box pressure caused by the subject's attempt to inspire against a closed airway result in small changes in box volume, which allow one to calculate the changes in lung volume. In addition, other instruments, such as: fully electronic spirometers, incentive spirometers, peak flow meters, windmill-type spirometers, tilt-compensated spirometers, and so on, are often used in clinical practice (for a review of pulmonary function tests, see [3]).

Lung volumes are affected by age and diseases such as emphysema, pulmonary fibrosis, Adult and Infant Respiratory Distress Syndromes (ARDS and IRDS), and so on. With age, VC and TLC decrease and RV increases. These changes start approximately after the age of twenty. The average VC can be estimated using the following relationships [4] (Eqs. 3 and 4):

$$\mathrm{VC}\ (\mathrm{ml, BTPS}) = [27.63 - (0.112 \times \mathrm{age})] \times \text{height in cm (for males)} \ldots \quad \textbf{(3)}$$

$$\mathrm{VC}\ (\mathrm{ml, BTPS}) = [21.78 - (0.101 \times \mathrm{age})] \times \text{height in cm (for females)} \ldots \quad \textbf{(4)}$$

Emphysema causes a loss of lung elasticity (increased compliance), resulting in increased RV and FRC. Pulmonary fibrosis reduces FRC as the lungs become stiffer (reduced compliance). The same occurs in ARDS and IRDS.

Mechanisms of Inspiration and Expiration

During inspiration, air flows into the lungs *via* a tree-like arrangement of airways. The trachea branches into twenty three sequential generations of airways of which the first sixteen are purely conductive, those from seventeenth to nineteenth are partly conductive and partly gas-exchanging and those from twentieth to twenty third are entirely gas-exchanging (See Chapter 2, Fig. **1**).

During inspiration, air is actively inhaled by the coordinated contraction of inspiratory muscles, represented primarily by the diaphragm and the external inter-costal muscles. The inspiratory muscles expand chest and lungs by exerting a force sufficient to overcome lung elasticity and airway flow resistance. During expiration, gases are passively exhaled by virtue of the elastic properties of the lungs (lung recoil), which tend to bring the system to its resting state (FRC).

Inspiration results from the flattening of the diaphragm and the raising of the rib cage. The contraction of the diaphragm (flattening) increases the vertical dimension of the thoracic cage and compresses the abdominal organs, generating a positive pressure within the abdomen that displaces outwardly the lower ribs - the result is an increase of both antero-posterior and lateral dimensions of the thorax (Fig. **2**). The contraction of external inter-costal muscles elevates the ribs (Fig. **2**), increasing the antero-posterior dimension of the chest and contributing to lung expansion.

Expiration is passive during normal (quiet) breathing, as it is caused by lung recoil, but it is active in pathological conditions, such as asthma or emphysema for example, and during heavy exercise. Active expiration results from the contraction of abdominal muscles (both internal and external obliques, and rectus abdominis; see Chapter 2, Fig. **2**), which lowers the ribs and shifts the diaphragm upward, and from the contraction of internal inter-costal muscles, which moves the ribs downward as well (Fig. **2**). Expiratory muscles are also essential for coughing and sneezing.

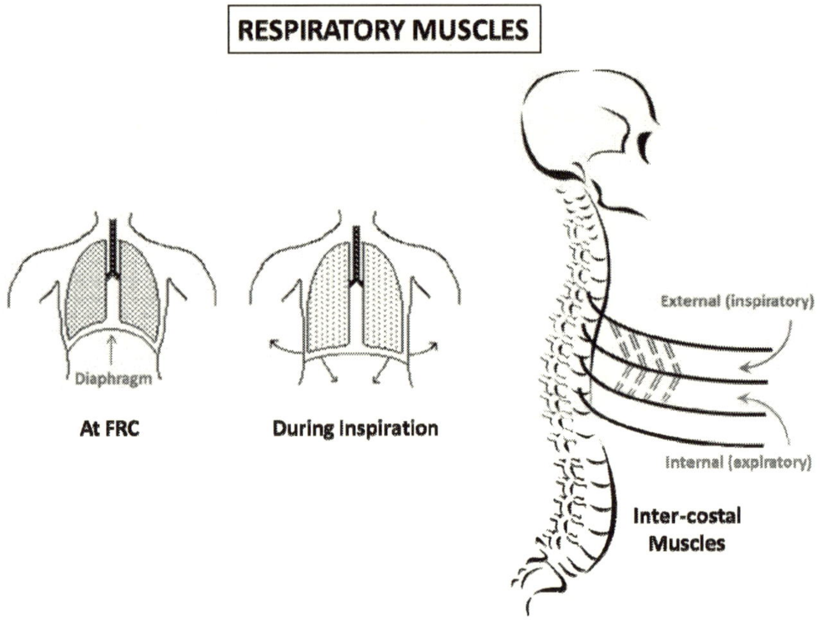

Figure 2: During normal (quiet) breathing, only inspiration is an active process involving contraction (flattening) of diaphragm and (minimally) of external inter-costal muscles. Forced inspiration and expiration involve additional (accessory) muscles (see text).

Accessory inspiratory muscles, which are active during heavy breathing (vigorous exercise, for example) and in diseased states that affect lung elasticity and/or flow resistance, include: scalenes, steronocleidomastoids, serratus anterior, serratus posterior-superior, levatores costarum, suprahyoid, trapezius, pectoralis major and minor, latissimus dorsi, sacrospinalis and subclavious. Accessory expiratory muscles, active during heavy exercise or in diseased conditions that increase expiratory flow resistance, include: transversus thoracis, serratus posterior-inferior and quadratus lumborum.

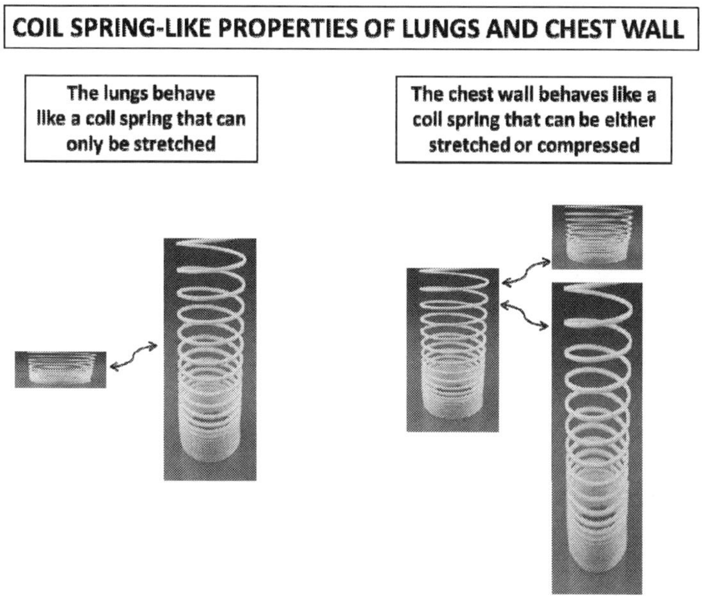

Figure 3: Coil spring images, adapted from MS-Word (Clip Art), simulating the elastic characteristics of lungs (left) and chest wall (right).

Respiratory mechanics is composed of two sections: "static" and "dynamic". The static section deals with the elastic properties of lungs, chest wall, and the combined lung + chest-wall system. The dynamic section deals with the physics of gas flow through airways during the breathing cycle.

Static Properties of Respiratory Mechanics

For understanding the mechanical properties of lungs and chest wall we need to keep in mind three fundamental rules, which are dictated by the specific elastic characteristics of lungs and chest wall:

1. ***At any volume the lungs always tend to collapse***

2. ***At volumes lower than ~70% of TLC the chest wall tends to expand***

3. ***At volumes larger than ~70% of TLC the chest wall tends to collapse***

Lungs and chest wall behaviors are based on their intrinsic elastic properties. Basically, lungs and chest wall behave like coil springs with different properties: the lungs are like a spring that can only be stretched (expanded), while the chest wall is like a spring that can be either stretched (expanded) or compressed (Fig. **3**).

Lungs

Elastic Characteristics

The lungs are roughly similar to a rubber balloon whose elastic properties can be described in terms of compliance (distensibility) or its reciprocal, elastance (resistance to distension). Compliance (C) is measured by the slope of the lung compliance curve (Fig. **4**, A, PL) - ratio of volume (V) over pressure (P) increments (Δ; see Eq. 5):

$$C = \frac{\Delta V}{\Delta P} \text{ (slope of pressure} - \text{volume curve) ...} \quad \textbf{(5)}$$

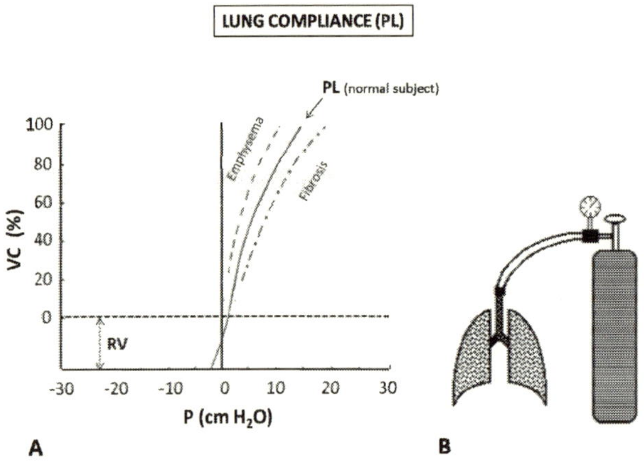

Figure 4: Lung compliance curve (A, PL). Its steepness decreases at larger volumes because the lungs become stiffer (less compliant) as it is stretched. Diseases that affect lung compliance shift the PL curve to the left (emphysema, increased compliance) or the right (fibrosis, decreased compliance). In isolated lungs, compliance could be measured by inflating the lungs with

incremental volumes of air and measuring the pressure needed to maintain the lungs inflated at each volume (B).

Each point in the lung compliance curve represents the pressure needed to maintain the lungs inflated at that particular volume; note that this curve describes the elastic properties of the lungs alone - it does not include the elastic properties of the chest wall. The lung compliance curve is not linear, as its steepness progressively decreases as the lungs expand - the lungs become stiffer as they approach their maximum volume. Therefore, at volumes near FRC increments in lung volume require small pressure increments, whereas at volumes close to TLC larger pressure increments are needed to expand the lungs by the same volume increments.

Certain lung diseases alter lung compliance. This is exemplified by the two additional curves drawn in Fig. **4A**, which represent compliance characteristics of emphysematous (dashed line) and fibrotic (dashed-dotted line) lungs. Emphysema increases compliance (decreases elastance), whereas fibrosis decreases compliance (increases elastance). Thus, an emphysematous lung is easier to inflate than a normal lung - less pressure is needed to produce the same volume increment; the opposite is true for a fibrotic lung, which is stiffer than normal.

The compliance curve of the lungs could be generated by inflating isolated lungs with increasing volumes (Fig. **4B**) and measuring the pressure (lung recoil pressure) necessary to maintain those volumes (Fig. **4A**). Obviously, *in vivo* one cannot inflate the lungs independently from the chest wall. Yet, also *in vivo* the compliance curve of the lungs can be drawn. This is done by measuring the intra-esophageal (same as intra-pleural) pressure while the subject holds the breath at different lung volumes with open glottis, and plotting the "negative" pressure values recorded with a "positive" sign (see below).

What Determines the Elastic Properties of the Lung

Three main factors determine the magnitude of lung compliance:

- *Surface tension (alveolar lining fluid/surfactant).*

- *Elastic characteristics of the lung tissue (elastic and collagen fibers).*

$ *Vascular pressure, interstitial fluid etc.*

Of these factors the most important is surface tension. This can be demonstrated by filling isolated lungs with either saline or air (Fig. **5**). When saline fills the alveoli, the surface tension generated by the air-liquid interface is eliminated. Consequently, lung compliance dramatically increases. In this condition, the elastic recoil of the lungs is entirely due to the elastic characteristics of the lung tissue. In contrast, when the saline is replaced with air, the lungs become much stiffer (less compliant) because of the surface tension generated by the air-liquid interface (Fig. **5**). In lungs filled with air there is also a greater hysteresis between inflation and deflation curves - at any given volume the pressure needed to maintain that volume is greater during lung inflation than during deflation (Fig. **5**). This is due to the presence of surfactant (see below).

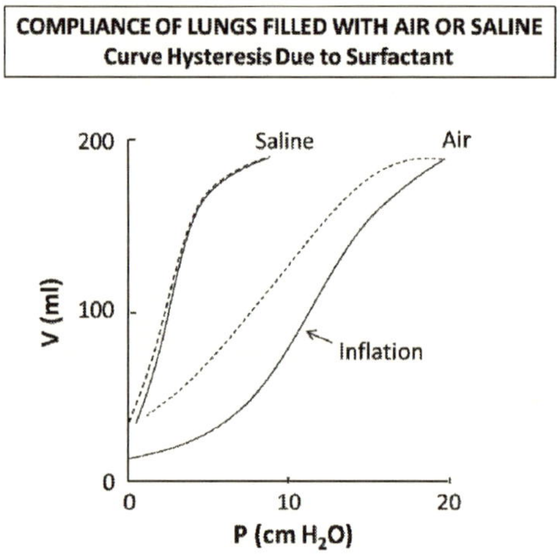

Figure 5: Compliance curves of isolated lungs filled with either air or water. Lungs filled with air are less compliant due to surface tension. The hysteresis (dotted curve) is caused by surfactant, whose effect in lowering surface tension is greater during lung deflation.

Surface Tension

Surface tension is defined as the tendency of a liquid surface to contract. The surface contraction is due to unbalanced attractive forces among the liquid molecules at the air-liquid interface. While H_2O molecules in solution attract each other with equal force in all directions, resulting in a net force of zero, at the air-water interface they are attracted to each other only laterally and downward.

This creates a downward force that tends to minimize the surface area. Surface tension is measured by the force exerted on a platinum strip dipped into the surface. Water has a surface tension of 72 dynes/cm.

Surfactant

An important property of surface tension, most relevant to the lungs, is its effect on curved surfaces. If the curved surfaces of the alveoli were lined with water without surfactant, surface tension would tend to collapse the alveoli with greater and greater force the smaller their volume.

This phenomenon is described by the law of Laplace (named after the French mathematician and astronomer Pier-Simon Laplace, 1749-1827) which states that the pressure (P) needed to maintain an alveolus inflated is equal to twice the surface tension (2T) over the radius (r) (Fig. **6**) - note that the Laplace law applies to any curved surface, not just the alveoli. Therefore, in the absence of surfactant the lungs would be extremely unstable - since the lungs are composed of over three hundred million alveoli communicating with each other, if at any time an alveolus were to become slightly smaller than its neighbors its tendency would be to empty its gases into the larger neighbors and rapidly collapse (Fig. **6**). The presence of surfactant at the alveolar surface prevents alveolar collapse.

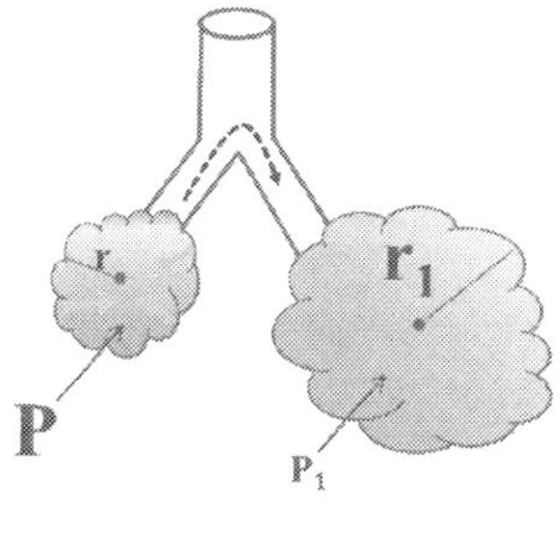

$$P = \frac{2T}{r} > P_1 = \frac{2T}{r_1}$$

Figure 6: Law of Laplace.

Surfactant is a substance that lowers surface tension and changes surface tension as the radius changes.

Surfactant is composed of a phospholipid (dipalmitoyl lecithin, DPL) produced by alveolar epithelial cells Type 2 (EP2, also known as type 2 granular pneumocytes). In EP2 cells (Fig. 7), surfactant is aggregated into lamellar bodies which are secreted into the alveoli's hypophase (liquid lining) where the surfactant unravels into tubular myelin (TM). The lipids of the surfactant are compressed into the "surfactant reservoir", which provides surfactant storage for resupplying the lipid monolayer that coats the alveolar surface. At the air-liquid interface, the charged end of DPL (lecithin) is in water and the hydrophobic end (fatty acid chain) is in air.

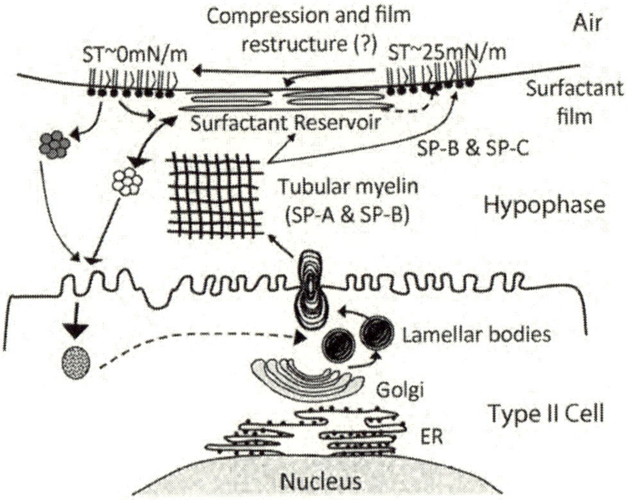

Figure 7: Schematic diagram of surfactant synthesis and secretion by alveolar epithelial cells type 2 (EP2 cells). Surfactant compression reduces surface tension (ST) - in this example, from ~25 to 0 milliNewtons per meter (mN/m, same as dynes/cm). SP = surfactant proteins; ER = endoplasmic reticulum. Reproduced from: Orgeig, S. *et al.*, Recent advances in alveolar biology: evolution and function of alveolar proteins. Respir. Physiol. Neurobiol. 173S:S43-S54, 2010. Permission granted by Elsevier.

In addition to lipids, surfactant contains proteins (SPs) which play a major role in lung protection by inhibiting and inactivating many foreign pathogens. There are two groups of SPs proteins (Fig. 7): large hydrophobic SPs (SP-B and SP-C), which regulate lipid adsorption at the air-liquid interface, and large hydrophilic SPs (SP-A and SP-D), which are "collectins" that inhibit foreign pathogens. The alveolar defense against foreign pathogens is also enhanced by peptides such as defensins and cathelicidins.

The behavior of the surfactant is shown in Fig. **8A**: flask "a" shows that in the absence of surfactant the surface tension at the air-water interface is 72 dynes/cm; flask "b" shows that by adding a few molecules of DPL (spread apart) the surface tension is significantly reduced (30 dynes/cm); flasks "c and d" show that the compression of DPL molecules on the surface, as it happens with decreasing alveolar volume, progressively lowers surface tension down to zero (d). Compression of DPL increases their two-dimensional pressure, which opposes the surface tension of the water-air interface and reduces the net surface tension of the water-surfactant complex down to zero. Therefore, surfactant serves two purposes: it lowers the surface tension, which reduces the work of breathing, and it reduces surface tension more and more the smaller the alveolar radius, which promotes alveolar stability – it prevents alveolar collapse. The reason for the greater efficiency of surfactant in deflation, which is reflected by the hysteresis of the compliance curve (Fig. **5**), is that while during inflation surfactant molecules become separated as the surface area increases, causing drop in compliance, during deflation surfactant molecules are squeezed together as the area decreases, causing an increase in compliance.

Lack of sufficient surfactant is the major cause of the respiratory distress syndromes (ARDS and IRDS). In these cases, surface tension is very high, which reduces lung compliance and greatly increases the inspiratory work load. Moreover, surface tension does not significantly decrease as alveolar volume decreases, so that many alveoli become unstable and collapse (become airless) at the end of expiration. This causes a conductive right-to-left blood shunt and consequential hypoxemia (see Chapter 7). Note that administration of surfactant helps in IRDS because premature infants don't make it. In contrast, in ARDS surfactant administration does not help because surfactant is being destroyed by inflammation which is the underlying cause.

Aside from reducing the work of breathing and providing alveolar stability, surfactant also helps maintaining the alveoli dry. The reason for this can be understood by examining the alveolar architecture. Being tightly packed together, the alveoli assume a polyhedral rather than spherical shape (Fig. **8B**) such that their surface-curvature varies (Fig. **8C**). At the corners where three alveoli meet the curvature's radius becomes very small. Therefore, in these regions, based on the

Laplace law, surface tension has its greatest effect (Fig. **8C**) – in other words, in these regions the alveolus, due to its shorter radius, would tend to recoil with greater force that in other regions with longer radius. The greater recoil of these short-radius regions creates a negative pressure at the alveolar inner surface which, in the absence of surfactant, would drive water into the alveolar airspace from the surrounding alveolar epithelium, interstitial fluid and capillary blood. By dramatically reducing the surface tension of these sharply curved regions the surfactant minimizes the negative pressure; this prevents water diffusion, so that the alveoli remain dry.

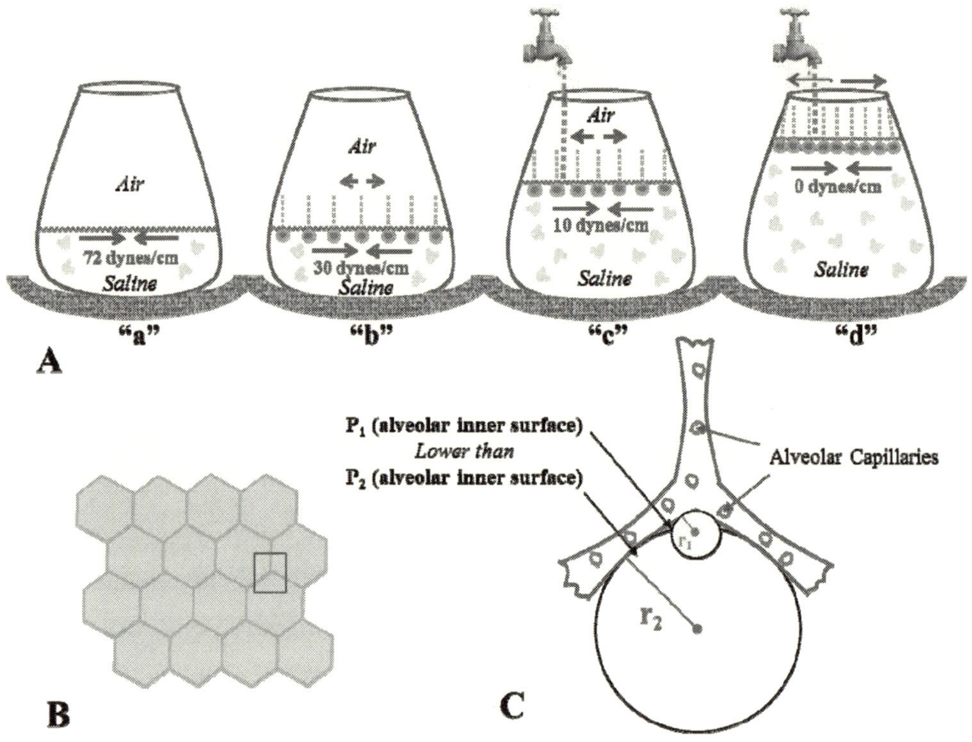

Figure 8: Surfactant properties. The water-air interface (A, "a") has a surface tension of 72 dynes/cm. Addition of DPL lowers the surface tension (A, "b"). Compression of DPL molecules has greater effect in reducing surface tension, down to 0 dynes/cm (A, "c" and "d") – in this example, DPL compression results from the reduction of air-water surface caused by addition of water to flasks "c" and "d" (A). Alveoli have polyhedral shape (B). Therefore, surface tension is greater at corners, where radius is shorter (C, enlarged view of square in B). Surfactant keeps alveoli dry – based on the law of Laplace, pressure is inversely related to alveolar radius (in C: P_1 is lower than P_2) such that, without surfactant, surface tension would cause water to diffuse into the alveoli from short-radius (r_1) corners.

Chest Wall

Elastic Characteristics of the Chest Wall

The chest wall has elastic properties as well but, unlike the lungs, it cannot be compared to a rubber balloon. Indeed, the chest wall is like a coil spring that can be either stretched (expanded) or compressed, an example being the coil spring of a car suspension (Fig. **3**). In cars, a wheel that hits a bump in the road moves upward and the coil spring is compressed. *Vice versa*, when the wheel falls into a pit it moves downward and the coil spring is expanded.

The elastic properties of the chest wall are described by the chest wall compliance curve (PC; Fig. **9**A). Note that, as in the case of the lungs, the pressure-volume relationship is not linear because the compliance of the chest wall changes with volume as well. However, unlike the lungs, the pressure needed for maintain a certain chest volume is positive at certain volumes and negative at others. This is due to the spring-like characteristics of the chest wall.

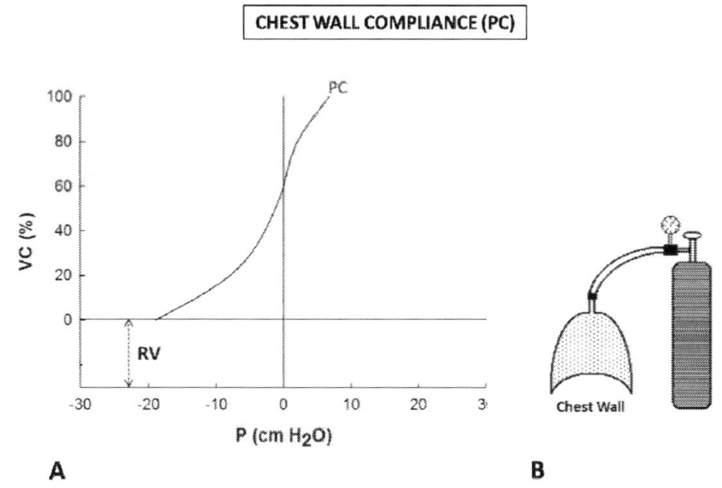

Figure 9: Compliance curve of the chest wall (A, PC). PC is positive or negative at volumes greater or smaller, respectively, than ~70% of TLC. In an isolated chest (lungs removed), compliance could be measured by inflating it (>70% TLC) and deflating it (<70% TLC) in steps, and measuring the pressure needed to maintain the chest volume at each step (B).

The resting point of the chest wall corresponds to a volume equal to approximately 70% of TLC; in Fig. **9A** this point is where the curve crosses the zero pressure line.

To expand the chest beyond 70% of TLC one needs inflate it (add positive pressure inside it), whereas to reduce the chest volume below 70% of the TLC one needs to remove gas from it, creating a negative (lower than atmospheric) pressure inside it.

The compliance curve of the chest wall (Fig. **9A**) could be obtained by inflating or deflating the chest cavity (after the lungs have been removed) to different volumes and measuring the pressure needed to maintain these volumes (Fig. **9B**). Obviously, in a living subject one cannot remove the lungs and inflate (or deflate) the chest cavity by itself. Yet, also in living subjects the compliance curve of the chest wall can be drawn. This is done by measuring the intra-esophageal (same as intra-pleural) pressure while the subject holds his/her breath at different volumes with closed glottis and relaxes the respiratory muscles (see below).

What Determines the Elastic Properties of the Chest Wall

Chest wall compliance is related to the rigidity and elastic properties of ribs, stern, spine and their joints, as well as to diaphragm and abdominal organs. Chest wall compliance is altered by abnormalities of thoracic bones and/or joints, caused by diseases such as kyphoscoliosis (abnormal curvature of the spinal column) or ankylosing spondylitis (arthritis of the spine), or by disorders that impose excessive weight on the chest, such as extreme obesity.

Combined Lung + Chest-Wall System

Compliance Characteristics of Lung + Chest-Wall

Lungs and chest wall are kept in contact with each other by the thin liquid layer that fills the very narrow intra-pleural space.

Therefore, the compliance of the lung + chest-wall system results from the combined effect of the elastic properties of each component. The compliance curve of the "total" (T) lung + chest-wall system (Fig. **10**A), can be drawn by measuring the pressure at the mouth (PT) while the subject holds the breath at different volumes with open glottis and relaxes the respiratory muscles. This curve can also be drawn by calculating the algebraic sum of the recoil pressures of lungs (PL) and chest wall (PC) at each lung volume (PT = PL + PC).

COMPLIANCE CHARACTERISTICS OF LUNGS (PL)
CHEST WALL (PC) AND LUNG + CHEST-WALL SYSTEM (PT)

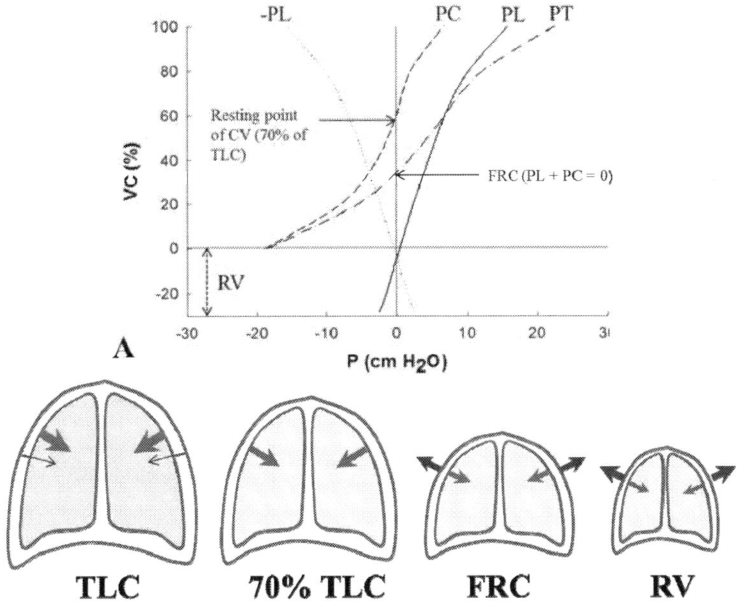

Figure 10: The compliance of the lung + chest-wall system (A, PT) results from the combined properties (algebraic sum) of PL and PC (PT = PL + PC). Pressure balance (PL + PC = 0) brings the system to its resting state (FRC). The lung + chest-wall system (PT) tends to expand or collapse at volumes smaller or greater that FRC, respectively (B). The curve labeled "-PL" (A) represents the lung compliance curve generated by measuring pressure in the intra-pleural (same as intra-esophageal) compartment.

Fig. **10B** shows that at volumes smaller than 70% of TLC (FRC and RV), lungs and chest wall exert opposing forces, because the lungs tend to collapse (pull inward) while the chest wall tends to expand (pull outward). At 70% of TLC the lungs tend to collapse even more, while the chest wall is at rest. At volumes larger than 70% of TLC both lungs and chest wall tend to collapse. At FRC, the lungs tend to collapse just as much as the chest wall tends to expand - the system is subjected to opposite forces (pressures) of equal strength (PT = PL + PC = 0). Therefore, at FRC the system is in balance such that, with relaxed muscles, the combined lungs + chest-wall system is static - it tends neither to expand nor to collapse. The volume at FRC depends on the strength of the two opposing forces: if lung compliance is abnormally increased, as in cases of emphysema, the FRC volume is greater than normal - the compliance curve of the lungs (PL) shifts to the left (Fig. **4**). The opposite is true in the case of pulmonary fibrosis (smaller volumes at FRC).

Since the lungs always tend to collapse, and so continuously tend to pull away from the chest wall, the intra-pleural pressure (PIP) is negative (lower than atmospheric) throughout the breathing cycle. This is true during normal (quiet) breathing, but it may become positive during expiration in vigorous exercise, or when airway flow-resistance in expiration increases, as with asthma or emphysema; it is also positive when one relaxes the respiratory muscles with closed glottis at volumes greater than 70% of TLC, or when one closes the glottis and "bears down" (Valsalva maneuver), as during defecation, parturition, coughing, sneezing, and so on.

The effects of different maneuvers on intra-pleural (PIP) and trans-pulmonary pressures are shown in Fig. **11**. Trans-pulmonary pressure (TPP) is the pressure gradient between intra-alveolar (PA) and intra-pleural (PIP) compartments. In any possible maneuvers (Fig. **11**) TPP is always the same as the lung recoil pressure (PL, Figs. **4** and **10A**), because it depends entirely on the lung's elastic properties - the larger the lung volume, the greater lung recoil and the greater TPP (Fig. **11**).

Method for determining the compliance characteristics of lungs, chest wall, and lung + chest wall system in a living subject.

Compliance Curve of the Lungs (PL)

The compliance curve of the lungs (PL) is generated by measuring the intra-esophageal pressure (same as the intra-pleural pressure, PIP) with an esophageal balloon [5] while the subject holds the breath at different lung volumes with open glottis. The pressure measured by this maneuver has negative values (lower than atmospheric pressure), because it is measured outside the recoiling lungs (-PL, Fig. **10A**, dotted line), but it is plotted with a positive sign (PL, Fig. **10A**, solid line), as if it had been measured inside the alveoli by inflating isolated lungs to different volumes. In other words, the curve with negative values reflects the tendency of the lungs to pull away (recoil) from the surrounding thoracic components: chest wall, mediastinum (heart, esophagus, and major vessels) and diaphragm; in contrast, the curve with positive sign represents the pressure needed inside isolated lungs to maintain them expanded. Intra-esophageal and intra-pleural pressures are virtually the same because both esophagus and intra-pleural space are subjected to the lung recoil - the esophagus is a sealed (floppy) compartment, as it is isolated from ambient and gastric gases by the upper esophageal sphincter (pharyngoesophageal sphincter) and the lower esophageal sphincter (cardias area), respectively. PL can also be calculated, as PL = PT – PC (Fig. **10A**, solid line).

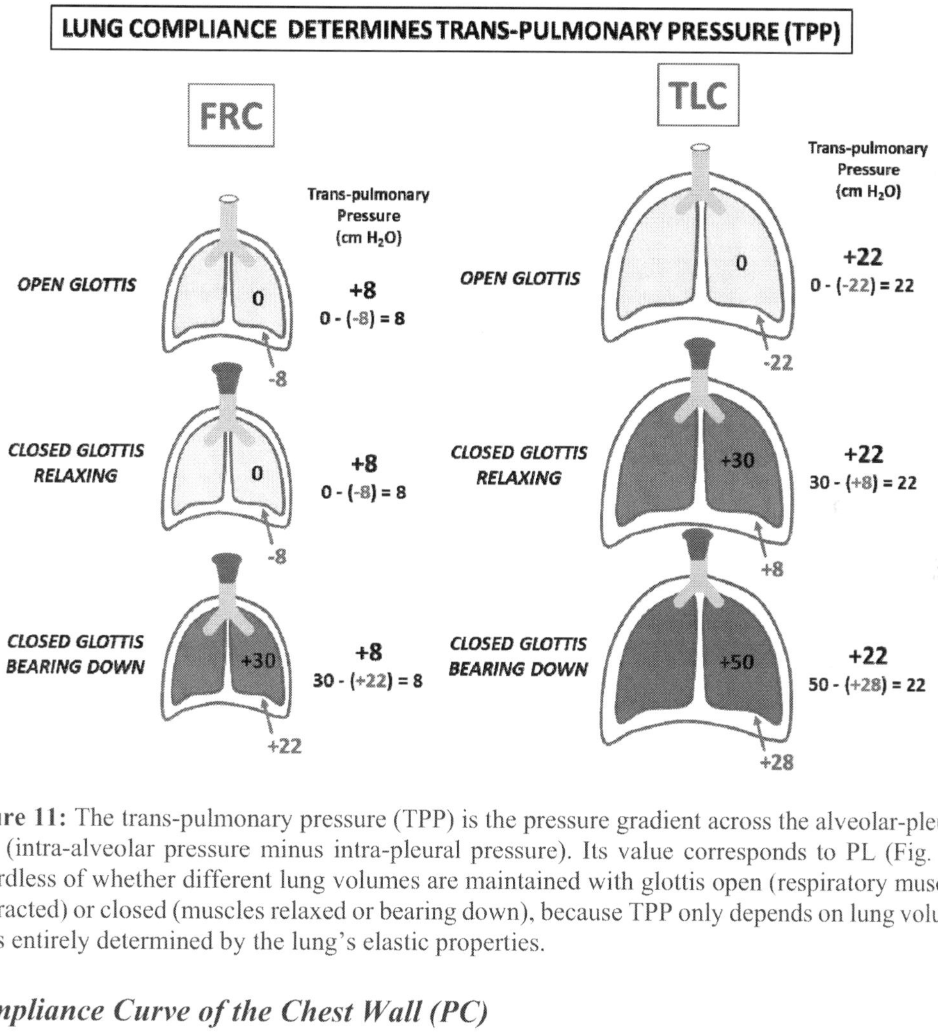

Figure 11: The trans-pulmonary pressure (TPP) is the pressure gradient across the alveolar-pleural wall (intra-alveolar pressure minus intra-pleural pressure). Its value corresponds to PL (Fig. **10**) regardless of whether different lung volumes are maintained with glottis open (respiratory muscles contracted) or closed (muscles relaxed or bearing down), because TPP only depends on lung volume - it is entirely determined by the lung's elastic properties.

Compliance Curve of the Chest Wall (PC)

The compliance curve of the chest wall (PC) is generated by measuring the intra-pleural pressure (PIP) with the esophageal balloon at different volumes while asking the subject to relax the respiratory muscles with closed glottis. PC can also be calculated, as PC = PT - PL (Fig. **10A,** dashed line).

Compliance Curve of the Lung + Chest Wall System (PT)

The compliance curve of the (total) lung + chest-wall system (PT) is generated by measuring at the mouth the pressure needed to maintain different lung volumes while asking the subject to relax the respiratory muscles with open glottis. PT can also be calculated, as PT = PL + PC (Fig. **10A,** dashed dotted line).

These measurements can be performed in living subjects because each of the described maneuvers allows one to isolate individual components. For example, when one measures PIP while the subject holds the breath with open glottis, the chest wall component (PC) is eliminated (Fig. **12**, lower panel); this gives the negative values of PL (-PL, Fig. **10A**, dotted line). By holding the chest wall at each volume with the respiratory muscles the chest wall is converted into what, metaphorically, one may call it: ***a "cast iron" chest wall*** (Fig. **12**, lower panel). Thus, in the intra-pleural (or intra-esophageal) space one monitors the negative pressure resulting from the tendency of the lung surface to pull away from the "cast iron" chest wall (Fig. **12**, lower panel).

Conversely, when one measures PIP with closed glottis at different volumes (respiratory muscles relaxed), just the pressure exerted by the chest wall component is monitored (PC; Fig. **10A**, dashed-dotted line), because by closing the glottis and relaxing the muscles the lung component (its elastic property) is eliminated. Since air cannot escape from the lungs (closed glottis), at each volume the lungs are converted into what one may call them: ***"cast iron" lungs*** (Fig. **12**, upper panel). Therefore, in the intra-pleural (or intra-esophageal) space one monitors only the pressure exerted by the chest wall, which presses onto the "cast iron" lungs at volumes greater than 70% of TLC, and pulls away from them at volumes smaller than 70% of TLC (Fig. **12**, upper panel).

As mentioned above, the elastic properties of lungs, chest wall and lung + chest-wall system are expressed in terms of compliance (C). Each point in the compliance curve represents the volume/pressure ratio. Compliance is measured statically (no air movement). The opposite of compliance, elastance (E), is the pressure/volume ratio. Therefore, C = 1/E and E = 1/C. If compliance is measured during the breathing cycle, resistive components due to gas flow through airways would be added to the elastic components being measured. Therefore, compliance must be measured at static conditions (no gas movement). Normal values of compliances for lungs (CL, Eq. 6), chest wall (CC, Eq. 7) and (total) lung + chest-wall system (CT, Eq.8) are:

$$\mathrm{CL} = 0.2\ \mathrm{l/cm\,H_2O}\ \ldots \tag{6}$$

$$\mathrm{CC} = 0.2\ \mathrm{l/cm\,H_2O}\ \ldots \tag{7}$$

$$\mathrm{CT} = 0.1\ \mathrm{l/cm\,H_2O}\ \ldots \tag{8}$$

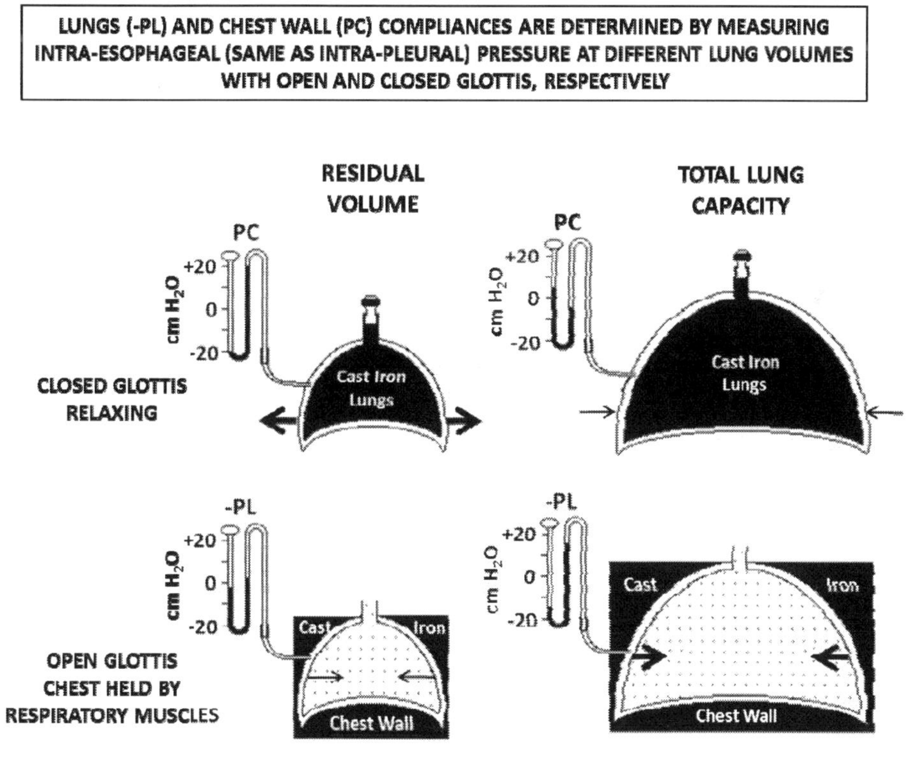

Figure 12: The compliances of lungs (PL) or chest wall (PC) can be measured in a living subject by asking him/her to hold different lung volumes with glottis open (respiratory muscles contracted) or closed (muscles relaxed), respectively, and measuring the intra-pleural (intra-esophageal) pressure at each volume. These maneuvers effectively convert lungs or chest wall into fixed volumes (*"cast iron" lungs or chest wall*), so that their elastic component is eliminated from the pressure measurements.

Note that the compliance of the lung + chest-wall system (CT) is a half the compliance of each component (CL and CC). This seems odd at first, but can easily be understood if we realize that compliance (C) and elastance (E) are comparable to conductance and resistance in electric circuits. Therefore, the elastance of the lung + chest-wall system (ET = 1/CT, Eqs. 9 and 10) is the sum of the elastance of each component (1/CC + 1/CL), just as the resistance of two resistors in series is the sum of the resistance of each resistor.

$$ET = \frac{1}{0.2} + \frac{1}{0.2} \ldots \quad \textbf{(9)}$$

$$ET = 10 \text{ cm } H_2O/l \ldots \quad \textbf{(10)}$$

Clinical Correlation: Pneumothorax

It is important to understand the elastic properties of chest wall, lungs and thorax because a number of diseases alter the balance among the interacting forces with significant functional consequences. In addition to the previously mentioned effects of emphysema, fibrosis and RDS, one should consider pneumothorax, a condition in which gas gains access to the intra-pleural space. This may occur as a result of lung rupture or chest-wall perforation (stabbing wound, for example), which causes alveolar gas or atmospheric air, respectively, to flow into the intra-pleural space; since the thin layer of liquid that occupies the intra-pleural space is what normally maintains the lung surface physically linked to the inner surface of the chest wall, gas flows in because intra-thoracic pressure is negative.

Gas flowing into the intra-pleural space frees lungs and chest wall from each other; this causes them to collapse and expand, respectively, according to their elastic properties. If enough gas diffuses into the intra-pleural space of both lungs, the lungs will collapse down to a volume lower than RV and the chest wall will expand to 70% of TLC (Fig. **10A**). A similar situation occurs when blood or other liquids accumulate in the intra-pleural space. With pneumothorax, PIP becomes progressively less negative and at complete lung collapse it becomes zero (same as atmospheric). In some cases it can even become positive; this is an acute and very dangerous condition, known as tension (or valvular) pneumothorax, which could cause rapid asphyxia if not treated immediately to allow gas to escape from the intra-pleural space (see Chapter 10: Restrictive Diseases - Pneumothorax).

Dynamic Properties of Respiratory Mechanics

Gases flow in and out of the lungs during the respiratory cycle because pressure gradients are created between alveoli and ambient. Chest expansion and diaphragm flattening during inspiration lowers the intra-alveolar pressure below atmospheric pressure, causing air to flow into the lungs. The reverse occurs in expiration.

Gases flow through the bronchial system, which is composed of upper and lower airways. Upper airways are located outside the chest and are subjected to atmospheric pressure; lower airways are inside the chest and are subjected to intra-pleural pressure. The anatomical location of the airways and other factors such as airway size, geometry and compliance determine the behavior of gas-flow in the bronchial tree.

Gas Flow Through Airways

Depending on velocity, gas-flow is either laminar or turbulent. Laminar flow occurs at low velocity and is characterized by a streamline movement of molecules parallel to the sides of the airway (Fig. **13, A**).

FOR THE SAME PRESSURE GRADIENT FLOW RATE IS GREATER WITH LAMINAR THAN TURBULENT FLOW

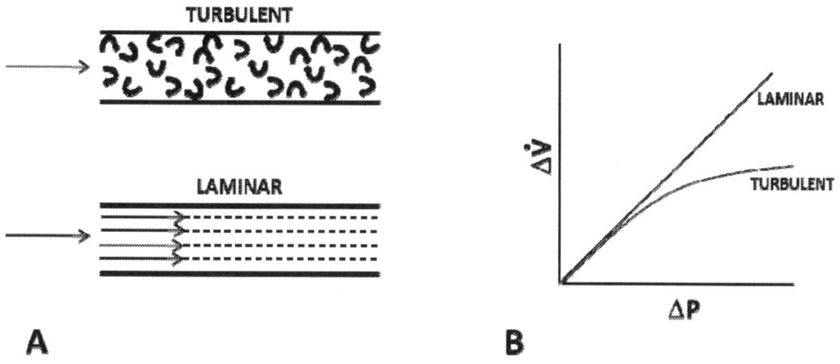

Figure 13: Examples of laminar and turbulent flows (A). Pressure increments (ΔP) generate larger flow-rate increments ($\mathbf{\Delta\dot{V}}$) with laminar than turbulent flow (B). Turbulent and laminar flows are typical of large and small airways, respectively, because flow velocity is greater in larger airways.

Turbulent flow develops at high gas velocity, or where airways branch out, and is characterized by complete disorganization of the stream lines (turbulence), with formation of swirls and eddies (Fig. **13A**). Laminar and turbulent flow are typical of small and large airways, respectively.

The laminar flow rate ($\overline{V}$) of a gas through a tube is described by the law of Poiseuille (named after the French physiologist Jean Louis Marie Poiseuille, 1797-1869), which is expressed in Eq.11:

$$\overline{V} = \frac{\Delta P \pi r^4}{8nl} \quad \ldots \qquad \textbf{(11)}$$

where, ΔP is driving pressure (pressure gradient), r radius, n viscosity and l length. Since flow resistance (R) is equal to driving pressure (ΔP) over flow rate ($\overline{V}$), Eq. 12:

$$R = \frac{\Delta P}{\overline{V}} \quad \ldots \qquad \textbf{(12)}$$

by rearranging the Poiseuille equation:

$$R = \frac{8nl}{\pi r^4} \quad \ldots \qquad \textbf{(13)}$$

Equation 13 shows that airway resistance (R) for laminar flow is proportional to airway length (l) and gas viscosity (n) but, most importantly, it is inversely related to the fourth power of the airway radius (r^4). This means that if the radius is reduced to 1/2 the resistance increases 16 times.

While in laminar flow the flow rate ($\overline{V}$) is proportional to driving pressure (ΔP), in turbulent flow $\overline{V}$ it is proportional to the square root of ΔP, and varies with gas density. Thus, with the same pressure gradient and gas type, turbulent flow is always slower than laminar flow (Fig. **13B**).

Whether gas flow in an airway is laminar or turbulent depends on the so called Reynolds number (R_e; named after the English mathematician Osborne Reynolds, 1842-1912), Eq. 14:

$$R_e = \frac{2rvd}{n} \quad \ldots \qquad \textbf{(14)}$$

where d is density, r radius, v average velocity and n viscosity. Turbulence occurs when R_e is greater than 2000. Thus, turbulence is more likely to occur where v and r have the greatest values (large airways).

Airway Resistance

As mentioned above, based on the law of Poiseuille airway resistance is inversely related to the fourth power of the airway radius. Therefore, one would expect that in the airway system most of the resistance is due to gas flowing through small airways. This is not the case, however, because what counts is not the radius of individual airways but the equivalent radius - the sum of the radii of all of the airways. Due to the large number of small airways, their equivalent radius is much larger than that of large airways, and it becomes progressively larger the closer the airways are to the alveoli (Fig. **14A**). Therefore, since airway resistances is inversely related to the fourth power of the radius (in this case the equivalent radius) the resistance (R) caused by small airways is smaller than that due to large airways (Fig. **14B**).

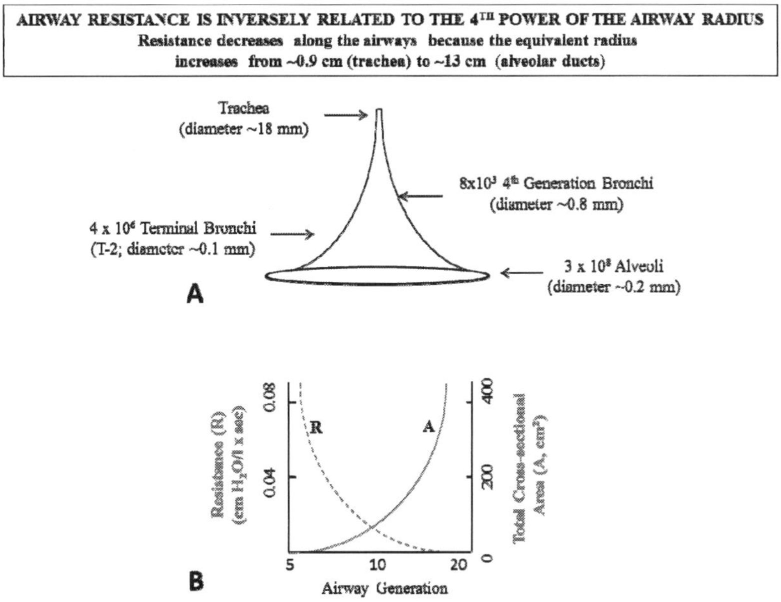

Figure 14: The airway diameter decreases from trachea to terminal bronchi, but the airway number increases from 1 to $4x10^6$, such that the equivalent diameter dramatically increases (A). Consequently, the equivalent (total) cross-sectional area progressively increases toward the alveoli (B, solid curve) and airway resistance greatly decreases (B, dashed curve).

Pressures During the Breathing Cycle

Figs. **15** and **16** show the changes in intra-pleural pressure during the breathing cycle. With quiet breathing, the intra-pleural pressure becomes more negative with inspiration, changing from ~ -5 cm H_20 at FRC to ~ -8 cm H_20 at the end of inspiration (FRC+VT; Fig. **15**, solid line), as lung's expansion needs to overcome both static (lung's elastic properties) and resistive forces.

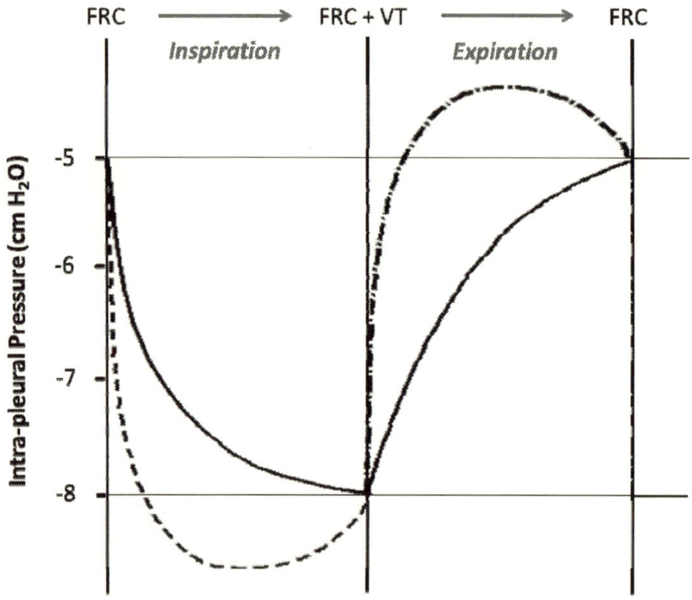

Figure 15: Changes in intra-pleural pressure (IPP) during the breathing cycle. During quiet breathing (at rest) and with normal airway resistance IPP changes following the solid line. In contrast, with forced inspiration and expiration, or with increased airway resistance, it becomes more negative in inspiration (dashed line) and less negative, or even positive, in expiration (dashed-dotted line) before returning to the same values (-8 and -5 cm H_2O, respectively).

This path depends on lung recoil, which increases at larger lung volumes as the lungs become stiffer and intra-pleural pressure is more negative. The kinetics (curve shape) of pressure-change during inspiration (Fig. **15** and **16**) depends on airway resistance. While with minimal airway resistance this curve follows the path depicted by the solid line (Fig. **15**, left), with increased resistance it might follow the path depicted by the dashed line (Fig. **15**, left). The area between the two lines represents the increase in the pressure gradient between alveoli and ambient that must be created to overcome airway resistance.

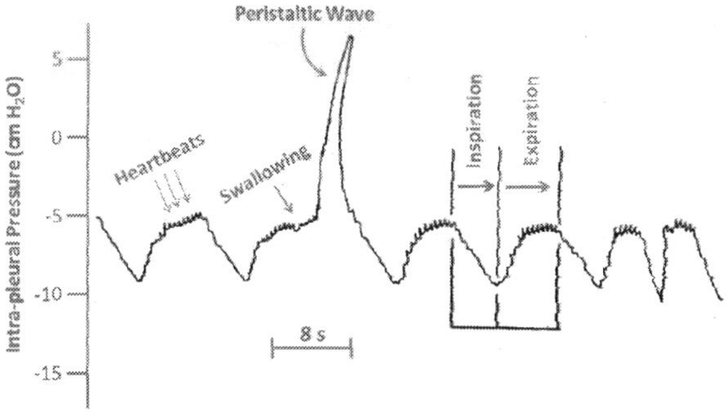

Figure 16. Changes in intra-pleural pressure (IP) changes during the breathing cycle, recorded from the author's esophagus with an esophageal balloon. During quite breathing, IP reversibly changes from -5 to -8 cm H_2O.

The opposite takes place during expiration. With normal airway resistance the intra-pleural pressure changes following the solid line (Fig. **15**, right); in forced expiration or in cases of increased airway resistance the intra-pleural pressure may follow the dashed-dotted line (Fig. **15**, right). In extreme cases the intra-pleural pressure may even become positive, eventually returning to -5 cmH_2O at the end of expiration (no gas flow).

Airway Dynamics During the Breathing Cycle

The intra-thoracic airways are subjected to the intra-pleural pressure, as they are linked to the interstitial framework of the lung tissue. Since the intra-pleural pressure is negative, the airway walls are stretched open during all phases of the breathing cycle (in normal, quiet, breathing), but the extent of stretching depends on lung volume. As shown in Figs. **15** and **16**, the intra-pleural pressure becomes progressively more negative during inspiration. Consequently, during this phase of the breathing cycle the airways are stretched open more and more, such that their diameter progressively increases and flow resistance decreases. The opposite is true in expiration. During expiration the intra-pleural pressure becomes progressively less negative (Figs. **15** and **16**) so that the diameter of the airways becomes smaller and airway resistance increases.

This phenomenon, studied in detail by Permutt and coworkers [6], does not create problems in normal subjects, but has serious consequences in patients with asthma and emphysema because in the former the small airways are already narrowed by the increased tone of the bronchial smooth muscle and other factors, and in the latter because the stretching of the airways is much reduced, due to less negative intra-pleural pressure of the emphysematous "floppy" lungs (reduced elasticity, increased compliance). Therefore, in patients with asthma and/or emphysema, expiration can be more demanding than inspiration, due to substantial increase in airway resistive work. Actually, while this is always true in asthma, patients with obstructive lung disease (emphysema) complain more in inspiration, because of increased lung volume (hyperinflation) and elastic work of breathing.

The mechanism of expiratory airway collapse in emphysematous patients can be understood by first studying flow rates during forced expiration in normal subjects. Fig. **17** shows the flow volume curve, which describes the relationship between flow rate and lung volume during inspiration and expiration (lower and upper curves, respectively), performed with different efforts. Note that during inspiration from RV to TLC, the greater the effort the greater the flow rate at any lung volume. This is also true for expiration, but only when the lungs are at their largest volumes (Fig. **17**, red arrow). As the lung volume decreases flow rate drops, reaching levels that cannot be increased regardless of effort (Fig. **17**, "effort independent" region). Expiratory flow limitation takes place when gas flow does not increase in spite of increased respiratory effort. This point is often referred to as "flow limit site or chock limit". The blue arrow in Fig. **17** indicates the difference in flow rate between inspiration and expiration, performed with different efforts, when the lung are at the same (relatively low) lung volume; note that flow rate is effort dependent only in inspiration (the greater the effort the greater the flow rate).

This suggests that some factors significantly limit flow rate below certain expiratory lung volumes. The reason for it is that flow rate depends not only on the gradient between intra-alveolar and ambient pressures, but also on the pressure gradient across the airways.

This phenomenon can be understood by monitoring the pressure gradients across the airway wall during forced inspiration and expiration in normal and emphysematous subjects (Fig. **18A and B**). While in normal subjects (Fig. **18A**) the pressure gradient across the airways during expiration may decrease down to zero (TPP = +10 - [+10] = 0), in emphysematous patients (Fig. **18B**) it may become inverted (TPP = +10 - [+15] = -5) such that pressure outside is greater than inside the airways. At this level the airway walls are still soft, and so begin to collapse. Consequently, flow resistance increases and flow rate decreases. Beyond this region, the airway wall becomes stiffer due to the bronchial cartilage, so that collapse is less likely to occur, even though TPP becomes negative even in normal subjects.

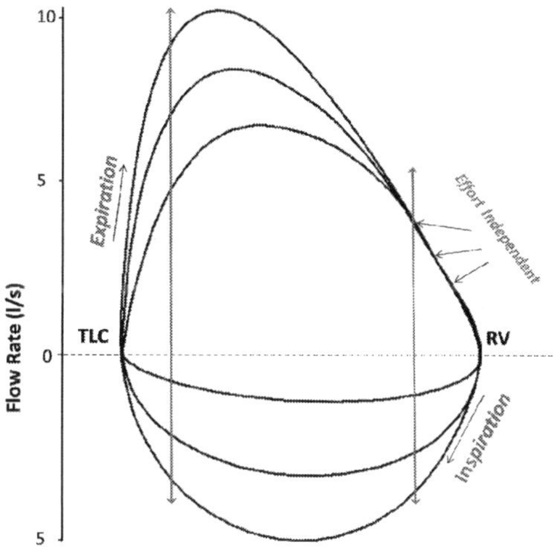

Figure 17: Flow volume curve - plot of flow rate *versus* lung volume. While at large volumes flow rate increases with increased effort both in inspiration and in expiration (red arrow). This is not the case during expiration at low lung volumes (blue arrow), due to airway collapse (effort independent region). Expiratory flow limitation takes place when gas flow does not increase in spite of increased respiratory effort. This point is often referred to as "flow limit site" or "chock limit."

The airway collapse is further potentiated in patients with emphysema, asthma, or bronchitis by a mechanism based on the "Bernoulli principle" (formulated by the by the Swiss physicist Daniel Bernoulli, 1700-1782). This principle states that "for the horizontal flow of a fluid (or gas) through a tube, the sum of the pressure exerted against the tube's wall and the kinetic energy per unit volume of fluid (or gas) is constant" (Fig. **18D**). Since the kinetic energy of a moving fluid (or gas) is directly related to the square of its velocity, as velocity increases kinetic energy increases and consequently the pressure against the wall decreases. This explains a phenomenon known as the "Venturi effect" (named after the Italian physicist Giovanni Battista Venturi, 1746-1822). Based on the Bernoulli principle, in regions where airways become narrower (partial collapse, bronchial spasm, mucous *etc.*)

the pressure against the airway wall drops because gas velocity increases. This may invert the normal pressure gradient across the airway wall, such that intra-pleural pressure becomes greater (more positive) than airway pressure, causing the airway to become even narrower (Fig. **18D**). Note that in emphysema and asthma the elastic work of breathing is also increased due to hyperinflation.

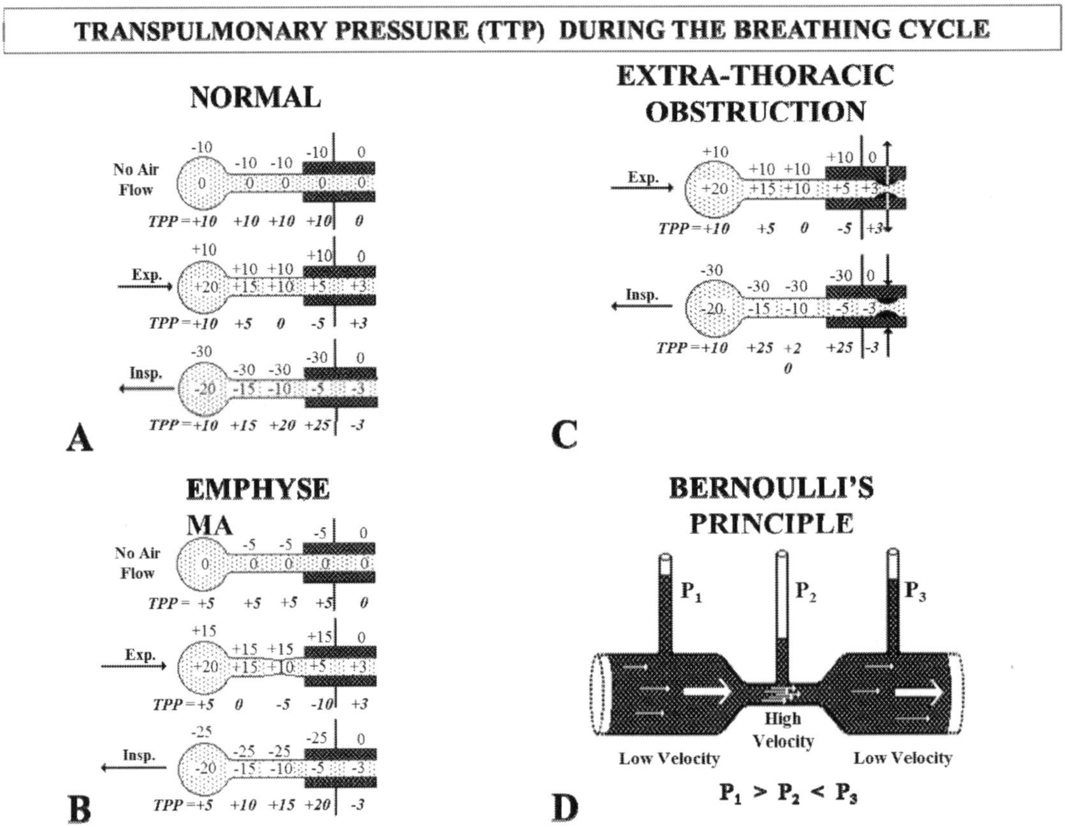

Figure 18: Examples of trans-pulmonary (trans-airway) pressures (TPP) in normal (A) emphysema (B) and extra-thoracic obstruction (C) conditions, at rest (no air flow) and during forced expiration or inspiration. During expiration, airway collapse begins to occur with emphysema where the airways' TPP assumes negative values (B, TPP = +10-[+15] = -5). Negative TPP may occurs also in normal subjects (A, TPP = +5-[+10] = -5), but only in upper bronchi, which are stiffer (non-collapsible) due to the presence of cartilage. With extra-thoracic obstruction (C), extra-thoracic airways tend to collapse with forced inspiration where trans-airway pressure is negative (TPP = -3+0 = -3). Airway collapse is potentiated by a mechanism based on the Bernoulli principle (D).

In contrast, in cases of extra-thoracic airway obstruction (Fig. **18C**), inspiration is much harder than expiration because these airways are surrounded by atmospheric pressure, such that the pressure gradient across the airway wall favors airway collapse during inspiration and airway dilation during expiration.

Work of Breathing

In a normal subject at rest, the work of breathing is only inspiratory and represents only a small fraction of the total energy turnover of the organism - muscular work in inspiration is needed to overcome two factors: lung's elastic recoil and airway resistance. Work of breathing, however, can be very significant in diseases that affect lung elasticity and/or airway resistance.

In emphysema, significant respiratory work is needed in expiration to overcome the airway resistance caused by reduced lung elasticity and consequential airway collapse. In pulmonary fibrosis, the inspiratory work is greatly enhanced because the lungs are stiffer than normal such that greater effort is required to expand them. In asthma, greater muscle effort is required in both inspiration and expiration to overcome the increased airway resistance, but work is greater in expiration because the already narrowed airways are further constricted by the unfavorable pressure gradient across their wall. Increased work is also needed in heavy exercise and in conditions of extreme obesity.

Respiratory work (W) is the product of pressure-change (ΔP) and volume-change (ΔV), expressed in cm H_2O per liter (Eq. 15):

$$W = \Delta P \times \Delta V \ldots \qquad \textbf{(15)}$$

In Fig. **19**, the area AECDA represents the total inspiratory work; of this, ABCDA represents the elastic work, and AECBA the resistive work, due to both airway and tissue resistances (viscous work). In cases of fibrosis, the inspiratory work in increased, but mostly to overcome tissue resistance. In this case, greater pressure increments are needed to generate the same volume increments, as compared to normal lung. Conversely, in obstructive lung diseases such as asthma, for example, the elastic work is normal, while the resistive work is greatly increased; in this case, both inspiratory and expiratory curves bulge out more prominently.

The work of breathing can be calculated by measuring the additional oxygen consumption ($\dot{V}O_2$) needed for breathing, making an assumption for efficiency (Eq. 16):

$$\text{Efficiency (\%)} = \frac{\text{Useful Work}}{\text{Total Energy Expended}} \times 100 \ldots \quad \textbf{(16)}$$

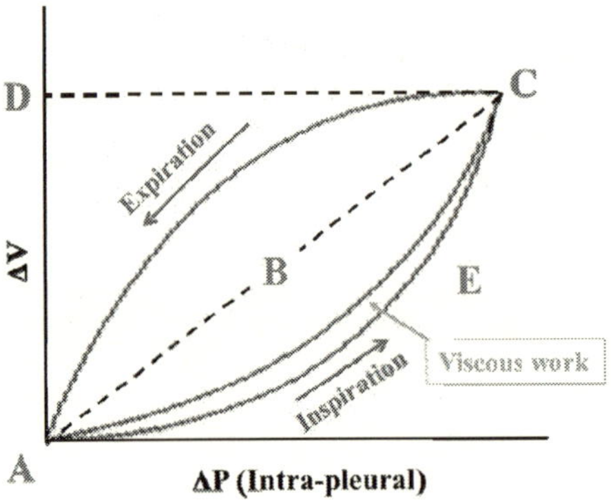

Figure 19: Plot of changes in intra-pleural pressure (ΔP) *versus* changes in lung volume (ΔV) during the breathing cycle. The total inspiratory work (W, area AECDA) is the sum of elastic work (area ABCDA) and resistive work (area AECBA). The resistive work is due mostly to airway resistance, as lung-tissue viscosity (viscous work) plays a minor role. W = ΔP x ΔV.

Efficiency is thought to range from 5% to 10%. At rest, the normal work of breathing is less than 5% of the total O_2 consumption of the organism.

Most Common Pulmonary Tests (For a Thorough Review of Pulmonary Function Tests, See [3]).

Forced Expiratory Volume in 1 Second (FEV_1)

FEV_1 is the volume expired in the first second of a forced expiration from total lung capacity (TLC) to residual volume (RV). FEV_1 significantly drops in patients suffering from emphysema, chronic bronchitis, asthma or fibrosis.

Forced Expiratory Volume in 1 Second Over Forced Vital Capacity (FEV_1/FVC)

FEV_1/FVC is the fraction of the forced expiration from TLC to RV (VC) exhaled in one second. In normal subjects, FEV_1/FVC = 83%. In patients suffering from emphysema or asthma it might be as low as 40%, due to airway collapse. In contrast, with fibrosis FEV_1/FVC is greater than normal, and could be as high as

90%, even though FEV_1 is lower than normal (reduced lung volume). The reason for it is that with fibrosis the airways are stretched by the more negative intra-pleural pressure, which lowers gas flow resistance.

Forced Expiratory Volume at mid-half expiration ($FEV_{25\text{-}75}$)

$FEV_{25\text{-}75}$ is the volume expired per second during in the mid portion (25-75%) of a forced expiratory volume, starting from TLC. In normal subjects $FEV_{25\text{-}75}$ = ~3.5 l/sec. In patients with emphysema, chronic bronchitis or asthma it might drop to values as low as 1.5 l/sec, whereas with fibrosis it is normal or even greater than normal.

Maximum Expiratory Flow Rate at 50% and 75% ($\dot{V}max_{50}$ and $\dot{V}max_{75}$)

$\dot{V}max_{50}$ and $\dot{V}max_{75}$ represent the maximum flow rates at 25% and 75%, respectively, of a forced expiration from TLC to RV. In normal subjects, $\dot{V}max_{50}$ may reach values as high as 6 l/sec, and $\dot{V}max_{75}$ 2.5 l/sec. Both parameters drop dramatically with emphysema and asthma.

Peak Expiratory Flow Rate (PEFR)

PEFR is the maximal expiratory flow rate reached during forced expiration from TLC. In normal subjects it is as high as 400-600 l/min. PEFR drops dramatically with emphysema, chronic bronchitis and asthma.

Peak Inspiratory Flow Rate (PIFR)

PIFR is the maximal inspiratory flow rate achieved during forced inspiration from RV to TLC. In normal subjects it is as high as 300-400 l/min. PIFR drops dramatically with extra-thoracic airway obstruction as well as with asthma and chronic bronchitis.

REFERENCES

[1] DuBois AB, Botelho SY, Bedell GN, Marshall R, Comroe (Jr) JH. A rapid plethysmographic method for measuring thoracic gas volume: a comparison with nitrogen washout method for measuring functional residual capacity in normal subjects. J Clin Invest 1956;35:322-326.

[2] DuBois AB, Botelho SY, Comroe (Jr) JH. A new method for measuring airway resistance in man using a body plethysmograph; values in normal subjects and in patients with respiratory disease. J Clin Invest 1956;35:327-335.

[3] Schlegelmilch RM, Kramme R. Pulmonary function testing. In: Kramme R, Hoffmann K-P, Pozos RS. Eds. "Springer handbook of medical technology". 2011;8:95-117.

[4] Baldwin ED, Cournand A, Richards DWJr. Pulmonary insufficiency; Physiological classification, clinical methods of analysis, standard values in normal subjects. Medicine 1948;27:243-278.

[5] The esophageal balloon can be a small, very compliant, rubber bag (the finger of a surgical glove, for example) tied to a narrow polyethylene tube which is connected to an amplifier *via* a stopcock and a pressure transducer (instrument that converts pressures into electrical signals). With some practice, the balloon can be inserted into a nostril, guided into the pharynx and then swallowed to reach the esophagus (a compartment subjected to intra-pleural pressure as it is isolated from atmospheric and abdominal pressures by the upper esophageal sphincter, also known as pharyngo-esophageal sphincter, and the cardias, respectively). An example of an intra-esophageal (same as intra-pleural) pressure record is shown in Fig. **16**.

[6] Pride NB, Permutt S, Riley RL, Bromberger-Barnea B. Determinants of maximal expiratory flow from the lungs. J Appl Physiol 1967;23:646-662.

CHAPTER 4

Gas Exchange

Camillo Peracchia

Abstract: This chapter focuses on the mechanisms of gas exchange between lungs and environment. In particular, it describes the changes in gas composition and physical property that take place as gases are flown in and out of the lungs. It explains the meaning of anatomical (conductive) dead space and describes methods for quantifying dead space, alveolar ventilation, oxygen consumption and carbon dioxide production. It introduces concepts of ideal *versus* average alveolar ventilation, alveolar dead space ventilation, right-to-left blood shunt (venous admixture), and body gas stores. It begins to explain how the complex relationship between alveolar ventilation and blood perfusion can be simplified into a "three compartment model" of the real lung. Finally, the relationship among alveolar ventilation, arterial PCO_2 and metabolic rate is discussed and presented quantitatively.

Keywords: Alveolar Dead-Space, Alveolar Gas-Equation, Alveolar-Ideal Gas, Ambient-Temperature-Pressure-Saturated (ATPS), Blood Shunt, Body Gas-Stores, Body-Temperature-Pressure-Saturated (BTPS), Carbon-Dioxide Production, Conductive Dead-Space, Exchange Ratio (R), Expiration, Gas Composition, Inspiration, O_2-CO_2 Diagram, Oxygen Consumption, Physiological Dead-Space, Respiratory Quotient (RQ), Standard-Temperature-Pressure-Dry (STPD), Steady-State Condition, Ventilation-PCO_2-Metabolism.

SYMBOLS, ACRONYMS AND NORMAL VALUES: See Appendix 3

Let's Take a Breath – Inspiration

Every time we take a breath a volume of ambient air enters the lungs flowing through a tree-like arrangement of airways (nose, larynx, trachea and bronchi), known as conductive (or anatomical) dead space (VCd), a region in which there is virtually no gas exchange with blood. Inspired air eventually reaches the alveolar space, the region where gas exchange with blood takes place. As mentioned in Chapter 3, the volume of air that enters the lungs at each breath is called tidal volume (VT). The alveoli receive only a portion of the inspired air because the first volume of gas that enters the alveoli is alveolar gas that has remained in VCd at the end of expiration (FRC), and some of the inspired air remains in VCd at the end of inspiration (FRC + VT; Figs. **1** and **2**). With normal breathing, approximately two thirds of VT reaches the alveolar space, while one third remains in VCd (Fig. **2**).

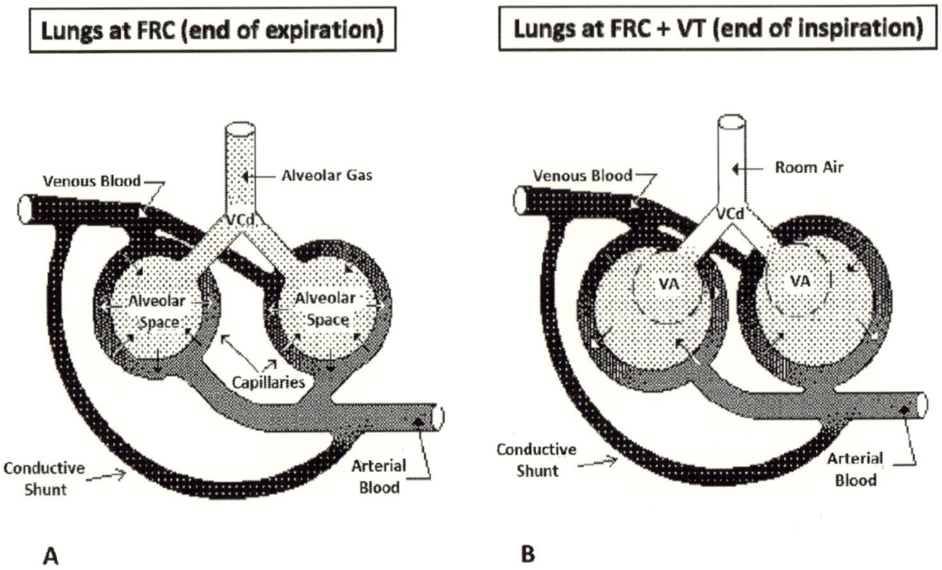

Figure 1: Schematic model of lungs at the end of expiration (A) and inspiration (B). At the end of expiration, alveolar gas fills the conductive (anatomical) dead space (A, VCd); this gas re-enters the alveolar compartment before fresh air during inspiration. Approximately 1/3 of the tidal volume (VT) inspired at each breath remains in VCd at end of inspiration (B). During normal breathing, one inspires ~500 ml (VT) ~10 times a minute (f), the total volume of air inspired being ~5 l/minute (**$\dot{V}$I**). The expired volume per minute (**$\dot{V}$E**) is slightly smaller, as the normal exchange ratio (R, $\dot{V}CO_2/\dot{V}O_2$) is less than one.

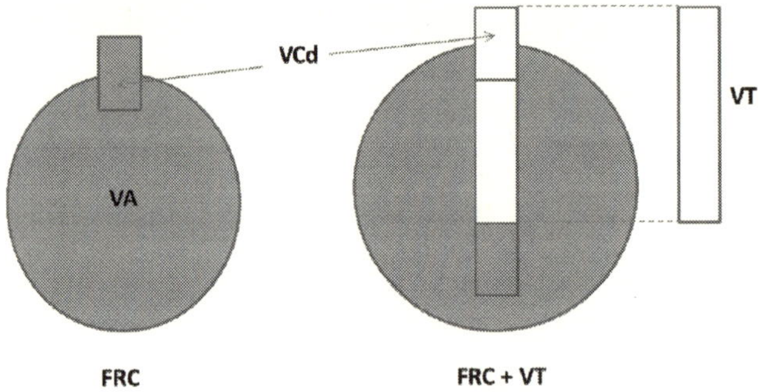

Figure 2: At the end of expiration (FRC) and inspiration (FRC + VT) VCd contains alveolar gas and room air, respectively. The alveoli only receive ~2/3 of VT's room air, because the last third remains in VCd.

During its travel from ambient to alveoli, inspired air undergoes important changes. As it flows through the conductive zone (airways) inspired air is warmed from ambient temperature (TA) to body temperature (TB, 37°C) and is humidified to saturation at body temperature (37°C). In the exchanging zone (VA), inspired air mixes with alveolar gas that has remained in the lungs at the end of the preceding expiration. As a result of all this, inspired air increases in volume, as it is heated and humidified, and changes in composition, as it mixes with alveolar gas (Fig. **3**).

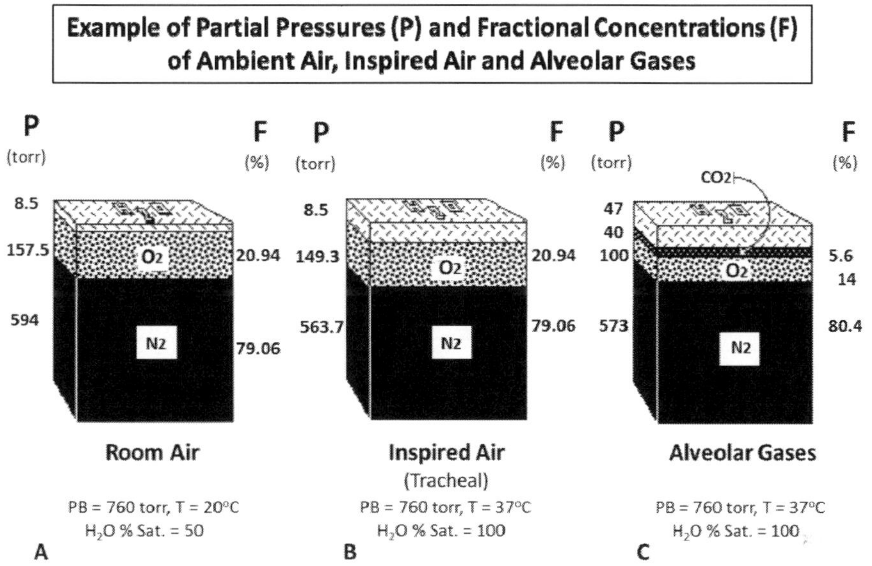

Figure 3: Composition of room air (A), inspired air (B) and alveolar gas (C). Inspired air (in VCd, B) is room air heated to 37^{0}C and humidified to saturation at 37^{0}C. Alveolar gas (C) is the same as inspired air in terms of temperature and humidity, but its composition reflects the alveolar gas exchange. The fraction of N_2 increases from B to C because R ($\dot{\mathbf{V}}\mathbf{CO_2}/\dot{\mathbf{V}}\,\mathbf{O_2}$) is normally less than one – the volume of O_2 diffusing into blood is greater than that of CO_2 exiting blood. Torr = mmHg.

The composition of a mixture of gases is defined in terms of fractional concentrations (F), or partial pressures (P). The fractional concentration of a gas "x" (Fx) in a gas mixture is the fractional volume occupied by gas "x" (**dry**) in the mixture of the (**dry**) gases. The partial pressure of gas "x" (Px) is the pressure exerted by gas "x" in the mixture of the gases, or the pressure gas "x" would exert if it were expanded to occupy the entire volume of the gas mixture in the absence of the other gases: Dalton's law (named after the English chemist and physicist John Dalton, 1766-1844). Px and Fx are calculated as follows (Eqs. 1 and 2):

$$\mathrm{Px} = \mathrm{Fx}(\mathrm{PB} - \mathrm{PH_2O}) \ ... \qquad \textbf{(1)}$$

$$Fx = \frac{Px}{PB - PH_2O} \quad \ldots \qquad (2)$$

where PB is the barometric pressure (in mmHg) and PH_2O the pressure of water vapor (in mmHg).

Let's blow air out – expiration

Upon exiting the lungs, expired gas undergoes changes in volume, as it cools and water condenses, and changes in composition, as alveolar gases mix with air that has remained in VCd at the end of inspiration (Figs. **1** and **2**). For quantifying gas exchange, respiratory gases are expired into a plastic bag. As gases enter the bag, they cool to ambient temperature (TA) and some of the water vapor condenses on the bag surface, although they remain 100% saturated with water vapor (but at TA). At ambient conditions (in the plastic bag) the expired gases are said to be at ATPS (Ambient Temperature and Pressure, Saturated with H_2O at TA). Conversely, the gases in the lungs are said to be at BTPS (Body Temperature and Pressure, Saturated with H_2O at 37°C). Examples of partial pressures and fractional concentrations of gases in the ambient, and in both inspired and alveolar compartments are given in Fig. **3**.

Lung volumes are always expressed at BTPS, whereas the volumes of O_2 consumed and CO_2 produced per minute ($\dot{V}O_2$ and $\dot{V}CO_2$, respectively) are always expressed at STPD (Standard Temperature, 273°K, standard Pressure, 760 mmHg, Dry). Examples of volume conversions are given in Appendix **1, A.** Fig. **4**, shows the changes in O_2 and CO_2 partial pressures as gases flow from ambient to cells and *vice versa*.

O_2 Consumption and CO_2 Production

Let's say that we inspire 700 ml of air (VT = 700 ml BTPS) ten times a minute (f = 10). The total inspired volume per minute (minute inspired ventilation, $\dot{V}I$) will obviously be 7,000 ml (BTPS), but will the total expired volume per minute (minute expired ventilation, $\dot{V}E$) also be 7,000 ml (BTPS)? It could, but most likely it will not! A more likely value for $\dot{V}E$ will be 6,950 ml (BTPS). Where did the missing 50 ml of $\dot{V}E$ go? The answer is simple:

$$\dot{V}I\ 7{,}000\ ml$$

$$-\ \dot{V}O_2\ 300\ ml$$

$$+\ \dot{V}CO_2\ 250\ ml$$

===============

$$=\ \dot{V}E\ 6{,}950\ ml$$

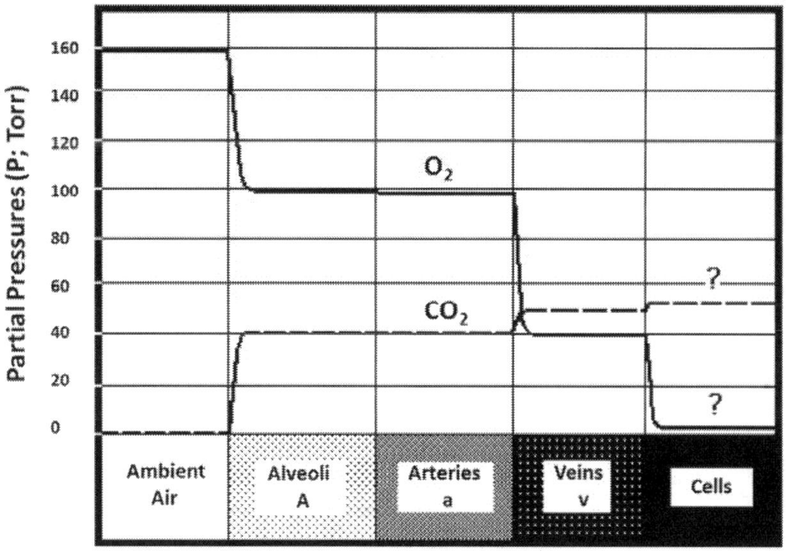

Figure 4: Gradual changes in PO_2 and PCO_2 (torr = mmHg) from ambient to tissue and *vice-versa*.

$\dot{V}I$ differs from $\dot{V}E$ because the Respiratory Quotient (RQ), the ratio between CO_2 produced and O_2 consumed (Eq. 3) at the cellular level is usually approximately 0.85, the result of burning a mixture of sugars, RQ = 1, and lipids, RQ = 0.7. This means that when respiration is in balance with the metabolism (steady state) the ratio between CO_2 production and O_2 consumption at the lung (R, respiratory exchange ratio, often symbolizes "RER" in exercise testing) and at the cellular level (RQ) is the same (R = RQ = 0.85) - for every liter of O_2 consumed 0.85 liters of CO_2 are produced. Thus, at steady state (R = RQ):

$$R = RQ = \frac{\dot{V}CO_2}{\dot{V}O_2} \quad ... \qquad \textbf{(3)}$$

The volume of oxygen consumed per minute ($\dot{V}O_2$) is the difference between the volume of inspired O_2 per minute ($\dot{V}I$ x FIO_2) and that of expired O_2 per minute ($\dot{V}E$ x FEO_2), thus:

$$\dot{V}O_2 = \dot{V}I \text{ x } FIO_2 - \dot{V}E \text{ x } FEO_2 \quad ... \qquad \textbf{(4)}$$

Equation 4 could be used to calculate $\dot{V}O_2$ but it would require measuring both inspired ($\dot{V}I$) and expired ($\dot{V}E$) ventilations (volumes per minute). A simple equation (Eq. 5, derived in Appendix **1, B1**) allows one to calculate $\dot{V}O_2$ by measuring just $\dot{V}E$:

$$\dot{V}O_2 = \dot{V}E\left(FIO_2 \frac{FEN_2}{FIN_2} - FEO_2\right) \quad ... \qquad \textbf{(5)}$$

If the expired gases are collected into a plastic bag, $\dot{V}E$ is the minute expired ventilation (expressed at STPD), $FIO_2 = 0.21$, $FIN_2 = 0.79$, and $FEN_2 = 1 - (FEO_2 + FECO_2)$. FEO_2 and $FECO_2$ are determined from gas samples taken from the bag, by means of O_2 and CO_2 meters.

The volume of CO_2 expired per minute ($\dot{V}CO_2$) is easier to calculate (Eqs. 6 and 7, Fig. **5**), because under normal conditions there is virtually no CO_2 in inspired air ($FICO_2 = 0$; see **Appendix 1, B**):

$$\dot{V}CO_2 = \dot{V}E \text{ x } FECO_2 \quad ... \qquad \textbf{(6)}$$

Since all of the CO_2 comes from the alveoli:

$$\dot{V}CO_2 = \dot{V}\bar{A} \text{ x } F\bar{A}CO_2 \quad ... \qquad \textbf{(7)}$$

Fig. **5** provides a graphic example of how the CO_2 production per minute is measured.

Conductive (Anatomical) Dead Space

As mentioned above (Figs. **1** and **2**), not all of the inspiratory tidal volume (VT) reaches the alveoli. With a normal breathing pattern (at rest) approximately two thirds of VT enter the alveolar compartment, while the last third remains in the conductive airways, which comprise all of the gas passageways that extend for the nose all the way down to the sixteenth generation of airways. In the conductive airways, there is virtually no gas exchange with blood, but for a minimal amount of exchange between air and the protoplasm of epithelial cells lining the airways. Therefore, in the conductive airways the composition of inspired air does not appreciably change.

GRAPHIC EXAMPLE OF METHOD FOR MEASURING CO_2 PRODUCTION PER UNIT TIME

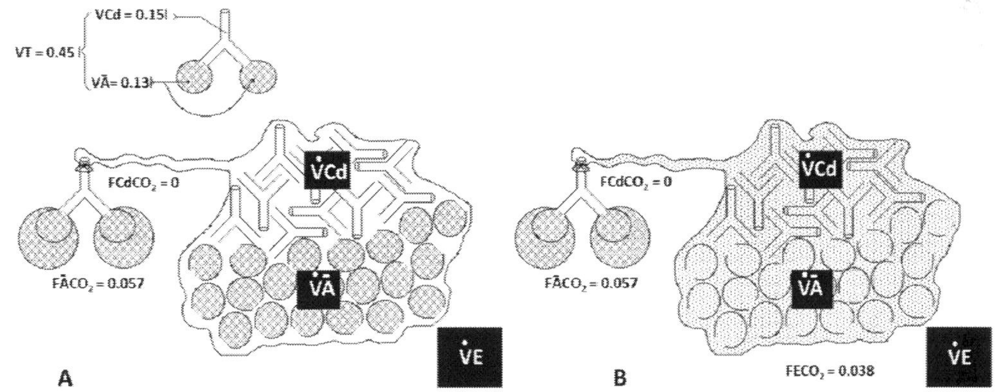

$$\dot{V}CO_2 = \begin{cases} \dot{V}\bar{A} \times F\bar{A}CO_2 = 3 \times 0.057 = \\ \dot{V}E \times FECO_2 = 4.5 \times 0.038 = \end{cases} \boxed{0.171\ l}$$

Figure 5: In this graphic example, the gases expired per minute (**$\dot{V}$E**), exiting from alveolar (**$\dot{V}$A**) and conductive (**$\dot{V}$Cd**, room air) compartments, are assumed to remain separated (A) or mixed (B) in the collecting bag. CO_2 production per minute (**$\dot{V}CO_2$**) is the product of the "smaller" **$\dot{V}$A** and "greater" $FACO_2$, which is the same as that of the "larger" **$\dot{V}$E** and smaller $FECO_2$.

While on the one hand the conductive (anatomical) dead space results in some wasted ventilation, as in this compartment there is no gas exchange with blood, on the other hand it provides several useful functions. As inspired air flows through the dead space compartment, it is heated and humidified to saturation at body temperature, such that the alveoli are well protected from exposure to cold and dry air - the system is amazingly efficient because even in very cold environments the gas that enters the alveoli is at body temperature and 100% saturated with H_2O vapor. Furthermore, the conductive (anatomical) dead space maintains the alveoli clean, as potentially dangerous environmental pollutants are trapped by the wet surface of the conductive airways and are eventually eliminated mixed with mucous by the activity of airway cilia.

Quantification of Conductive (Anatomical) Dead Space Ventilation

The conductive (anatomical) dead space volume can be directly measured by the Fowler's method (named after the American physiologist Ward S. Fowler). With this method (Fig. **6**), the subject is asked to breathe through a one-way breathing valve (a system that prevents mixing of inspired and expired gases), and PCO_2 of expired gases is continuously measured at the mouth by a CO_2 analyzer; simultaneously, the expired volume is also continuously monitored. At the beginning of expiration no CO_2 is detected because the first volume expired is air exiting from VCd. As alveolar gases start exiting, PCO_2 rapidly increases and eventually reaches a fairly constant value, often called alveolar "plateau". Actually, the plateau is not quite flat (horizontal), as PCO_2 continuously increases during expiration, but in normal subjects at rest the increase in PCO_2 is small (Fig. **6**).

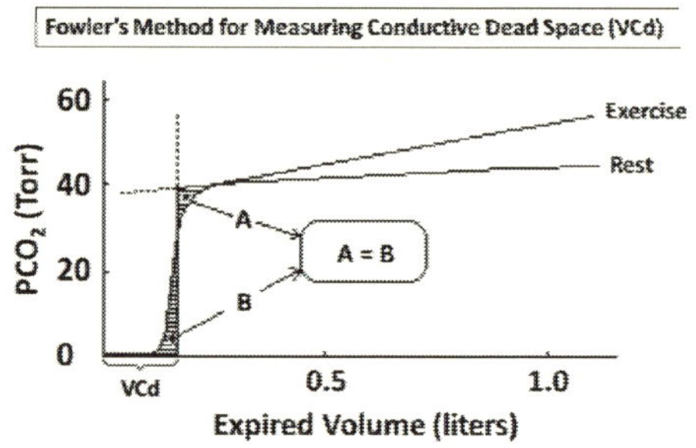

Figure 6: Plot of expired volume *versus* PCO_2. The first volume expired contains room air from dead space (VCd). Its volume is estimated by drawing a vertical line which transects the plotted curve such that areas A and B are of equal size. The origin of the dotted-line on the X-axis corresponds to VCd.

In contrast, during exercise PCO_2 increases at a faster rate - the stronger the exercise, the faster the rate and the steeper the slope of the curve (Fig. **6**). In certain lung diseases the rate of increase may be quite variable as alveoli with different PCO_2 empty at different times, due to different compliances. Therefore, individual samples of end-expiratory gases give reliable values of the average alveolar gas composition only in normal subjects, at rest.

VCd can also be indirectly calculated by the Bohr's method (invented by the Danish physiologist Christian Bohr, 1855-1911). This method determines the amount of VCd by measuring the drop in PCO_2 that takes place as the volume of average alveolar gas ($V\bar{A}$) mixes, during expiration, with gas (room air) that had remained in VCd at the end of the inspiration. The conductive (anatomical) dead space ventilation ($\dot{V}Cd$), which represents the total volume of gas that ventilates VCd per unit time (minute), is expressed in Equation 8, when $FICO_2 = 0$ (derived in Appendix **1, C1**):

$$\dot{V}Cd = \dot{V}E\frac{P\bar{A}CO_2 - PECO_2}{P\bar{A}CO_2} \quad ... \qquad \textbf{(8)}$$

where $\dot{V}E$ is the minute expired ventilation (expressed at BTPS), $P\bar{A}CO_2$ is the average alveolar PCO_2, obtained from samples of end tidal (mixed alveolar, $\bar{A}$) gases taken at the mouth, and $PECO_2$ is the mixed expired PCO_2 obtained from samples of mixed expired gases in the expiratory collecting bag.

The conductive (anatomical) dead space per breath is expressed by Equation 9:

$$VCd = \frac{\dot{V}Cd}{f} \quad ... \qquad \textbf{(9)}$$

where "f" is respiratory frequency (breaths per minute).

Equation 10 expresses the conductive (anatomical) dead space fraction, which is a measure of the fraction of total minute ventilation "wasted", in terms gas exchange with blood, in the conductive dead space compartment:

$$\frac{\dot{V}Cd}{\dot{V}E} = \frac{P\bar{A}CO_2 - PECO_2}{P\bar{A}CO_2} \quad ... \qquad \textbf{(10)}$$

In normal subjects, breathing at rest, $\dot{V}Cd/\dot{V}E \approx 1/3$ (~33%). $\dot{V}Cd$ can also be calculated by subtracting $\dot{V}\bar{A}$ from $\dot{V}E$ (Eq. 11).

$$\dot{V}Cd = \dot{V}E - \dot{V}\overline{A} \ ... \ (\mathbf{11})$$

Physiological Dead Space Ventilation

In normal subjects virtually all of the dead space ventilation is conductive (anatomical, $\dot{V}Cd$), being restricted almost exclusively to conductive airways (Figs. **1, 2** and **5**). In contrast, in patients affected by certain chronic lung diseases, such as emphysema for example - a condition that leads to disruption of alveolar septa greatly reducing the capillary circulation of some of the alveoli - the affected alveolar regions behave almost like dead space regions (Fig. **7A**). This additional dead space ventilation, known as alveolar dead space ventilation ($\dot{V}Ad$), takes place in alveoli that are ventilated but lack significant blood perfusion. Therefore, these alveoli contain gas with a composition very similar to that of room air, as gas exchange with blood is minimal. The sum of conductive ($\dot{V}Cd$) and alveolar ($\dot{V}Ad$) dead space ventilations is called physiological (or total) dead space ventilation ($\dot{V}Pd$, Fig. **7A**). Obviously, in emphysematous patients $\dot{V}Pd$ is always greater that $\dot{V}Cd$, while in normal subjects $\dot{V}Pd$ and $\dot{V}Cd$ are virtually the same, as $\dot{V}Ad$ is only 1-2% of $\dot{V}\overline{A}$.

The opposite condition is the alveolar (right-to-left) blood shunt ($\dot{Q}As$, Fig. **7B**) - the equivalent of dead space on the blood side. The alveolar shunt is caused by venous blood that, after exiting from alveoli well perfused but unventilated or very poorly ventilated (maldistribution shunt-like effect), mixes with oxygenated blood exiting from well ventilated and well perfused alveoli. While the presence of significant alveolar shunt always reflects a pathological condition, a small amount of venous admixture, known as anatomical or conductive shunt ($\dot{Q}Cs$), is also present in normal people (see Chapter 7). The sum of $\dot{Q}As$ and $\dot{Q}Cs$ is called physiological shunt ($\dot{Q}Ps$, Fig. **7B**).

Quantification of Physiological Dead Space Ventilation

The physiological dead space ventilation ($\dot{V}Pd$) can be indirectly calculated by measuring the drop in PCO_2 that takes place as gas coming from well perfused and well ventilated alveoli – the so called "alveolar ideal" compartment ($\dot{V}Ai$, see below) – mixes, during expiration, with room air coming from both alveoli ventilated but virtually unperfused ($\dot{V}Ad$) and the conductive (anatomical) dead space compartment ($\dot{V}Cd$; Fig. **8**). The physiological dead space ventilation ($\dot{V}Pd$) is expressed by Equation 12 (derived in Appendix **1, C2**):

$$\dot{V}Pd = \dot{V}E\frac{PaCO_2 - PECO_2}{PaCO_2} \; ... \qquad \textbf{(12)}$$

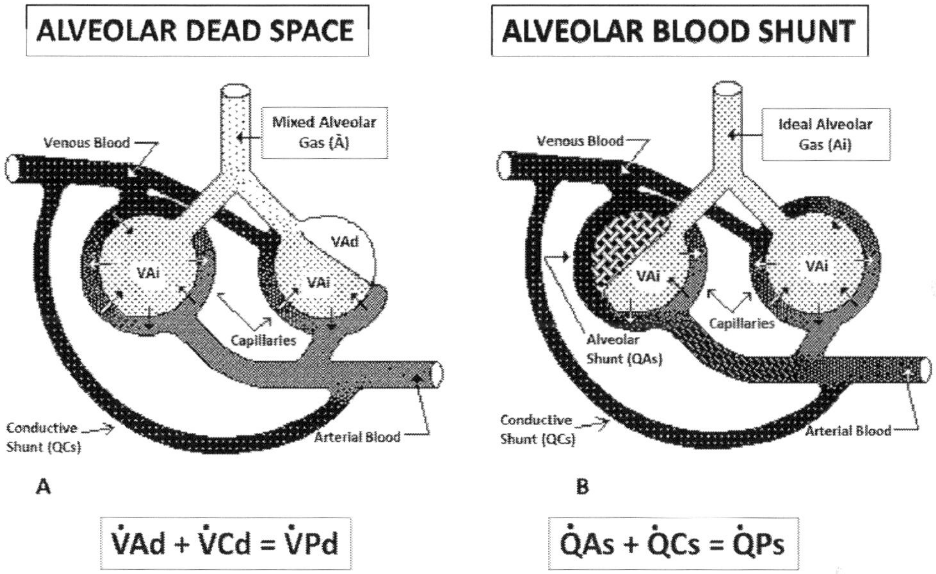

Figure 7: Graphic representation of alveolar dead space (VAd, A) and alveolar shunt (QAs, B). VAd is shown as an alveolar compartment ventilated but unperfused (A). Similarly, QAs is shown as a compartment perfused but unventilated (B). Note, however, that these are functional equivalent models of the real lung (see Chapter 7).

$\dot{V}E$ and $PECO_2$ are measured as described above ($\dot{V}E$ should be converted from ATPS to BTPS because $\dot{V}Pd$ is a lung volume), and $PaCO_2$ is obtained from arterial blood samples.

The physiological dead space per breath is expressed by Equation 13:

$$VPd = \frac{\dot{V}Pd}{f} \; ... \qquad \textbf{(13)}$$

Equation 14 expresses the physiological dead space fraction, which is a measure of the fraction of total ventilation "wasted", in terms of gas exchange with blood, in both conductive and alveolar dead space compartments:

$$\frac{\dot{V}Pd}{\dot{V}E} = \frac{PaCO_2 - PECO_2}{PaCO_2} \ldots \quad \textbf{(14)}$$

In normal subjects, breathing at rest, $\dot{V}Pd/\dot{V}E = \dot{V}Cd/\dot{V}E = 1/3$ (~33%).

$\dot{V}Pd$ can also be calculated by subtracting the alveolar ideal ventilation ($\dot{V}Ai$) from $\dot{V}E$ (Eq. 15).

$$\dot{V}Pd = \dot{V}E - \dot{V}Ai \ldots \quad \textbf{(15)}$$

For a graphic example of conductive and physiological dead spaces, see Appendix **1**, Fig. **1**.

Alveolar Dead Space and Right-to-Left Blood Shunt

In the previous section we have defined the alveolar dead space as a lung region ventilated but unperfused and the alveolar shunt as a region perfused but unventilated. This seems pretty simple, but it isn't quite so. In most cases neither $\dot{V}Ad$ nor $\dot{Q}As$ are clear cut compartments; rather, most often they result from the presence of a myriad of lung regions with widely different ventilation/perfusion ($\dot{V}/\dot{Q}$) ratios. What we call alveolar dead space ventilation ($\dot{V}Ad$) is actually the functional equivalent of alveolar regions with abnormally high $\dot{V}/\dot{Q}$. What we call alveolar shunt is the functional equivalent of regions with abnormally low $\dot{V}/\dot{Q}$ (maldistribution shunt-like effect), plus some potential conductive shunt regions (alveoli with $\dot{V}/\dot{Q} = 0$).

While material dealing with the consequences of $\dot{V}/\dot{Q}$ maldistribution in terms of shunt and alveolar dead space will be discussed in detail in Chapter 7, it is important to start introducing some elements of the so called "three-compartment-model" [1], a model which allows one to quantify the "functional equivalent" magnitudes of venous admixture (conductive shunt plus maldistribution shunt-like effect) and alveolar dead space ventilation. This approach simplifies the complexity of the real lung, with its wide spectrum of $\dot{V}/\dot{Q}$ ratios, into a functionally equivalent model that lumps together all of the regional contributions to venous admixture, wasted alveolar ventilation, and ideal gas exchange into three compartments: one with $\dot{V}/\dot{Q} = 0$ (shunt), one with $\dot{V}/\dot{Q} = \infty$ (alveolar dead space) and one with a perfectly efficient $\dot{V}/\dot{Q}$ (alveolar ideal), respectively. By definition, the alveolar ideal compartment ($\dot{V}Ai$) is composed of alveoli whose exchange ratio ($R = \dot{V}CO_2/\dot{V}O_2$) matches the cellular respiratory quotient (RQ, usually ~0.85), and whose CO_2 partial pressure is virtually the same as that of arterial blood ($PAiCO_2 \approx PaCO_2$; see Chapter 7).

Alveolar Ideal PO_2 ($PAiO_2$), Alveolar Gas Equation and $(Ai\text{-}a)PO_2$ Gradient

For evaluating quantitatively venous admixture (conductive shunt plus maldistribution shunt-like effect) and alveolar dead space by means of the three-compartment-model, one needs to know the O_2- and CO_2-compositions of each compartment. The composition of shunt and alveolar dead space compartments can be easily determined because the shunt compartment is unventilated (contains no gas) and the blood perfusing it is mixed venous blood, and the alveolar dead space compartment is unperfused and the gas it contains has the composition of ambient air. A bit harder is to determine the composition of the alveolar ideal compartment (Ai), because its blood and gas cannot be sampled. However, based on the "three-compartment-model" we know that $PAiCO_2$ and $PaCO_2$ are virtually the same (Eq. 16):

$$PAiCO_2 \approx PaCO_2 \ ... \qquad \textbf{(16)}$$

In contrast, this isn't the case for the alveolar ideal PO_2 because, due to the effect of blood shunts, $PAiO_2$ cannot be equated to PaO_2 (Eq. 17):

$$PAiO_2 \neq PaO_2 \ ... \qquad \textbf{(17)}$$

This is due to the presence of hemoglobin (Hb) in blood. As Hb approaches O_2-saturation, the curve describing the relationship between gas tension and gas content for O_2 in blood is much less steep than that for CO_2 (Appendix **1, D,** Fig. **2**), such that a decrease in blood O_2-content caused by the admixture of shunted blood causes a sizable drop in PaO_2, while an increase in CO_2 content of similar amounts minimally increases PCO_2. Thus, PaO_2 is always significantly lower than $PAiO_2$. This difference, known as the $(Ai\text{-}a)PO_2$ gradient (also symbolized as $AaDO_2$), reflects the magnitude of venous admixture (conductive shunt plus maldistribution shunt-like effect), albeit with some limitations (see Chapter 7). In normal subjects at rest $(Ai\text{-}a)PO_2$ = 2-4 mmHg, while in old people at rest values as high as 10 mmHg are still within the normal range. An estimate of the normal (Ai-a)PO_2 can be obtained by calculating the following: (Age+10)/4.

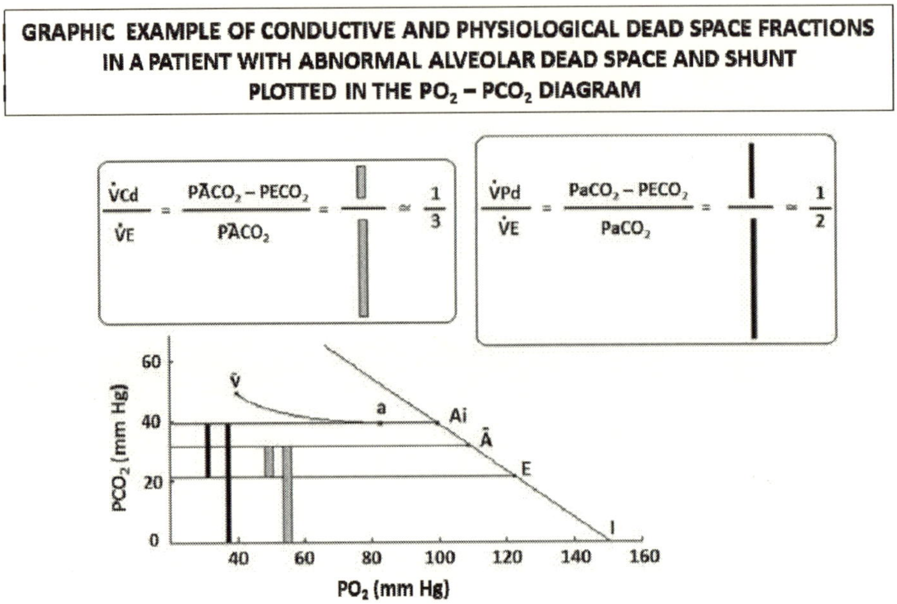

Figure 8: O_2-CO_2 diagram plotting PO_2 and PCO_2 in end-tidal ($\bar{A}$, mixed alveolar), expired (E) and inspired (I) gases, and in mixed venous ($\bar{v}$) and arterial (a) blood. This diagram allow one to readily appreciate the magnitudes of conductive (**$\dot{V}$Cd**, top left), physiological (**$\dot{V}$Cd**, top right) and alveolar (**$\dot{V}$Ad**) dead space fractions, as well as that of both the (Ai-a)PO_2 gradient and the exchange ratio (R, the slope of the oblique line originating at I). In this example, 50% of **$\dot{V}$E** is wasted in **$\dot{V}$Pd** and ~33% in **$\dot{V}$Cd**. There is also a sizable right-to-left blood shunt because the (Ai-a)PO_2 is almost 20 mmHg (see Chapter 7). Note that "Ai" and "a" have virtually the same PCO_2 but different PO_2.

This being the case, how can we determine $PAiO_2$, and with that the O_2 content of alveolar ideal blood? We do so by capitalizing on the concept that $PAiCO_2 \approx PaCO_2$, which allows us to obtain $PAiO_2$ by means of an important equation known as the "*alveolar gas equation*" [2, 3] (Eq. 18) - note that in order to understand how this equation determines the value of $PAiO_2$ one needs to understand how it has been derived (see Appendix **1, E**):

$$PAiO_2 = PIO_2 - \frac{1-FIO_2(1-R)}{R} PaCO_2 \;... \qquad \textbf{(18)}$$

in this equation PIO_2 is the inspired PO_2 at BTPS, FIO_2 = 0.2094, and R is the exchange ratio, which in the ideal alveolar compartment (Ai), at steady state, is the same as RQ. Since the term "1-FIO_2(1 - R)" is usually close to one, a short form of the alveolar gas equation is most often used (Eq. 19):

$$PAiO_2 \approx PIO_2 - \frac{PaCO_2}{R} \ldots \quad \textbf{(19)}$$

When R =1, or when breathing 100% FIO_2, the equation is even simpler (Eq. 20):

$$PAiO_2 = PIO_2 - PaCO_2 \ldots \textbf{(20)}$$

O_2-CO_2 Diagram

A convenient way of graphically representing the partial pressures of alveolar and blood gases, their relationship to the exchange ratio (R), and their changes in relation to a variety of physiological and pathological states, is provided by a diagram in which PO_2 and PCO_2 are plotted on horizontal and vertical axes, respectively. The O_2-CO_2 diagram, also known as Fenn-Rahn diagram [4] (Fig. **8**), is the most representative map of gas exchange.

Body Gas Store

Oxygen, carbon dioxide and nitrogen are stored in different amounts in various areas of the body (Fig. **9**). In a normal male (~70 kg, 155 lb.) the total amount of O_2 is approximately 1.5 liters (at end of normal inspiration), whereas the total amount of CO_2 is approximately 6 liters. Most of the O_2 is in lungs, arteries and veins, whereas most of the CO_2 is in the tissue. The amount of gas stored in different regions of the body is quite constant at rest, but can dramatically change with acute changes in metabolic rate and/or respiration.

Acute Changes in Ventilation Affect the Exchange Ratio (R ≠ RQ)

An interesting phenomenon related to the properties of gas stores takes place during acute hyper- or hypo-ventilation. These are transient conditions in which one starts breathing above or below the metabolic needs, respectively - acute hyperventilation may occur at the onset of a hysteric/panic attack or during fast ascent to high altitudes in unpressurized airplanes; acute hypoventilation may occur in COPD or asthmatic patients at the onset of sudden respiratory distress.

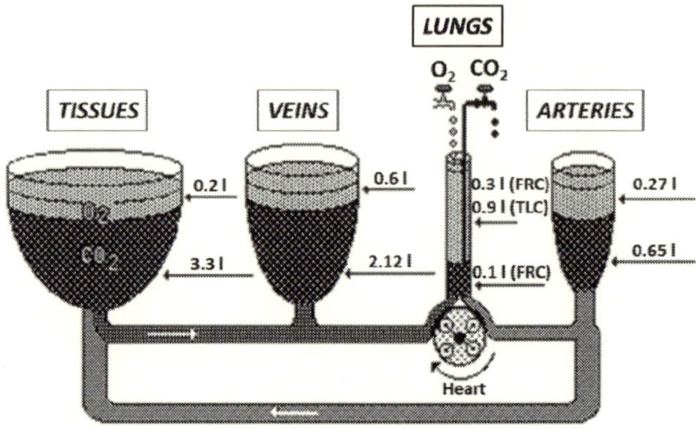

Figure 9: Body gas stores in different body compartments. The total amount of stored CO_2 is approximately four times that of O_2.

To understand the consequences of these transient conditions, let's assume that a subject who is breathing at steady state (R = RQ) has PAO_2 = 102 mmHg, $PACO_2$ = 40 mmHg and R = 0.8 (point A in Fig. **10**). Now let's assume that hi/she starts hyperventilating (for example: doubling VT at constant "f" or *vice versa*).

Obviously, this acute hyperventilation will cause a drop in $PACO_2$ and an increase in PAO_2, such that eventually point A will move to point A'. Curiously, however, point A will not shift downward along the R = 0.8 line but it will follow a curved path, such as the one indicated by the arrow in Fig. **10**, moving toward greater and greater exchange ratio (R-lines > 0.8), finally to return to steady state (R = 0.8) at point A'. The opposite phenomenon will take place in acute hypoventilation (Fig. **10**).

In spite of the changes in R we know that RQ did not change from its original value of 0.8. So, why does R transiently change? The reason is that the much greater solubility of CO_2 than O_2 in body fluids enables CO_2 to be added to, or removed from, blood and other body fluids in much larger quantities than O_2, for similar changes in partial pressure gradients, at least at O_2 pressures at which Hb approaches 100% O_2-saturation. This explains the changes in R when respiration is not at steady state with the metabolism. At the very beginning of hyperventilation the fast rate of CO_2 removal from the lungs causes a large increase in PCO_2 gradient between alveolar gas and mixed venous blood entering the alveolar capillaries. This gradient allows for large CO_2 volumes to diffuse out of the capillary blood into the alveoli (large increase in $\dot{V}CO_2$). In contrast, the simultaneous increase in inspired O_2 results in only a small increase in O_2 diffusion from alveolar gas to capillary blood (small increase in $\dot{V}O_2$). This adds only a small amount of dissolved O_2 in the blood, because before hyperventilation, with PAO_2 = 102 mmHg, the hemoglobin of end-capillary blood was already 98% saturated - at this PAO_2 the curve that relates O_2 content to O_2 partial pressure (O_2 dissociation curve) is almost flat, meaning that relatively large changes in O_2 partial pressure result in small changes in O_2 content (see Appendix **1**, Fig. **2**). The consequence of this is that at the lungs $\dot{V}CO_2$ transiently becomes significantly greater than $\dot{V}O_2$ (R > 1; Fig. **10**), such that, transiently, R ≠ RQ. If hyperventilation continues at the same rate, eventually the $P\bar{v}CO_2$ of blood entering the alveolar capillaries will have significantly dropped to a steady state level, such that the $\dot{V}CO_2/\dot{V}O_2$ gradient will return to normal - $\dot{V}CO_2$ at the lungs will again match the $\dot{V}CO_2$ at the tissue, such that the original R value (0.8) will be reestablished (point A' in Fig. **10**, R = RQ). The opposite will take place with acute hypoventilation.

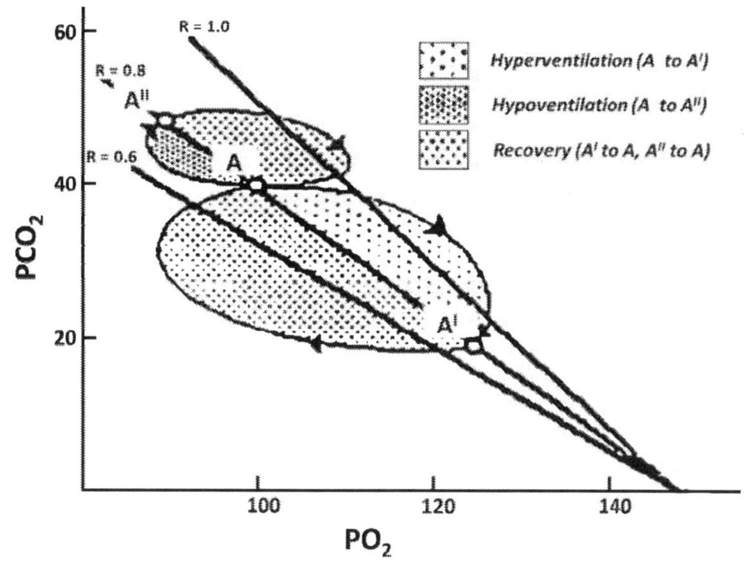

Figure 10: Acute hyper- or hypo-ventilations cause respiration to be transiently out of steady-state with the metabolism (R ≠ RQ). With acute hyperventilation, transiently R becomes greater than RQ, while with acute hypoventilation R becomes lower than RQ.

Note that recoveries from hyper- or hypo-ventilation behave like acute hypo- or hyper-ventilation, respectively. The reason for it is found in the chemical control of breathing (see Chapter 8). With hyperventilation, $PACO_2$ has dropped from 40 to 20 mmHg, and PAO_2 has increased from 102 to 125 mmHg (Fig. **10A** and **A^I**, respectively). The sharp drop in $PaCO_2$ dramatically decreases the stimulation of peripheral and central chemo-receptors, which are sensitive to $PaCO_2$-induced pH change (see Chapter 8). Therefore, transiently there will be hypoventilation. Hypoventilation will cause PaO_2 to drop – in this example down from ~125 to ~85-90 mmHg (Fig. **10**) – but this drop will affect only minimally the O_2 receptors (see Chapter 8), as they are strongly activated only when PaO_2 drops below ~70 mmHg. During this transient period, $PACO_2$ rises very slowly, remaining just above 20 mmHg for quite some time, as hyperventilation removed large quantities of CO_2 from the stores, while only increased slightly the O_2 stores. The result is that the drop in PCO_2 stimulus allows the system to become slightly hypoxemic (Fig. **10**). Similar reasoning applies to recovery from acute hypoventilation (Fig. **10A^{II}** to **A**).

Relationship Among Ventilation, Arterial PCO_2 and Metabolic Rate

At steady state conditions (R = RQ) the system maintains ideal alveolar ventilation and arterial PCO_2 precisely matched to metabolic rate. Due to feedback mechanisms of the control of breathing (see Chapter 8), at constant metabolic rate the arterial PCO_2 is inversely related to the ideal alveolar ventilation ($\dot{V}Ai$), such that, after reaching steady state, a doubling of $\dot{V}Ai$ reduces $PaCO_2$ to 1/2, whereas a reduction of $\dot{V}Ai$ to 1/2 will double $PaCO_2$ (Fig. **11**). This precise relationship is expressed by Equation 21 (derived in Appendix **1, E**):

$$PaCO_2 = \frac{K \times \dot{V}CO_2}{\dot{V}Ai} \quad \ldots \qquad \textbf{(21)}$$

where K is a constant (863, at 37°C) which is independent of barometric pressure, but only varies with changes in body temperature (see Appendix **1, F**). At constant metabolic rate, $\dot{V}CO_2$ will not change, and so the ratio $PaCO_2/\dot{V}Ai$ will remain constant.

Equation 21 is represented graphically in Fig. **11**.

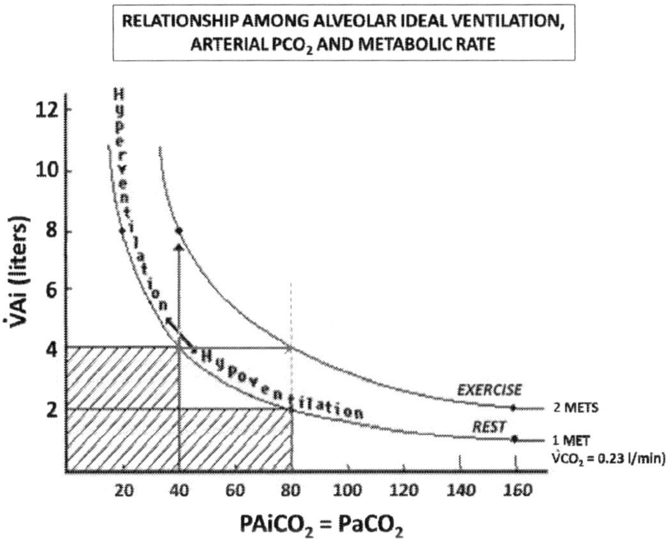

Figure 11: Plot of $PaCO_2$ *versus* **V̇Ai** at normal or increased metabolic rate. $PaCO_2$ is inversely related to **V̇Ai** and directly related to metabolic rate (**V̇CO₂** → $\dot{V}CO_2$). At steady state, doubling **V̇Ai** halves $PaCO_2$, and halving **V̇Ai** doubles $PaCO_2$. When $\dot{V}CO_2$ doubles (2 METS), **V̇Ai** has to double for $PaCO_2$ to remain at 40 mmHg. If **V̇Ai** does not change, $PaCO_2$ will double (80 mmHg, red arrow).

This relationship reflects a fundamental function of the regulation of breathing, a mechanism that allows the organism to maintain the rates of CO_2 removal at pace with the metabolic rate of CO_2 production (see Chapter 8). Indeed, as shown in Fig. **11**, at steady state (R = RQ) V̇Ai and metabolic rate are precisely matched, such that when metabolic rate doubles (from 1 MET to 2 METS), during exercise for example, V̇Ai has to double (from 4 to 8 l/min, hyperpnea) to maintain $PaCO_2$ at 40 mmHg; if V̇Ai does not double, $PACO_2$ will double (from 40 to 80 mmHg; Fig. **11**, red arrow). Similarly, if V̇Ai doubles at the same metabolic rare (hyperventilation), after reaching steady state $PaCO_2$ will drops to a half (from 40 to 20 mmHg). This relationship is particularly relevant for determining the proper amount of "ideal" alveolar ventilation need to regulate $PaCO_2$ and arterial pH in patients mechanically ventilated.

REFERENCES

[1] Riley RL, Cournand A. "Ideal" alveolar air and the analysis of ventilation-perfusion relationships in the lungs. J Appl Physiol 1949;1:825–847.

[2] Fenn W O, Rahn, H, Otis AB. A theoretical study of the composition of the alveolar air at altitude. Am J Physiol 1946;146:637-653.

[3] Riley RL, Counrand A. "Ideal" alveolar air and the analysis of ventilation-perfusion relationship in the lungs. J Appl Physiol 1949;1:825-847.

[4] Rahn H, Fehn WO. A graphical analysis of the respiratory gas exchange. Washington, DC, Am Physiol Soc; 1955.

Lung Function In Health And Disease, 2014, 100-121

CHAPTER 5

Gas Transport

Nasr H. Anaizi

Abstract: The primary function of the respiratory system is to supply oxygen (O_2) and eliminate carbon dioxide (CO_2), a task that is accomplished in conjunction with the circulatory system, which transports these gases between the lungs and peripheral tissues. This chapter covers the principles and mechanisms involved in the transport of O_2 and CO_2 in the blood. In particular, it discusses the passive diffusion of gases across the alveolar blood-gas barrier and related factors, and the physical laws and gas properties; it provides a comparison of gas transfer profiles among O_2, CO_2, carbon monoxide, and nitrous oxide; it defines the lung diffusion capacity (transfer factor) and its measurement; it describes the function of hemoglobin in the transport of O_2, the hemoglobin-oxygen dissociation curve, and the factors that regulate hemoglobin oxygen affinity; and finally, it describes the transport of CO_2 in the blood, the role of carbonic anhydrase, and the Haldane effect.

Keywords: Blood-Gas Barrier, Bohr Effect, Carbon Dioxide, Carbon Monoxide, Carbonic Anhydrase, Chloride Shift, Diffusion Capacity, Diffusion Constant, Dissociation Curve, 2,3-Diphosphoglycerate (2,3-DPG), Fick's Law, Gas Transport, Graham's law, Haldane Effect, Hemoglobin, Nitrous Oxide, Oxygen, Partial Pressure, Transfer Coefficient, Transfer Factor.

The focus of this chapter is on the principles and mechanisms involved in the transport of oxygen and carbon dioxide in the blood between the lungs and the peripheral tissues. The primary function of the respiratory system is to supply oxygen and eliminate carbon dioxide, a task that is accomplished in conjunction with the circulatory system which transports O_2 and CO_2 between the lungs and peripheral tissues. As blood flows through the alveolar capillaries it is separated from the alveolar space by an extremely thin barrier made up of flattened endothelial-epithelial cells often referred to as the blood-gas barrier. Thus, the blood in the alveolar capillaries comes into virtual contact with fresh air allowing for the gases to diffuse and equilibrate between the two compartments (gas exchange).

Net gas transfer is determined mainly by three factors:

- The rate of net **diffusion** of the gas which is driven by the difference in its partial pressure between the two compartments, *i.e.*, the partial pressure gradient (ΔPx).

- The gas carrying **capacity of the blood**. For example, as discussed later under "Oxygen Transport", the oxygen carrying capacity of the blood is determined by the concentration of functional hemoglobin and the partial pressure of oxygen in the blood (PO_2).

- The rate of **perfusion** (blood flow). This factor is important when gas transfer is perfusion-limited as it is normally the case for most gases including O_2 and CO_2.

DIFFUSION

Gas molecules move and collide randomly owing to their inherent kinetic energy. Diffusion is the net movement of like molecules down their concentration or partial pressure gradient, *i.e.* from areas of higher rates of collision to areas of lower rates of collision. Net diffusion across a barrier is governed by Fick's law (Fig. **1**) which states that the rate of net diffusion of substance *x* is directly proportional to:

1. The **concentration gradient** (ΔCx) or partial pressure gradient (ΔPx) between the two sides of the diffusion barrier. Fig. **2** shows PO_2 and PCO_2 values at different points in the circulation. At the level of the alveoli, the ΔPO_2 at the beginning of the capillary is normally ten times greater than ΔPCO_2 (60 *vs.* 6 mm Hg). However, despite this ten-fold difference in the gradient CO_2 diffuses more easily in body fluids and through biological membranes than does O_2 because of other factors (discussed below)

2. The **surface area** (**A**) available for diffusion: the greater the surface area the greater is the diffusion rate. In other words, the greater the number of functional alveoli the greater is the diffusion surface available for gas exchange and the greater is the rate of diffusion. The subdivision of the lung into a large number of very small chambers for gas exchange (alveoli) greatly increases its surface-to-volume ratio and provides an immense surface area for gas exchange. It is estimated that the lungs of a young healthy adult comprise about 300 million alveoli with an estimated surface area of approximately 70 m^2.

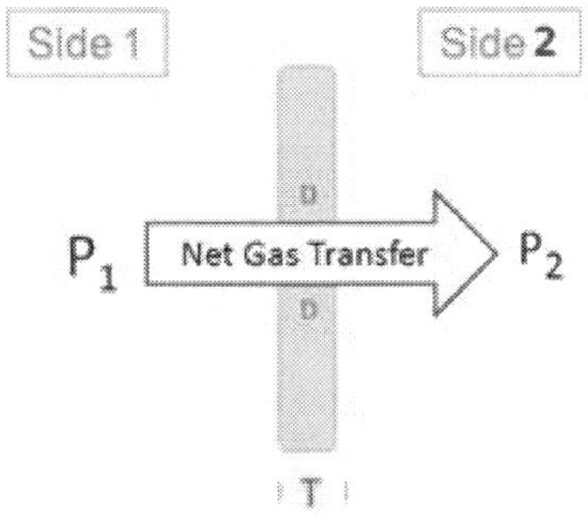

Figure 1: Gas Diffusion through a membrane from side 1 to side 2 driven by the partial pressure difference ($P_1 - P_2$). A= Surface area available for diffusion. T = thickness of diffusion barrier. D = diffusion constant which is directly proportional to the solubility and inversely related to the square root of the gas's molecular mass. The quantity $\frac{D*A}{T}$ = the diffusion capacity. Net Gas Transfer = Partial pressure gradient x Diffusion Capacity

3. The **diffusion constant** (D) (aka coefficient of diffusion) of the gas through the diffusion barrier. This is determined, for any given temperature, by the solubility (S) of the gas and the square root of its molecular mass (D ᾱ S/$\sqrt{MM}$; Graham's law). Gases in general are highly lipid soluble and move with ease through the lipid core of biological membranes. However, gases differ in terms of their solubility in water. At body normal temperature (37°C) the solubility of CO_2 in normal saline or plasma is 21 times higher than that for O_2 (0.65 *vs*. 0.031 ml/l/mmHg), and the CO_2 diffusion constant (D) through biological membranes is approximately 18 times greater than that for O_2 as can be easily derived by applying Graham's law (Eq. 1):

$$\frac{CO_2 \text{ diffusion constant}}{O_2 \text{ diffusion constant}} = 21 \text{ x } \sqrt{\frac{32}{44}} = 18 \ldots \quad \textbf{(1)}$$

As a result of these differences it has been estimated that the overall net diffusion rate in body fluids and membranes is approximately 20 times higher for CO_2 than for O_2. In summary, CO_2 diffuses much more readily than O_2 and therefore its transfer by diffusion does not require as high a driving force (ΔPx) as does O_2.

Diffusion rate is also affected by the diffusion distance; it is inversely related to the thickness (T) of the diffusion barrier (diffusion distance). In healthy alveoli, the thickness of the gas-blood barrier averages about 0.5 μm and constitutes virtually no resistance to gas exchange. However, under certain pathological conditions, the alveolar-capillary membrane can become too thick to the point of impeding gas diffusion. Several components make up the gas-blood barrier: 1- the alveolar epithelium, its basement membrane, and the surfactant layer that lines it; 2- the interstitial space; 3- the capillary endothelium and its basement membrane; 4- the plasma; 5- the erythrocyte membrane.

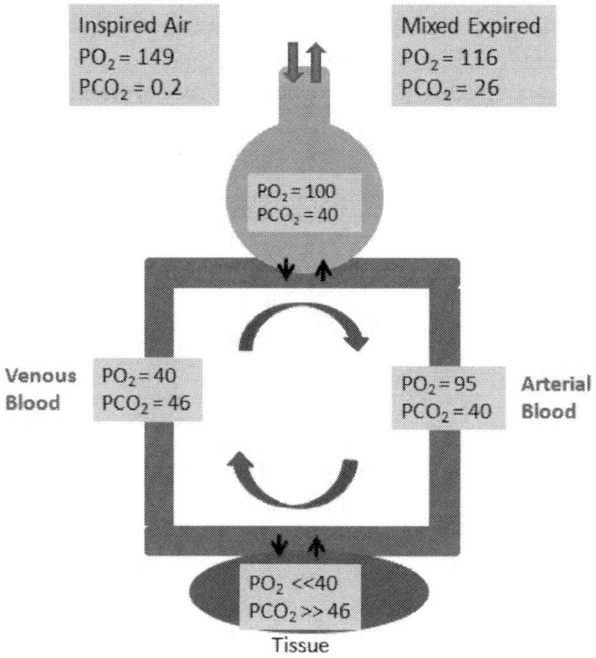

Figure 2: The partial pressures of O_2 and CO_2 at various points in the respiratory system. Note the favorable gradients for the diffusion of O_2 from the alveolar gas into the alveolar capillary blood and the diffusion of CO_2 in the opposite direction ($\Delta P_{O_2} = 100 - 40 = 60$ mm Hg and $\Delta P_{CO_2} = 46 - 40 = 6$ mm Hg). At the level of the tissue, gas exchange is driven by similarly favorable gradients. At rest, the average ΔP_{O_2} along the alveolar capillaries is estimated at 12 mmHg and pulmonary diffusion capacity for O_2 at 21 ml/min/mmHg. Net O_2 transfer = $\mathbf{\dot{V}O_2}$ = 12 x 21=252 ml/min = resting O_2 consumption.

In addition to the resistance offered by the multilayered gas-blood barrier, gas transfer rate is affected in equal measure by the rate of chemical interaction of the gas with hemoglobin (Hb). The rate of this chemical interaction is in turn determined by the rate constant (θ) of the chemical reaction (between the gas and

Hb) and the blood volume in the capillary (V_c). These two barriers may be thought of as two resistances in series [D_M and ($\theta * V_c$)].

The three determinants of gas diffusion rate [diffusion coefficient (D), surface area (A), and diffusion distance (T)] can be lumped into one term called ***lung diffusion capacity*** or ***transfer factor*** and Fick's law may now be expressed as follows:

Rate of net gas transfer = Partial pressure gradient * lung diffusion capacity (DL*x*, Eq. 2)

$$\Delta Px \frac{\mathrm{D\,x\,A}}{\mathrm{T}} = \Delta Px * \mathrm{DL}x \; \ldots \tag{2}$$

The lung diffusion capacity (DL*x*) varies from gas to gas even under normal conditions, and the profile of the partial pressure of a given gas in the blood along the alveolar capillary is determined in part by its DL*x* and partly by its interaction with blood components, particularly hemoglobin (Hb). A gas with favorable diffusion properties and limited or no interaction with Hb will equilibrate rapidly across the diffusion barrier so that its partial pressure in the alveolar capillary blood and alveolar gas phase will become equal early along the alveolar capillary. The net transfer of the gas in this situation will be limited only by the rate of blood flow and the gas transfer is described as ***perfusion-limited***. Under normal conditions, this is the case for most gases including O_2, CO_2, and N_2O (nitrous oxide) [1].

While O_2 and CO_2 have significant degrees of interaction with Hb, N_2O has none and at the same time it is able to cross the alveolar membranes easily. The PN_2O in the blood rises rapidly reaching its level in the alveolar gas within the first quarter of the capillary length. On the other hand, because of their interactions with Hb, the equilibrium points for O_2 and CO_2 are reached a little farther along the capillary (Fig. **3**). The net rate of transfer for each of these three gases is perfusion-limited because they all reach equilibrium well before the blood reaches the end of the alveolar capillary.

An entirely different picture is encountered in the case of carbon monoxide (CO). Because of the avidity with which hemoglobin binds CO, the CO molecules are removed from the liquid phase almost as rapidly as they enter and the PCO in the blood hardly rises as the blood flows along the alveolar capillary. At the end of the alveolar capillary the blood PCO is only a fraction of the PCO in the alveolar gas phase (see Fig. **3**). Therefore, the rate of CO transfer is clearly limited by diffusion rather by blood flow.

Lung Diffusion Capacity (Transfer Factor)

The surface area of the lungs (A), the diffusion constant (D), and the diffusion distance or thickness (T) are difficult to measure individually and are usually lumped together in one constant known as the **lung diffusion capacity** [2] for the gas in question (DLx). Considering the diffusion of oxygen in the alveoli:

Oxygen lung diffusion capacity (Eq. 3):

$$DLO_2 = \frac{A*DO_2}{T} \ldots \quad \textbf{(3)}$$

Net O_2 diffusion rate (Eqs. 4 and 5):

$$\dot{V}O_2 = \Delta PO_2 \text{ x } DLO_2 \ldots \quad \textbf{(4)}$$

$$DLO_2 = \dot{V}O_2 / \Delta PO_2 = \dot{V}O_2 / [PAO_2 - PcO_2] \ldots \quad \textbf{(5)}$$

where PAO_2 is the alveolar PO_2 and PcO_2 the mean pulmonary capillary (c) PO_2.

Since it is not possible to directly measure the PO_2 in the pulmonary capillaries, the DLO_2 can only be estimated indirectly. This is accomplished by measuring pulmonary diffusion capacity for carbon monoxide (DLCO) and multiplying its value by 1.23 which is the estimated ratio of DLO_2 to DLCO resulting from the differences between the two gases in terms of their molecular masses and solubility (Graham's law). Using this technique, the normal, resting pulmonary diffusion capacities for CO and O_2 (in a young adult male of average height) have been estimated at 25 and 31 ml/min/mm Hg respectively.

DLCO Measurement

The method employed in the measurement of carbon monoxide lung diffusion capacity (DLCO) takes advantage of the extremely high affinity of hemoglobin (Hb) for CO which is 210 times that of O_2. In the presence of a small amount of CO in the inspired gas virtually all the CO molecules that diffuse across the alveolar-capillary membrane into the blood are immediately bound to Hb and virtually none remains free in pulmonary capillary blood. Therefore, in practice PcCO ≈ 0. Consequently, the pulmonary diffusion capacity equation for CO is reduced to (Eq. 6):

$$\mathrm{DLCO} = \frac{\dot{\mathrm{V}}\mathrm{CO}}{\mathrm{PACO}} \cdots \quad \textbf{(6)}$$

Both numerator and denominator are easily determined. The subject takes a few breaths from a gas mixture containing 0.1% to 0.3% CO. The PACO is measured in the end-tidal expired gas, and then a 10-second breath hold is performed at maximal inflation. Helium (~10%) is included in the gas mixture in order to measure the volume of the lungs by the dilution technique. The CO concentration in alveolar gas is measured and the amounts of CO in the lungs at beginning and at end of the breath hold are determined; the difference between these two quantities represents the amount of CO transferred from the alveoli to the blood during the 10 seconds of breath hold. $\dot{V}CO$ is then calculated using Eq. 7 and the result may be plugged in Eq. 8 to obtain an estimate of DLO_2. However, this last step is usually unnecessary since DLCO value is the more commonly reported by lung function testing laboratories. Also, the DLCO value is often factored for lung volume to give what is called carbon monoxide ***transfer coefficient*** (KCO), a rate constant also known as the transfer factor or diffusion capacity per unit alveolar volume. Unlike DLCO, KCO is independent of gender, and is affected mainly by age.

$$\dot{\mathrm{V}}\mathrm{CO} = [(\mathrm{VL} \times \mathrm{FCO})_{\mathrm{i}} - (\mathrm{VL} \times \mathrm{FCO})_{\mathrm{f}}]\frac{60}{10} \cdots \quad \textbf{(7)}$$

where VL= lung volume, FCO= CO fraction in the alveolar gas mixture; i denotes the initial value (at the beginning of the 10 second breath hold), and f denotes the final (at the end of breath hold)

$$\mathrm{DLO_2} = 1.23 * \mathrm{DLCO} = 1.23\left(\frac{\dot{\mathrm{V}}\mathrm{CO}}{\mathrm{PACO}}\right) \cdots \quad \textbf{(8)}$$

The lung diffusion capacity for O_2 (Eq. 8) varies with age, gender, and height and ranges from 20 to 30 ml/min/mmHg. It also changes with physical activity and it is altered by pulmonary disease. During exercise, alveolar surface area available for diffusion is increased significantly because of the larger tidal volumes and greater expansion of the alveoli, as well as the recruitment (*i.e.*, opening and perfusion) of a greater number of alveolar capillaries. Greater alveolar ventilation rate during heavy exercise can raise alveolar PO_2 as high as 120 mm Hg whereas greatly increased O_2 consumption by muscle fibers can reduce mixed venous PO_2 to as low as 20 mmHg. As a result, the partial pressure gradient driving diffusion is greatly elevated. Thus, the net O_2 diffusion rate is increased by the combination of increased DLO_2 and ΔPO_2. However, during heavy exercise the blood transit time in the alveolar capillaries is markedly shortened because of the marked rise in cardiac output. Consequently, despite the elevated diffusion rate, the blood, as it rapidly passes through the lungs, will not fully equilibrate with alveolar gas. The result is a significantly lower arterial PO_2 during heavy exercise than under resting conditions (*e.g.*, 85 *vs.* 100 mmHg).

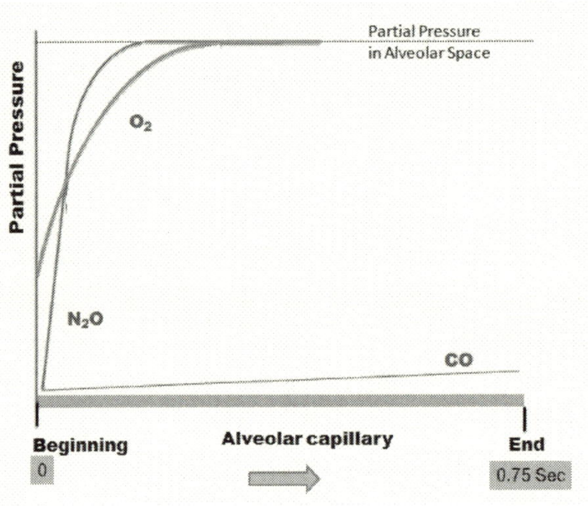

Figure 3: Changes in the partial pressures of oxygen, nitrous oxide, and carbon monoxide along the alveolar capillary. The O_2 curve shows that under resting conditions O_2 equilibrates relatively rapidly across the alveolar-capillary membrane so that equilibration is complete by the end of the first third of the capillary. This leaves nearly two thirds of the capillary as a physiologic reserve to ensure complete equilibration of gas exchange under different physiological conditions such as exercise.

Conditions such as diffuse parenchymal lung disease, idiopathic pulmonary fibrosis, and lung edema thicken the alveolar blood-gas barrier and increase the diffusion distance impeding gas diffusion and lowering the DLO_2. Similarly, alveolar collapse (atelectasis) or destruction of alveolar septa (as occurs in emphysema) reduces alveolar surface area and DLO_2 resulting in a significant degree of hypoxemia even at rest. This is easily exacerbated further by stresses such a respiratory infection or ascent to high altitude (low inspired PO_2) or physical activity. In virtually all cases where DLO_2 is reduced and gas diffusion is impaired there exists a wide gap in the PO_2 between the ideal alveolar gas and the systemic arterial blood [(Ai-a)PO_2 gradient].

OXYGEN TRANSPORT

In an adult human the blood has to carry some 500 liters of O_2 from the lungs to the periphery. Oxygen is carried in two forms: bound to hemoglobin (Hb) (>98%) and as physically dissolved gas (<2%). The blood O_2 content or concentration ($[O_2]_{total}$; expressed as milliliters of O_2 per deciliter of whole blood) is calculated as the sum of the Hb-bound and the dissolved oxygen (Eqs. 9-11):

$$[O_2]_{total} = [O_2]_{bound} + [O_2]_{dissolved} \ldots \quad \textbf{(9)}$$

$$[O_2]_{bound} = O_2 \text{ bound to Hb} = [Hb] \times 1.34 \times \frac{\%\,Sat}{100} \ldots \quad \textbf{(10)}$$

$$[O_2]_{dissolved} = PO_2 \times \text{Solubility Coefficient } (\alpha O_2) \ldots \quad \textbf{(11)}$$

where:

- [Hb] = the hemoglobin concentration in blood in grams per deciliter (g/100 ml)

- 1.34 (ml/g) = the maximum O_2 carrying capacity of hemoglobin, *i.e.*, the maximum volume of O_2 that can be bound to 1 gram of hemoglobin when fully saturated with oxygen (The absolute maximum O_2 carrying capacity of pure Hb is estimated at 1.39 ml/g,; the use of the lower value of 1.34 reflects largely the fact that 3 to 4% of Hb molecules are tied up by carbon monoxide, CO).

- % Sat = Percent saturation of Hb with oxygen.

- αO_2 = the O_2 solubility coefficient in blood. At 37°, αO_2 has a value of 0.003 ml of O_2 per 100 ml of blood per mmHg of PO_2. The concentration of the physically dissolved O_2 is determined in accordance with Henry's law which states that the concentration of physically dissolved gas equals the product of the gas' partial pressure times its solubility coefficient (Eq. 12). Therefore, using normal values of arterial PO_2 (100 mm Hg) and body temperature (37°):

$$[O_2]_{dissolved} = 0.003 \times 100 = 0.3 \text{ ml } O_2/100 \text{ ml} \ldots \quad \textbf{(12)}$$

This means that under normal conditions, each liter of arterial blood can carry only 3 ml of O_2 in the dissolved form. This amount would be woefully inadequate to satisfy the metabolic needs of the body. This remains true even when breathing pure O_2 and the physically dissolved O_2 concentration increases seven fold in proportion to the rise in PO_2. These considerations highlight the importance of hemoglobin (Hb) in O_2 transport. Considering that under normal conditions the total O_2 concentration in the pulmonary venous blood (or systemic arterial blood) is approximately 20 ml/100 ml (or 200 ml/l) it is clear that hemoglobin increases the O_2 carrying capacity of the blood nearly 67 fold (200/3).

Assuming an [Hb] of 15 g/100 ml and $\%SaO_2$ of 98% (Eq. 13):

$$[O_2]_{bound} = 1.34 \times 15 \times 0.98 = 19.70 \text{ ml}/100 \text{ ml} \ldots \quad \textbf{(13)}$$

Therefore the total arterial oxygen content = 19.70 + 0.3 = 20 ml/100 ml = 200 ml per liter of blood. In anemic patients the $[O_2]_{total}$ decreases in direct proportion to the fall in Hb concentration triggering adaptive, compensatory mechanisms to ensure adequate tissue oxygenation; these include increased cardiac output and tissue perfusion and a greater O_2 extraction by the tissues due to the greater drop in tissue PO_2 and increased O_2 gradient between blood and tissue.

Hemoglobin

Hemoglobin (Hb) is a globular protein macromolecule (molecular weight = 6.5 kD) consisting of 4 subunits (Fig. **4**). Each subunit is composed of a peptide chain and a heme group. The heme, in turn, consists of a protoporphyrin ring with a ferrous ion (Fe^{++}), which is anchored in the center of the ring by chemical bonds to 4 nitrogen atoms of the pyrrole groups of the protoporphyrin ring (Fig. **5**). Each Fe^{++} ion is capable of binding one molecule of oxygen. Therefore, each Hb tetramer is capable of binding up to four O_2 molecules. The globin portion of adult hemoglobin consists of two alpha and two beta polypeptide chains ($\alpha_2\beta_2$). The peptide chains are responsible for binding protons (H^+) and carbon dioxide (CO_2). Protons bind mainly to the nitrogen in the amino groups and in the imidazole groups of histidine residues. Some protons bind to the carboxylate groups. CO_2 binds to the terminal amino groups of the Hb polypeptide chains to form a carbamate group (Eq. 14):

$$R\text{-}NH_2 + CO_2 \Rightarrow R\text{-}NH\text{-}COO^- + H^+ \ldots \tag{14}$$

The binding of protons and CO_2 is accompanied by the formation of ionic bonds (aka salt bridges or links) within the polypeptide chain and between chains of deoxyhemoglobin. These bonds result in conformational changes in the Hb molecule referred to as the ***tense state (T form)***. According to a model proposed by Jacques Monod & co-workers in 1965 to describe the behavior of allosteric enzymes, the quaternary structure of allosteric proteins, including hemoglobin, exists in two states: stressed (T form) and relaxed (R form). These states represent conformational shifts brought about by the presence of the substrate and/or allosteric modulators and involve readjustment of interactions between the subunits of the macromolecule. The T form is structurally more taut and constrained than the R form and has a lower affinity for the substrate. In the case of deoxyhemoglobin (the T form) the conformational stress stems from non-covalent, electrostatic interactions between oppositely charged groups resulting in 8 salt bridges or links which are responsible for the T form being more stable than the R form which lacks such links [3].

This T form (deoxyhemoglobin) is structurally more stable but characterized by the bending of the protoporphyrin ring so that the Fe^{++} lies outside the plane of the ring. This tense conformational state is further stabilized in the presence of 2,3-diphosphoglycerate (2,3-DPG) ions which form additional ionic bonds between the two β chains and prevent the binding of oxygen. Thus the binding of 2,3-DPG and O_2 to the β subunits are mutually exclusive.

$$Hb \xrightarrow{O_2} HbO_2 \xrightarrow{O_2} Hb(O_2)_2 \xrightarrow{O_2} Hb(O_2)_3 \xrightarrow{O_2} Hb(O_2)_4$$

In the lungs, O_2 binding and the release of H^+ and CO_2 lead to the breaking of the ionic bonds including those between the two β chains releasing 2,3-DGP and causing the Hb molecule to assume a ***relaxed state (R form)*** in which the protoporphyrin ring straightens and the F^{++} returns to lie in the plain of the ring. This conformational change allows O_2 to bind the β subunits.

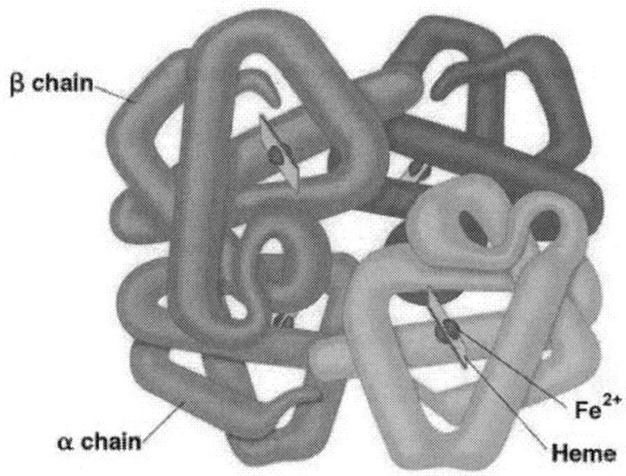

Figure 4: Hemoglobin A is a tetramer with a molecular weight of 67 kD. It is made up of 4 subunits – two α chains and two β chains. Shown at the center of each subunit is the heme group with its ferrous ion that is responsible for binding oxygen.

Hemoglobin accounts for approximately one third of the weight of a red blood cell, which is estimated to contain 250 million hemoglobin molecules. When fully saturated each molecule of Hb binds 4 molecules of O_2. The dynamics of O_2 binding to hemoglobin is such that the binding of the first O_2 facilitates the binding of the second which in turn facilitates the binding of the third and so on. The binding of the 1st O_2 molecule results in the disruption of many of the ionic bonds between the subunits of deoxyhemoglobin and increases the affinity of Hb for the 2nd O_2 molecule 500-fold. This phenomenon of heme-heme interaction is referred to as ***positive cooperativity*** and is reflected in the sigmoid or ***S*** shape of the oxyhemoglobin dissociation curve (Fig. **6**).

Positive cooperativity is due to the conformational changes that occur in the Hb structure and in its oxygen affinity as O_2 molecules are successively bound. Since this process is reversible, the unloading of O_2 at the tissue level is made gradually easier as successive O_2 molecules are released.

Examining the sigmoid shape of the oxyhemoglobin (HbO_2) dissociation curve (Fig. **6**) two main areas are readily distinguishable:

1. The steep portion of the curve (PO_2 <70 mm Hg) ensures that O_2 is promptly loaded onto Hb as the PO_2 rises in the alveolar capillaries. The steep portion of the curve also allows for O_2 extraction to be increased as necessary to meet the metabolic needs of the more active tissues such as the skeletal muscle fibers during exercise; it ensures that an adequate amount of O_2 is promptly released (unloaded) to the cells as the PO_2 drops.

2. The flat portion of the curve (PO_2 >70 mm Hg) indicates that changes in PO_2 between 70 and 200 mmHg result in negligible changes in the blood total oxygen content ($[O_2]_{total}$). For example doubling PO_2 from 80 to 160 mmHg increases the blood $[O_2]_{total}$ by less than 1.5 ml/100 ml as illustrated by the following calculations.

Assume: [Hb]= 15 g/100 ml, Hb maximum O_2 carrying capacity = 1.34 ml/g, $\%SaO_2$ at PO_2 of 80 mm Hg = 94%, $\%SaO_2$ at PO_2 of 160 mm Hg = 100%, and O_2 solubility coefficient = 0.003 ml/100 ml/mm Hg.

Therefore:

At PO_2 = 80 mm Hg (Eqs. 15-17):

$[O_2]_{bound} = 15 \times 1.34 \times 0.94 = 18.894$ ml/100 ml ... **(15)**

$[O_2]_{dissolved} = 80 \times 0.003 = 0.24$ ml/100 ml ... **(16)**

$[O_2]_{total} = 18.894 + 0.24 = 19.134$ ml/100 ml ... **(17)**

At PO_2 = 160 mm Hg (Eqs. 18-20):

$[O_2]_{bound} = 15 \times 1.34 \times 1.00 = 20.10$ ml/100 ml ... **(18)**

$[O_2]_{dissolved} = 160 \times 0.003 = 0.48$ ml/100 ml ... **(19)**

$[O_2]_{total} = 20.1 + 0.48 = 20.58$ ml/100 ml ... **(20)**

The $[O_2]_{bound}$ increased by 1.206 ml/100 ml (6.4%) whereas the $[O_2]_{dissolved}$ doubled as a result of the doubling of the PO_2 in accordance with Henry's law. However, the absolute increase in the total O_2 concentration in the blood ($[O_2]_{total}$) is too small (1.446 ml/100 ml) to contribute significantly to the process of O_2 transport. The physically dissolved oxygen concentration ($[O_2]_{dissolved}$) can be increased significantly by raising the fraction of oxygen in the inspired gas mixture and/or exposing the organism to hyperbaric conditions to elevate PO_2 in the blood. Breathing oxygen enriched gas mixtures for prolonged periods can result in tissue damage (see Chapter 7: Oxygen Toxicity).

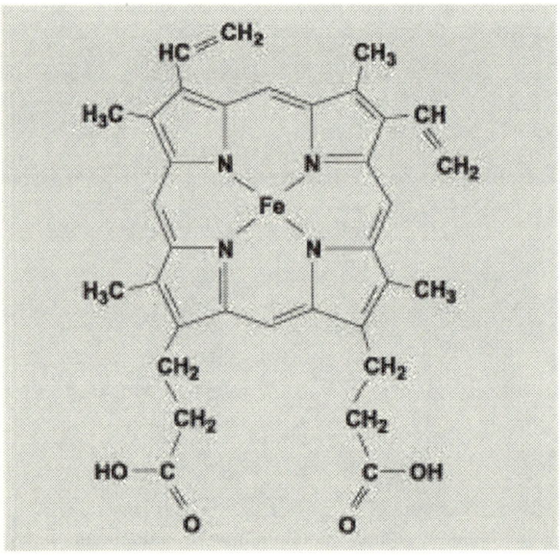

Figure 5: The heme group with the F^{++} ion anchored in the center to the N of the 4 pyrrole groups that make up the skeleton of the protoporphyrin ring.

As a result of minor variations in amino-acid composition of the polypeptide chains, several types of Hb subunits exist including α, β, γ and δ. The two principal types of functionally normal hemoglobins are the adult hemoglobin (HbA or HbA_1) and the fetal hemoglobin (HbF). The adult type has two alpha and two beta peptide chains ($\alpha_2\beta_2$), whereas HbF has two alpha and two gamma chains ($\alpha_2\gamma_2$). During gestation, HbF is the predominant type in the fetus from approximately the 3rd to the 9th months and persists for a few months after birth until HbF is replaced by HbA. Because the gamma (γ) subunits have a higher affinity for oxygen than the beta (β) subunits, HbF has a greater affinity for O_2 than HbA, a characteristic that facilitates the oxygen transfer from mother to fetus. Also, because it lacks the β subunits, the HbF does not bind 2,3-DPG and therefore it does not respond allosterically to changes in 2,3-DPG concentration. These differences explain the leftward shift of the HbF oxygen dissociation curve relative to that of HbA. However, HbF-O_2 responds to changes in pH much more strongly than HbA-O_2. This elevated response to the Bohr effect more than compensates for the lack of response to 2,3-DPG.

Regulation of Hb-O_2 Affinity

The S shape of the oxyhemoglobin (HbO_2) dissociation curve is considered as a molecular adaptation to ensure optimal uptake and unloading of O_2 at the appropriate tissue site. Oxygen transport *via* Hb is further regulated by changes in PCO_2, pH, temperature, and 2,3-bisphosphoglycerate (2,3-BPG) (aka 2,3-diphosphoglycerate or 2,3-DPG) concentration within the red blood cells. These factors can have profound effects on the affinity of Hb for O_2 and the ease with which O_2 is picked up in the alveoli or the ease with which it is released into the peripheral tissues where it is consumed. These effects manifest as shifts of the HbO_2 dissociation curve either to the right or the left as illustrated in Fig. **7**. Alterations in Hb-O_2 affinity are quantified by the change in the value of the P_{50}, which is the PO_2 required for achieving a 50% saturation of Hb with O_2. In a healthy, resting adult the P_{50} is 26 mm Hg for arterial blood (PCO_2 = 40 mm Hg, pH = 7.40) and 28 mm Hg for the venous blood (PCO_2 = 46 mm Hg, pH = 7.37). These values are in sharp contrast with the low P_{50} (2 mm Hg) for the monomeric myoglobin, which lacks the constraints of the ionic bonds between the subunits of Hb and therefore displays no cooperativity. Increases in PCO_2, $[H^+]$, 2,3-DPG, and body temperature all cause the HbO_2 dissociation curve to shift rightward ($\uparrow P_{50}$, $\downarrow$affinity) as a consequence of the formation of ionic bonds within Hb molecule and the resultant conformational changes (stressed state). The shift of the curve to the right because of acidosis ($\uparrow[H^+]$, $\downarrow$pH) is known as the **Bohr Effect**. The increase in $[H^+]$ is also responsible for the influence of hypercapnia ($\uparrow PCO_2$) on Hb affinity for oxygen.

DIPHOSPHOGLYCERATE (2,3-DPG)

2,3-DPG is a byproduct of glycolysis, which is the sole energy pathway in the red blood cell, and its intracellular concentration increases markedly under certain conditions characterized by high glycolytic rates due to insufficient oxygen delivery to peripheral tissues (hypoxia, lung disease, congestive heart failure, anemia, *etc.*). One molecule of 2,3-DPG binds to one molecule of Hb wedging itself in the central cavity where the 4 subunits of the Hb tetramer come together. Respiratory alkalosis (↓PCO_2) associated with high altitude hyperventilation stimulates glycolysis causing an increase in erythrocyte [2,3-DPG], which in turn tends to push the HbO_2 dissociation curve rightward. This rightward shift becomes manifest under chronic conditions of high-altitude hypoxia when the effect of increased 2,3-DPG prevails over the effect of hypocapnia (↓PCO_2, ↓$[H^+]$) (leftward shift). Under these conditions, the net shift is decidedly rightward which facilitates the offloading of oxygen.

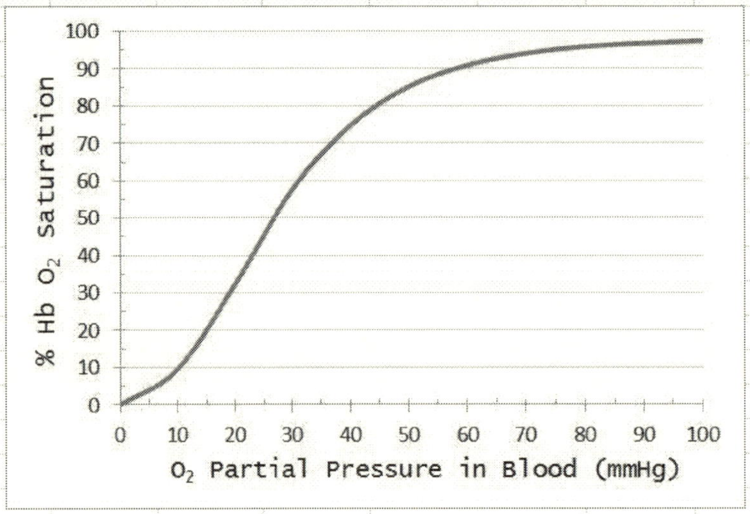

Figure 6: Oxyhemoglobin dissociation curve showing its characteristic S shape (or sigmoid shape). The sigmoid shape of the curve is caused by the heme-heme interactions (cooperativity). Note that: At the normal arterial blood PO_2 of 100 mm Hg, Hb is virtually fully saturated with O_2 (*i.e.*, all heme groups are occupied by O_2 molecules); the %Sat is nearly 100%., The PO_2 in mixed venous blood is normally around 40 mmHg and the %Sat ≈ 75%. The PO_2 at which Hb is 50% saturated (the P_{50}) (which is normally 26 mm Hg) helps to show whether the curve is shifted to the left or to right and it is a way to quantify the extent of the shift (*i.e.*, the change in Hb O_2 affinity).

At the level of peripheral tissue, the β subunits easily release their O_2 whereas the α subunits continue to hold tightly on to theirs. After O_2 is released from the β subunits 2,3-DPG moves into the space between the two β chains in the central cavity of the tetramer forming strong ionic bonds between the two β peptide chains and changing the shape of the Hb molecule thereby facilitating the release of O_2 from α subunits. The adaptive value of the influence of 2,3-DPG on the HbO_2 dissociation curve lies clearly in facilitating O_2 release at the peripheral tissues level under hypoxemic conditions. The importance of 2,3-DPG is highlighted by *in vitro* findings that the P_{50} in the complete absence of 2,3-DPG is only 1 mm Hg compared to 26 mm Hg in its presence. In other words, 2,3-DPG reduces the Hb-O_2 affinity 26 fold.

In order for O_2 to bind to deoxyhemoglobin the microenvironment in terms of pH and ionic composition must be such that the salt links stabilizing the deoxyhemoglobin molecule (the T form) including those between 2,3-DPG and the β chains are broken. Such conditions are encountered at the level of the alveoli.

CARBON DIOXIDE TRANSPORT

Under resting conditions, approximately 300 liters of CO_2 are transported daily in the blood from the periphery to the lungs. This is the same rate at which CO_2 is being produced by metabolism (200 ml/min). CO_2 is carried in the blood in three forms: (1) physically dissolved (~10%); (2) carbamino compounds (~25%); (3) bicarbonate (~65%).

CO_2 diffuses from the cells (where it is produced in the course of energy metabolism) into the plasma, where a small amount (5%) remains and is carried as dissolved gas in the plasma and the rest enters the erythrocytes (RBCs) where most of it undergoes chemical transformations, as shown in Fig. **8**, while a small amount (5%) is carried in physical solution within the cell. The CO_2 solubility coefficient in the blood at 37°C is twice as high that for O_2 (0.065 *vs*. 0.030 ml/100 ml/mmHg) and significantly greater volume of CO_2 is carried in the dissolved form as illustrated by the following calculations (Eq. 21):

$$(P\bar{v}CO_2 - PaCO_2)(0.065\ x10)(\dot{Q}) = (46 - 40)(0.65)(5) = 3.9 \times 5 = 19.5 \text{ ml of } CO_2/\text{min} \ldots \quad \textbf{(21)}$$

Assuming a total of 200 ml/min, the fraction carried as dissolved is approximately 10% (19.5/200 = 9.80%).

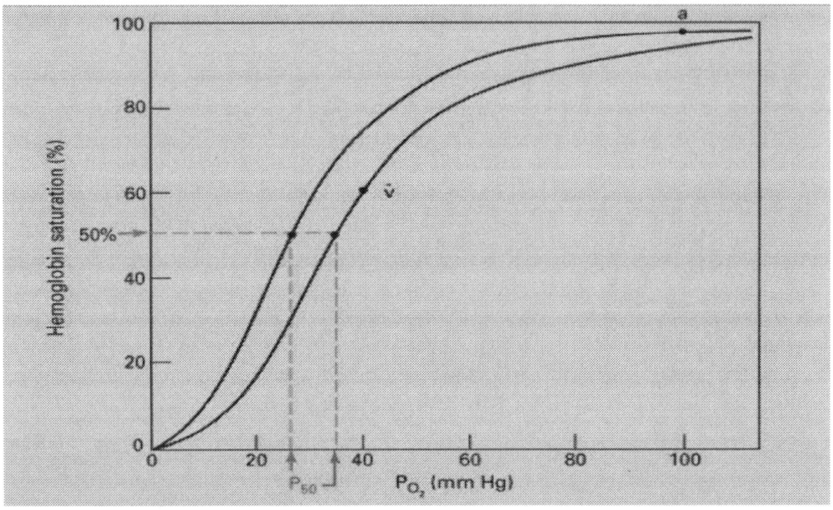

Figure 7: Changes in hemoglobin-oxygen affinity. Factors that cause the oxyhemoglobin dissociation curve to shift to the right (↑P_{50}) are:, Increased H^+ concentration (↓ pH)(acidosis), Increased P_{CO_2} (↓pH) (*the Bohr effect*), Increased temperature (fever), Increased concentration of 2,3-DPG (aka 2,3-BPG), These conditions which favor the offloading of O_2 are found at the level of the peripheral tissues., Factors that cause the curve to shift to the left (↓P_{50}) are:, Decreased H^+ concentration (↑pH)(alkalosis), Lowered temperature (hypothermia), Reduced concentration of 2,3-DPG, Carbon monoxide (CO) poisoning, These conditions which favor the loading of O_2 are found at the level of the lungs.

Inside the RBC, the largest fraction (≈65%) of CO_2 is combined with H_2O to form carbonic acid (H_2CO_3) in a reversible hydration reaction (Eq. 22) catalyzed by alpha carbonic anhydrase (αCA):

$$CO_2 + H_2O \Leftrightarrow H_2CO_3 \Leftrightarrow \mathbf{HCO_3^-} + H^+ \ldots \qquad \textbf{(22)}$$

The generated protons (H^+) are picked up (buffered) by the globin of Hb whereas the $\mathbf{HCO_3^-}$ is transported across the erythrocyte membrane into the plasma compartment in exchange for Cl^- *via* a highly specific *anion exchanger*. This exchange is known as *the chloride shift*. The hydration of CO_2 is highly dependent on the catalytic activity of carbonic anhydrase (αCA) which is one of the most efficient enzymes in nature. It is estimated that in the presence of αCA nearly 100 thousand molecules of CO_2 are hydrated every second. By contrast, the un-catalyzed reaction is so slow that it would take nearly 3.9 months to hydrate as many molecules of CO_2. In the blood, carbonic anhydrase is found almost exclusively inside the erythrocytes [4]. An additional fraction of CO_2 (25%)

combines with Hb to form carbamino-Hb or carbamate as shown in Eq 14. The binding of CO_2 and H^+ to hemoglobin lowers its affinity for O_2 which favors the unloading of O_2 in the peripheral tissue (Bohr Effect).

Fig. **8** illustrates the modes of CO_2 transport.

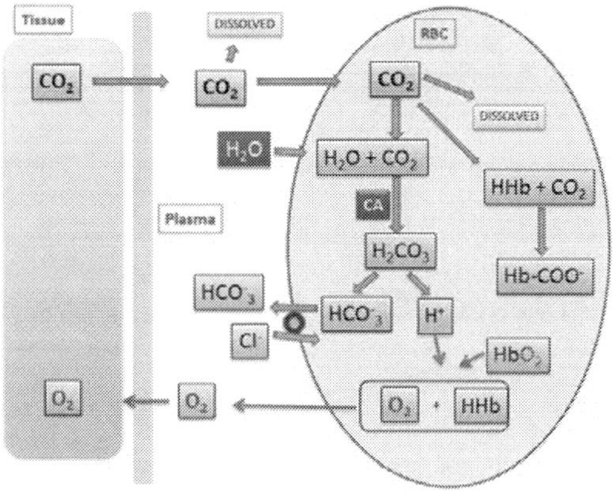

Figure 8A: Depicted are the three forms in which CO_2 is transferred in the blood and the processes that take place in the capillaries of the peripheral tissues where CO_2 is produced. Some 65% of CO_2 molecules are hydrated within the red blood cell (RBC) by carbonic anhydrase (CA) and the resultant $\mathbf{HCO_3^-}$ ions are transferred into the plasma in exchange for Cl^- ions *via* the anion exchanger in the RBC membrane Shown also are the buffering of H^+ by hemoglobin and the formation of carbamino hemoglobin (Hb-COO^-).

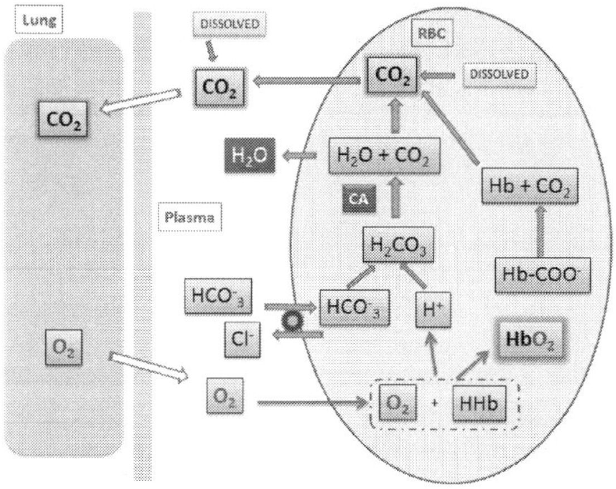

Figure 8B: Transfer of CO_2 from blood to lung. The processes involved are the same as shown in Fig. **8A** except they occur in the opposite direction.

The Haldane Effect

When the CO_2 content in the blood is plotted against its partial pressure in the physiological range (20 – 80 mm Hg), the resultant "dissociation curve" is virtually linear indicating that in contrast to the HbO_2 dissociation, there is no cooperativity in the binding of CO_2 to hemoglobin. Blood has no CO_2 saturation point in part because CO_2 can be stored in different forms throughout the body. The body CO_2 stores are estimated at 100 liters of which only 2.5 liters are in the blood (the remainder is mostly found in bone and adipose tissue). By contrast, the total body oxygen content is approximately 1.5 liter and virtually all of it is located in the blood and lungs.

The binding of O_2 to hemoglobin has a significant effect on its affinity to bind CO_2. A higher PO_2 (*i.e.*, higher Hb O_2 saturation) shifts the Hb-CO_2 dissociation "curve" downward and rightward indicating reduced affinity and *vice versa.* This phenomenon is called the **Haldane Effect** (Fig. **9**) which is not to be confused by the Bohr Effect mentioned above which describes the influence of CO_2 and H^+ on Hb-O_2 dissociation curve.

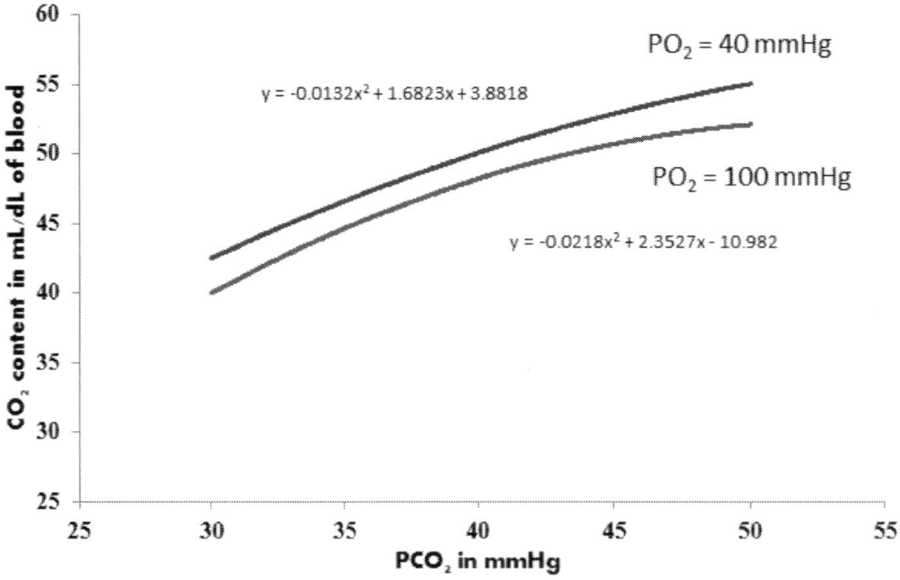

Figure 9: Haldane Effect. The effect of PO_2 and hemoglobin O_2 saturation level on the blood CO_2 carrying capacity as indicated by the total CO_2 concentration in the blood. The blue line represents venous blood.

The underlying mechanism for the Haldane Effect is the change in the shape of the Hb molecule to the *relaxed state* (R form) as it binds O_2 and the resultant decrease in the pKa of the imidazole groups of the histidine residues. As a result, HbO_2 becomes a stronger acid, releasing protons (H^+) and less able to bind CO_2 as carbamino compounds. The opposite occurs at the tissue level when HbO_2 loses its O_2 and deoxyhemoglobin being a weaker acid (stronger base) is able to bind more H^+ driving the carbonic anhydrase-catalyzed CO_2 hydration reaction toward the formation of more HCO_3^- (Eq. 23) thereby permitting the transport of a greater amount of CO_2 in the form of bicarbonate..

$$CO_2 + H_2O \leftrightarrows H_2CO_3 \leftrightarrows H^+ + HCO_3^- \ \ldots \qquad \textbf{(23)}$$

In Summary, hemoglobin transports O_2 from the lungs to the peripheral tissues and CO_2 in the opposite direction. The affinity of Hb for O_2 is regulated by key factors that act as allosteric modulators. These include $[H^+]$, PCO_2, [2,3-DPG], and temperature. At the tissue level (*e.g.*, in exercising muscle) all these factors are elevated altering the shape of the Hb molecule and causing a decrease in O_2 affinity which is seen as a rightward shift in the oxyhemoglobin dissociation curve. Such conditions favor the offloading and delivery of O_2 to the tissues where it is consumed. The exact opposite takes place at the level of the lungs.

REFERENCES

[1] Nitrous oxide (N_2O, "laughing gas") is a colorless, non-flammable oxide of nitrogen with a slightly sweet odor and taste. It is used as an anesthetic in surgery and dentistry. It is not to be confused with nitric oxide (NO), a naturally occurring free radical, powerful vasodilator and an important signaling molecule in the mammalian organism.

[2] "Transfer Factor, TL" is the preferred expression used in European literature instead of "Diffusion Capacity, DL", which is widely used in the US. Macintyre N, Crapo RO, Viegi G, *et al.* Standardization of the single-breath determination of carbon monoxide uptake in the lung. Eur Respir J 2005; 26:720-35.

[3] "Oxygen binding markedly changes the quaternary structure of hemoglobin"; pages 201-205 in the 7th edition (2012) of Stryer, L., Biochemistry, W.H. Freeman & Co., New York. Also, Hemoglobin Structure and Mechanism pages 332-341 in the 4th edition (2011) of Voet & Voet Biochemistry, Wiley & Sons

[4] However, at least in skeletal muscles, carbonic anhydrase is also found attached to the capillary wall and accessible to plasma (Geers C, Gros G. Carbon dioxide transport and carbonic anhydrase in blood and muscle. Physiol Rev 2000;80:681-715). In general, carbonic anhydrase is found inside the cells of tissues that elaborate secretions that have a pH that is different than that of the blood. Examples include salivary glands, stomach, pancreas, renal tubule cells, aqueous humor producing cells in the eye, CSF-producing cells in the brain.

CHAPTER 6

Acid-Base Balance

Nasr H. Anaizi

Abstract: This chapter deals with acid-base homeostasis with special emphasis on the role of the respiratory system. After explaining why maintaining a relatively constant proton activity is critical to optimal cellular function we define acid-base balance and describe the basic mechanisms responsible for acid-base homeostasis. After describing the unique role of the HCO_3^-/CO_2 buffer pair in acid-base regulation the four primary acid-base disturbances are defined. Finally an extensive outline is presented of the various approaches for the evaluation of acid-base disorders followed by examples and a few clinical cases.

Keywords: Acid-Base Disorders, Acid-Base Homeostasis, Acidemia, Acidosis, Alkalemia, Alkalosis, Anion Gap, Base Excess, Buffering Capacity, Davenport Diagram, Henderson-Hasselbalch, Hydrogen Ions, Imidazole Group, Metabolic Acidosis, Metabolic Alkalosis, pH, pKa, Respiratory Acidosis, Respiratory Alkalosis, Standard Bicarbonate.

The respiratory system plays a vital role in acid-base homeostasis. Its contribution is critical to the moment-to-moment control of blood pH. Normal cellular function requires that the concentrations of free protons ($[H^+]$) in body fluids both inside and outside the cells be maintained within certain limits.

Vital proteins such as enzymes, transporters, ion channels, ionic pumps, peptide hormones, receptors, growth factors, signaling molecules, and mediator proteins are sensitive to changes in the hydrogen ions concentration ($\Delta[H^+]$) in their microenvironment. The imidazole groups and N-terminal amine groups are the primary proton-binding sites in protein molecules (Fig. **1**).

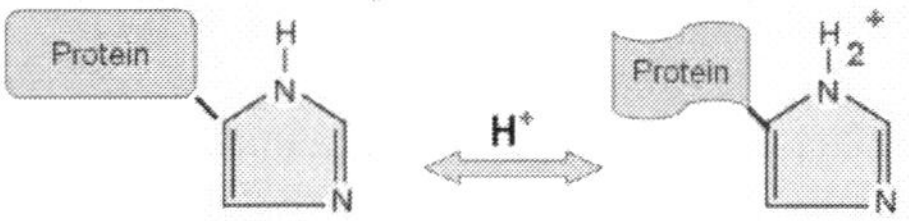

Figure 1: Reversible binding of protons to the imidazole group. Note the resulting conformational change in the protein molecule.

The small radius of H^+ (10^{-9} m) enables it to reach and interact with reactive sites within a protein molecule, altering its conformation and function. Consequently marked fluctuations in $[H^+]$ associated with acid-base disorders (ABD) can result in a wide variety of serious clinical manifestations. Disruption of acid-base homeostasis is common, particularly accompanying acute cardiovascular, pulmonary, metabolic, and/or renal complications.

Normal acid-base values in different body fluids are shown in Table **1**. Deviations of $[H^+]$ outside the normal range can have profound effects on cell metabolism and membrane function. Both acute and chronic acid-base abnormalities are associated with a variety of serious disorders including impaired cellular metabolism and electrolyte imbalance leading to cardiac arrhythmias, weak vascular tone, myocardial failure, and skeletal muscle weakness. Severe deviations of $[H^+]$ from the normal range cause severe cardiac and neural dysfunction and may lead to coma and death. The range of $[H^+]$ compatible with life is approximately 16-160 nanomoles/l (pH: 6.8 - 7.8). It should be emphasized that the pH value *per se* is of limited significance unless seen in the context of the patient's clinical condition. For instance, an arterial pH of 7.1 resulting from a transient seizure is not as dangerous a sign as the same value resulting from the ingestion of a toxic substance such as methanol.

Table 1: Normal Acid-Base Values (for simplicity, in each case, a single average value is given in bold numbers with the corresponding range between parenthesis)

	Arterial Blood	Arterial Plasma	Mixed Venous Blood	Mixed Venous Plasma	CSF[a]	ICF[b]
pH	**7.4** (7.37-7.42)	**7.38** (7.35-7.40)	**7.36** (7.33-7.39)	**7.34** (7.30-7.36)	**7.32** (7.29-7.32)	**7.00** (6.80-7.34)
[H+], nanomol/l	40 (38-43)	42 (40-45)	44 (41-47)	46 (44-50)	48 (48-51)	100 (48-158)
PCO_2, mmHg	40 (37-43)	39 (35-45)	46 (44-48)	45 (40-50)	46 (45-50)	50 (45-55)
$[HCO_3^-]$, mEq/l	24 (22-26)	22 (20-24)	27 (22-26)	25 (22-27)	22 (20-24)	12 (8-22)

[a]CSF = Cerebrospinal Fluid
[b]ICF = intracellular fluid. Here, values vary widely depending on the tissue type and its function; compare for instance skeletal muscle fibers during strenuous exercise ($pH_i \approx 6.8$) and proximal tubule cells ($pH_i \approx 7.30$).
MADSHUS I. H. Regulation of intracellular pH in eukaryotic cells. Biochem. J. (1988) 250, 1-8

Ventilation has the dual function of supplying O_2 for cell metabolism and removing the CO_2 produced in the course of the complete oxidation of metabolic fuel. In order for ventilation to meet the body's metabolic needs, a dynamic relationship exists among three key variables: metabolic rate ($\dot{V}CO_2$), arterial blood PCO_2 ($PaCO_2$) and ideal alveolar ventilation ($\dot{V}Ai$) [1]. $PaCO_2$ is a major determinant of $\dot{V}Ai$. Primary changes in $\dot{V}Ai$ manifest themselves as changes in $PaCO_2$ and these in turn translate into changes in $[H^+]$ (or ΔpH) in arterial blood. Therefore, ventilation may be viewed as a pH control mechanism, as well as a mechanism for ridding the body of waste CO_2 and supplying it with O_2.

To see how this pH-control system works, we should first review a few fundamental concepts in acid-base chemistry. Advances in medical technology have made the measurement of arterial blood gases, which include PaO_2, pHa and $PaCO_2$, simple and readily available. However, integration of this information in the overall clinical picture and the correct interpretation and use of these values in the diagnosis and treatment of acid-base disorders remain elusive. Poor understanding of acid-base chemistry and physiology stems in part from the confusing terminology and mathematical expressions (negative logarithms, inverted fractions, *etc.*) that are commonly used in this field. The problem is further complicated by the rote memorization and use of vague, derived parameters such as "base excess". A good grasp of the fundamental principles of acid base chemistry and physiology is both necessary and sufficient to correctly diagnose and quantify acid-base disturbances.

IONIZATION OR DISSOCIATION CONSTANT

Consider acetic acid (HA, Eqs. 1 and 2) as an example:

$$HA \rightleftharpoons H^+ + A^- \ldots \quad \textbf{(1)}$$

$$Ka = \frac{[H^+][A^-]}{[HA]} = 1.8 \times 10^{-5}\ \text{moles/l} \ \ldots \quad \textbf{(2)}$$

This relationship can also be expressed using the Henderson-Hasselbalch (HH) equation (Eq. 3):

$$pH = pK_a + \log\frac{[A^-]}{[HA]} \ \ldots \quad \textbf{(3)}$$

where pH = -log[H^+] and pK_a = -logK_a. For acetic acid, pK_a = 4.75. This equation shows the direct relationship between pH and the ratio of the un-protonated to protonated forms of the acid. The level of protonation of acid as a function of the pH of the solution is illustrated in Fig. **2**. The pKa of 4.75 corresponds to a level of 50%. Thus, the pKa value is the same as the value of the pH of the solution at which protonated and un-protonated forms of the acid exist in equal concentrations. The pKa value of an acid is inversely related to its strength; the lower the pKa the stronger is the acid.

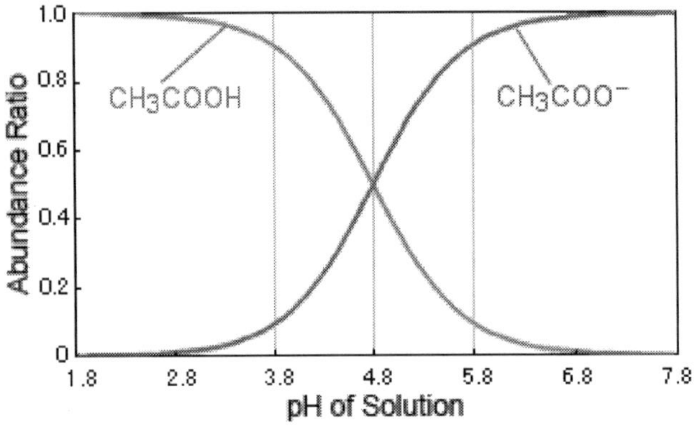

Figure 2: Relationship between the dissociation status of acetic acid and the pH of the solution. When pH is about 4.76, which corresponds to the pKa of acetic acid, the two forms exist in identical amounts, [Acetic Acid] = [Acetate]. Adapted from: http://www.shimadzu.com/an/hplc/support/lib/ lctalk/29/29intro.html

BUFFERING pH

Buffers prevent or minimize the change in the activity of free protons ($\Delta[H^+]$), *i.e.* in the pH of the solution resulting from addition of acid or base. Fig. **3** compares the pH in pure water and in a buffer solution as HCl is added. A buffer pair is made up of a weak acid and its conjugate base. Ideally, the pK_a of this buffer system should be equal or close to the desired pH of the solution. The addition of 100 mEqs of HCl to one liter of water containing 200 mEqs of acetate ion causes conversion of about half the acetate to acetic acid, thereby neutralizing much of the added H^+ ion and minimizing $\Delta[H^+]$ (*i.e.*, buffering the pH). In a buffer system composed of HA and A^-, the un-dissociated acid (HA) protects the pH of the solution against the addition of bases (or OH^-) while the conjugated base (A^-) guards against the addition of acid (H^+).

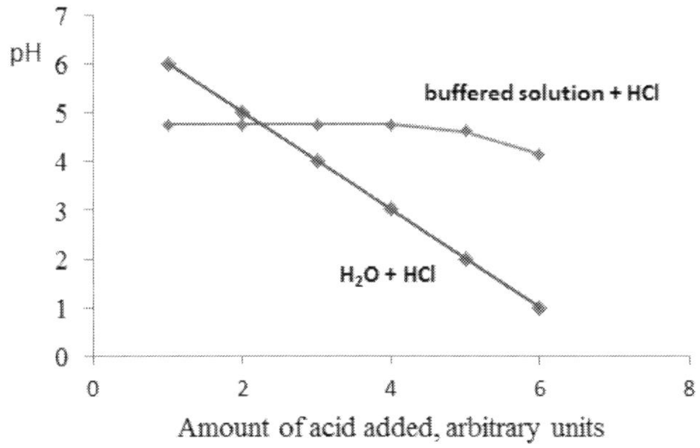

Figure 3: Effect of adding acid to pure water or a buffered solution.

The ***buffering capacity*** of a pH buffer system is a quantitative measure of the ability of the buffer to produce or absorb protons, and it is determined by two factors - the total **amount** of buffer available ($HA+A^-$) and the fraction of buffer in its protonated form (HA), which is determined by the **pK_a** of the buffer system relative to the pH of the solution. The **CO_2 / HCO_3^-** system is the main buffer system in the extracellular fluid despite the fact that its pK_a (6.1) is relatively far removed from the desired blood pH (7.4). We shall see that it is mainly the volatility (or "*openness*") of this buffer system that makes it a very effective buffer.

THE CO_2/HCO_3^- BUFFER

HCO_3^- is the most abundant base in the blood with a normal arterial $[HCO_3^-] \approx 24$ mEq/l. The concentration of HCO_3^- is related to the concentration of dissolved CO_2 as follows (Eq. 4):

$$CO_2 + H_2O \rightleftharpoons H_2CO_3 \rightleftharpoons H^+ + HCO_3^- \ldots \quad \textbf{(4)}$$

This relationship can be described using the Henderson-Hasselbalch equation (Eq. 5):

$$pH = pK_a + \log\frac{[HCO_3^-]}{[H_2CO_3]} = 6.1 + \log\frac{[HCO_3^-]}{0.03 \text{ x } PCO_2} \ldots \quad \textbf{(5)}$$

where pKa is 6.1 and the concentration of carbonic acid, or dissolved CO_2, is expressed as the product of CO_2 partial pressure times CO_2 solubility coefficient at 37° C ($\alpha = 0.03$ mEq/l per mmHg). $[HCO_3^-]$ is given in mEq/l.

Judging by its pK_a value (6.1), the **CO_2/HCO_3^-** buffer pair appears to be a poor system for buffering blood pH (arterial ≈ 7.40; venous ≈ 7.36). However, what this system lacks in terms of an ideal pKa it compensates for in other ways because it possesses three important attributes:

- **Openness**: The acid component (**CO_2**) of the buffer pair is gaseous and its level is controlled by alveolar ventilation - this makes it an open system.
- **Flexibility**: The base component (**HCO_3^-**) is controlled primarily by the kidney. Therefore, the two components are controlled independently by two different organ-systems - this allows a greater flexibility in the overall pH-control system.
- **Abundance**: The total quantity of the buffer is relatively large, which translates into a large buffering capacity.

To understand how ventilation makes this buffer system very effective, we need to consider the difference between an ***open system*** and a ***closed system*** following the addition of acid load.

ADDING AN ACID LOAD TO A CLOSED SYSTEM

Let's look at 1 liter of a solution containing 24 mEq/l of HCO_3^- and 5.6% dissolved CO_2, which are typical physiological values in arterial blood. At 37° C and a barometric pressure (PB) of 760 mmHg (Eqs. 6 and 7):

$$PaCO_2 = 0.056\,(760 - 47) = 40 \text{ mmHg} \ldots \quad \textbf{(6)}$$

$$\text{dissolved } [CO_2] = 0.03PaCO_2 = 1.2 \text{ mEq/l} \ldots \quad \textbf{(7)}$$

substituting these values into the Henderson-Hasselbalch equation (Eq. 8):

$$pH = 6.1 + \log([HCO_3^-]/[CO_2]) = 6.1 + \log(24/1.2) = 6.1 + 1.3 = 7.4 \ldots \quad \textbf{(8)}$$

What happens when we add an acid load to this closed system? The addition of 11 mEqs of HCl converts 11 mEqs of HCO_3^- to CO_2 and water. This increases dissolved [CO_2] to: 11+1.2 = 12.2 mEq/l. By using the Henderson-Hasselbalch equation:

$$pH = 6.1 + \log (13/12.2) = 6.13 \ldots \quad \textbf{(9)}$$

This new pH value (Eq. 9) would be lethal to the organism. Thus, in a closed system $PaCO_2$ rises following the addition of acid leading to a marked and possibly dangerous drop in the pH.

ADDING AN ACID LOAD TO AN OPEN SYSTEM WITH A FIXED [CO_2]

In an open system we can maintain a constant $PaCO_2$ (and therefore a constant [CO_2]) by bubbling through the solution a gas mixture containing 5.6% CO_2 ($PaCO_2$ = 40 mmHg). If $PaCO_2$ is maintained constant at 40 mmHg, adding an 11 mEq acid load to a 1 liter of solution will still reduce the bicarbonate concentration by 11 mmoles, but will cause a much smaller drop in pH (Eq. 10):

$$pH = 6.1 + \log (13/1.2) = 7.13 \ldots \quad \textbf{(10)}$$

The ΔpH is now only -0.27 (relative to 7.40) compared to -1.27 in the closed system where CO_2 cannot escape and $PaCO_2$ is allowed to rise following the addition of the non-volatile acid load. What if we can go a step further by reducing $PaCO_2$ below its normal value, as it normally occurs *in vivo* with metabolic acidosis? This compensatory response reduces the dissolved [CO_2] below its normal level and brings the [HCO_3^-]/[CO_2] ratio closer to the normal value of 20, thereby minimizing ΔpH. The quantitative example below should further clarify this point.

ADDING AN ACID LOAD TO AN OPEN SYSTEM WITH A VARIABLE [CO_2]

If we drop $PaCO_2$ in the equilibrating gas from 40 to 30 mmHg, so that the dissolved [CO_2] is reduced from 1.2 to 0.9 ([CO_2] = 0.03 x 30 = 0.9), the addition of 11 mEqs of acid per liter will decrease the pH by only 0.14 units relative to the normal value (Eq. 11):

$$pH = 6.1 + \log (13/0.9) = 7.26 \ldots \quad \textbf{(11)}$$

Our body behaves like an open system, as we control the blood concentration of dissolved CO_2 by altering the ventilation rate. Changes in alveolar ventilation aimed at minimizing the change in pH in the face of an acid or base load are referred to as ***respiratory compensation***. As described later there are many ways to graphically display changes in acid-base equilibrium. The Davenport diagram (**HCO_3^-** *vs.* **pH**) is one of the more traditional ways of illustrating the acid-base status. This famous diagram was developed in 1974 by the American physiologist Horace W. Davenport (1913-2005).

DAVENPORT DIAGRAM

To better visualize the dynamic relationships among the traditional elements of "the acid-base picture", a simple bicarbonate-pH diagram is used. In this diagram, HCO_3^- values are plotted on the y axis against pH values on the x axis, according to the following version (Eq. 12) of the Henderson-Hasselbalch equation:

$$[HCO_3^-] = 0.03\ PaCO_2 \times 10^{(pH - 6.1)} \ldots \quad \textbf{(12)}$$

Let's use the Davenport diagram to examine our example of an acid load in an open system with a fixed $PaCO_2$ value of 40 mmHg. If we plot $[HCO_3^-]$ *versus* pH at a fixed $PaCO_2$, as shown in Fig. **4**, an exponential curve called **isobar** is defined. This curve includes *all* possible values for $[HCO_3^-]$ and pH at a particular $PaCO_2$. The ***normal point*** on the diagram corresponds to a $[HCO_3^-]$ of 24 mEq/l and a pH of 7.4, and lies on the $PaCO_2$ = 40 mmHg isobar. If we keep $PaCO_2$ fixed and apply a load of acid or base we shift from the normal point to a new point on the *same* isobar. The exact location of the point will depend on the amount of acid or base added.

However, if after the addition of an acid load we allow $PaCO_2$ to drop to a new level (*e.g.*, isobar 30) the pH drop will be smaller than if we maintained $PaCO_2$ fixed at 40 mmHg. In our example of an open system with a variable $PaCO_2$, an acid load of 11 mEq/l will reduce pH by only 0.14 unit (from 7.40 to of 7.26) because we now can shift to and remain at the $PaCO_2$ = 30 mmHg isobar (Fig. **5**).

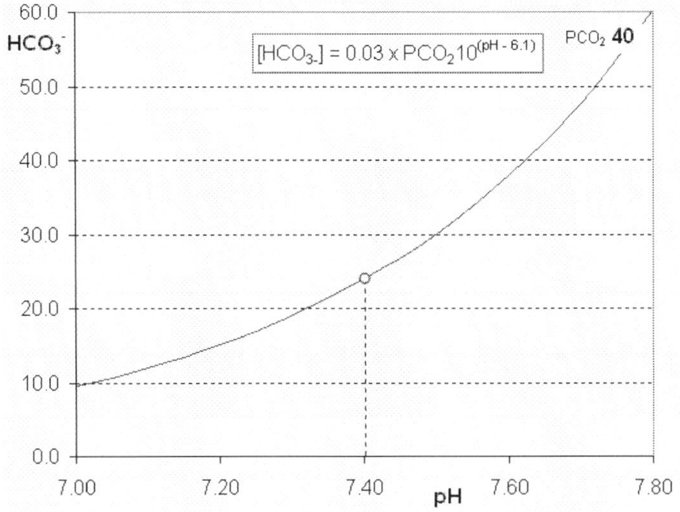

Figure 4: Davenport Diagram. In this diagram, the HCO_3^- values (mEq/l) are plotted (on the y axis) against the pH values (on the x axis) according to the following version of the Henderson-Hasselbalch equation shown on the graph above. The normal arterial blood pH corresponds to a HCO_3^- level of 24 mEq/l

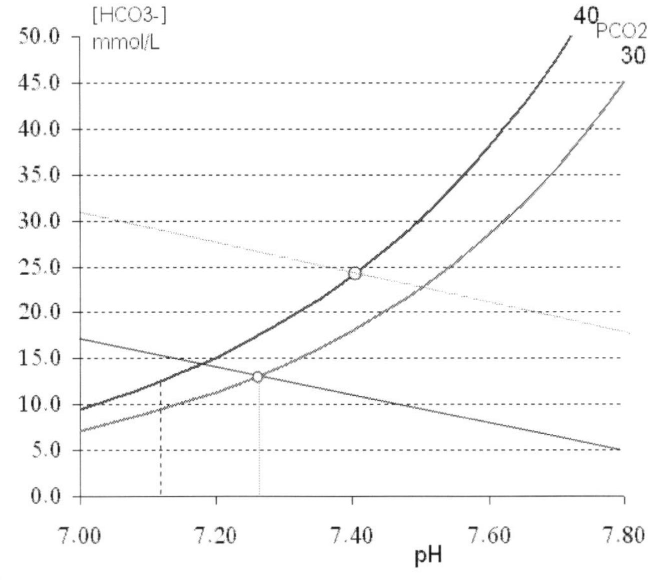

Figure 5: Davenport Diagram showing the advantage of lowering $PaCO_2$ following the addition of an acid load. A lower $PaCO_2$ mitigates the drop in pH (compare the pH values corresponding to the same HCO_3^- level in the two isobars). Depicted in this diagram are also two parallel blood-buffer lines each describing the changes in pH and HCO_3^- level (mEq/l) as we vary $PaCO_2$ and move from one isobar to another.

BLOOD-BUFFER LINE

When we examine the behavior of the $\mathbf{CO_2/HCO_3^-}$ buffer system in simple aqueous solutions or *separated plasma* [2] we notice that varying $PaCO_2$ does not significantly affect

$[HCO_3^-]$. However, in whole **blood**, varying $PaCO_2$ alone significantly changes $[HCO_3^-]$ because a significant amount of protons are absorbed by **hemoglobin** [3]. Therefore, unless we know that $PaCO_2$ is being maintained constant, we cannot simply assume that the change in $[HCO_3^-]$ is due to the addition of a non-volatile acid or base.

MODEL SYSTEM

To understand why in a simple aqueous system a change in the $PaCO_2$ has a negligible effect on the HCO_3^- concentration, we need to use the equilibrium relationship for the CO_2/ HCO_3^- buffer system (Eq. 13):

$$Ka = \frac{[H^+][HCO_3^-]}{0.03 \text{ x } PCO_2} \ \ldots \qquad \mathbf{(13)}$$

Table **2** shows the normal acid-base values of arterial blood. If $PaCO_2$ doubles, both H^+ and HCO_3^- concentrations increase by $40\text{x}10^{-9}$ M, which doubles the numerator and maintain the equilibrium. Although this doubles the $[H^+]$ (from 40 to 80 nanoEq/l), it results in only a miniscule, negligible increase in $[HCO_3^-]$. Thus, changing $PaCO_2$ in a protein-free, aqueous system, results in negligible $[HCO_3^-]$ change.

Table 2: Normal arterial acid-base values.

pH	7.40
$[H^+]$	$40 \text{ x } 10^{-9}$ M
$[HCO_3^-]$	$24 \text{ x } 10^{-3}$ M
α $PaCO_2$	$1.2 \text{ x } 10^{-3}$ M

$\alpha = 0.03$ (CO_2 solubility coefficient at 37°).

BUFFERING OF H^+ BY HEMOGLOBIN DEFINES THE *IN VITRO* BLOOD-BUFFER LINE

Although based on its pKa alone hemoglobin (Hb) would a poor buffer in normal physiological pH range, it can bind a considerable amount of H^+ inside the erythrocyte. This is also where most of the conversion of CO_2 into HCO_3^- occurs, as it is catalyzed by the carbonic anhydrase, which is present in abundance inside the erythrocyte but not in the plasma. In order for the CO_2 hydration reaction (Eq 4) to continue as blood PCO_2 increases the generated protons (H^+) are bound (buffered) by Hb resulting in increased production of HCO_3^- ions. For the same reason, blood $[HCO_3^-]$ decreases as the PCO_2 drops and H^+ ions are released by Hb as it binds oxygen. As a result of this dynamics, significant changes in $[HCO_3^-]$ occur when the blood PCO_2 is altered. The buffering capacity (BC) of blood is the amount of H^+ that can be absorbed or released by 1 liter of blood for each unit change in pH. The blood BC *in vitro* can be defined as the ratio of change in $[HCO_3^-]$ to change in pH (Eq. 14):

$$BC = \Delta[HCO_3^-] / \Delta pH \ldots \quad \textbf{(14)}$$

BC, expressed in *slykes* (mEq/l per pH unit), can be estimated from the hemoglobin concentration
([Hb]) (g/100 ml blood) as follows (Eqs. 15 and 16):

$$BC\ (\textit{in vitro}) = 8.2 + 1.56[Hb] \ldots \quad \textbf{(15)}$$

$$BC'\ (\textit{in vivo}) = 2.5 + 0.5[Hb] \ldots \quad \textbf{(16)}$$

In a subject with normal [Hb] (15 g/100 ml blood), the estimated BC value *in vitro* is -30 slykes. Anemic patients are expected to have lower than normal BC because of their reduced [Hb].

As we vary the $PaCO_2$ in whole blood *in vitro*, the $[HCO_3^-]$ changes in a linear fashion forming a buffer line with a slope of approximately 30 slykes. This relationship can be graphically represented as shown in Fig. **6** (*in vitro* blood-buffer line). However, in contrast to the *in vitro* situation, in the body *in vivo* HCO_3^- distributes into plasma, interstitial fluid, and to some extent intracellularly with an overall volume of distribution equivalent to 50% of body weight. Consequently, the change in $[HCO_3^-]$ associated with a given change in $PaCO_2$ *in vivo* is only about 1/3 of what is observed *in vitro* (Fig. **6**). Therefore, the slope of the *in vivo* normal blood-buffer line is only -10 (*i.e.*, BC' = -10 slykes). BC' (*in vivo*) = 1/3 BC (*in vitro*)

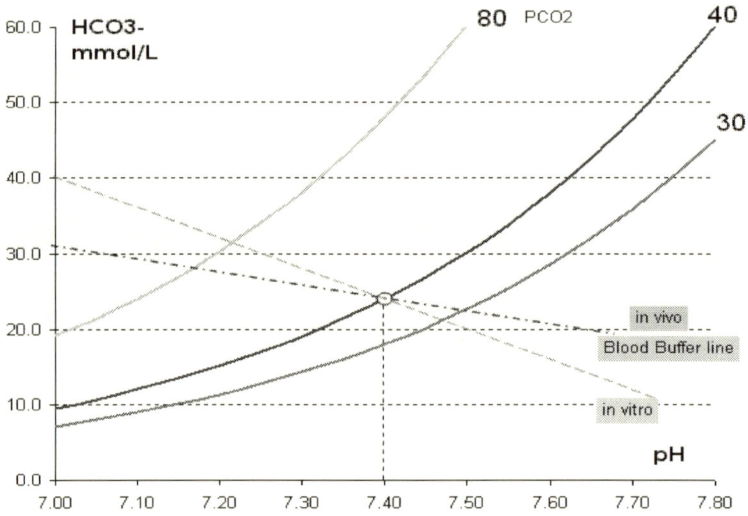

Figure 6: Davenport Diagram showing three isobars and the blood buffer lines (*in vitro* and *in vivo*) defined by the course of pH-$[HCO_3^-]$ relationship as a result of the change in $PaCO_2$. The absolute value of the slope of the blood buffer line equals the blood buffering capacity. Notice the difference in the slopes of the two blood buffer lines (see text for explanation)

RESPIRATORY ACID-BASE DISORDERS

Hyperventilation, whether voluntary or due to disease, causes a drop in $PaCO_2$ and a rise in pHa, plus a small *decrease* in arterial $[HCO_3^-]$. This condition is referred to as an acute respiratory alkalosis. The opposite changes occur with hypoventilation causing acute respiratory acidosis. The predicted bicarbonate concentration ($[HCO_3^-]_{predicted}$), due to a pure, uncompensated, respiratory alkalosis - a change in pH under these conditions due solely to changes in $PaCO_2$ and to the buffering effects of proteins - can be calculated according to the following equation, which simply says in mathematical terms that *purely respiratory changes are associated with movement along the normal blood buffer line away from the normal point.*

$$[HCO_3^-]_{predicted} = 24 + BC'(7.4 - pH) = 24 + (2.5 + 0.5\,[Hb])(7.4 - pH) \ldots \quad \textbf{(17)}$$

The differences between predicted and the actual ($[HCO_3^-]_{actual}$) or observed bicarbonate levels is referred to as base excess (BE):

$$BE = [HCO_3^-]_{actual} - [HCO_3^-]_{predicted} \cdots \quad \textbf{(18)}$$

Base Excess (BE) is defined as the amount of acid or base that must be added to one liter of arterial blood to restore its pH to 7.4. When defined in this way, **BE** indicates the change in plasma $[HCO_3^-]$ that cannot be accounted for by the combined effects of $\Delta PaCO_2$ and blood buffers and points to the additional involvement of a non-respiratory (renal) component.

There is a second definition of **BE** based on the concept of **standard bicarbonate** which is the level of bicarbonate in the plasma when a fully oxygenated sample of whole blood is equilibrated (*in vitro*) at 37°C with a $PaCO_2$ of 40 mmHg. **BE** is calculated as the difference between the measured (actual) and the normal values for the standard bicarbonate multiplied by an empirical factor (1.2) related to the buffering capacity of hemoglobin (Eq. 19):

$$BE = 1.2\,([HCO_3^-]_{40} - 24) \ldots \quad \textbf{(19)}$$

where $[HCO_3^-]_{40}$ denotes the actual (observed) standard bicarbonate whereas 24 is the value of the normal, standard, plasma $[HCO_3^-]$.

METABOLIC ACID-BASE DISORDERS

Pure, uncompensated respiratory disorders would have zero base excess (BE = 0). The presence of a significant BE indicates the presence of a non-respiratory component. This may be primary or may simply represent a compensatory renal response to primary respiratory ABD ($\Delta PaCO_2$). On the Davenport diagram the normal blood buffer line passes through the ***normal point*** (pHa = 7.4, $[HCO_3^-]$ = 24 mEq/l plasma). If we add or eliminate HCO_3^- while maintaining the $PaCO_2$ fixed at 40 mmHg, we will move up or down along the isobar away from the normal point. This will produce either a positive or negative BE. The value of BE at any point on the Davenport diagram is equal to the vertical distance between that point and the normal blood buffer line, and corresponds to the change in [HCO_3^-] that is *not* due to changes in the buffering of CO_2 following $\Delta PaCO_2$. A negative BE which indicates a base deficit may be due to the consumption of HCO_3^- in the process of buffering (neutralizing) a non-volatile (fixed) acid load and would indicate the presence of a non-respiratory component, in this case a primary ***metabolic acidosis***. Alternatively, a negative BE may be caused by renal compensation for a drop in $PaCO_2$ *i.e.*, for a primary respiratory alkalosis.

To differentiate between the two possibilities we rely on clinical assessment and clinical data and experience (see Conceptual Method later).

BY CONTRAST, AN ALKALI

load causes ***metabolic alkalosis*** and a positive BE. Examples of metabolic (non-respiratory) acid-base disorders are shown in Tables **3** and **4**.

Table 3: Causes of Non-Respiratory (Metabolic) Acidosis

Failure to dispose of usual metabolic acid load
Renal failure;
Proximal Renal Tubular Acidosis (pRTA);
RTA4
Increased acid load
Endogenous: lactic acidosis; keto-acidosis
Exogenous: NH_4Cl, $CaCl_2$, Lysine HCl
Toxic Ingestion: Aspirin, methanol, ethylene glycol, *etc.*
Loss of HCO_3^-
Via the GIT (acute diarrhea)
Via the Kidney

Thus, the presence of a significant BE indicates the presence of a non-respiratory acid-base process. This could be primary or compensatory. The normal value of BE ranges from -2 to +2 mEq/l.

On the Davenport diagram (Fig. 7) we can define a series of parallel blood buffer lines depending upon the BE. If we superimpose a respiratory disorder on a non-respiratory (metabolic) one, we will move along a blood buffer line that is displaced from the normal line by a distance equal to the BE value, but whose slope is still equal to -BC'.

Table 4: Causes of Non-respiratory (Metabolic) Alkalosis

Net gain of HCO_3^-
Administration of $NaHCO_3$
Massive blood transfusion (citrate $\Rightarrow HCO_3^-$)
Milk-alkali syndrome
Magnesium Depletion
Contraction Alkalosis
Loop or thiazide diuretics
Sweat losses in cystic fibrosis
Gastric fluid losses.
Net loss of H^+ through of the GI: vomiting, NG-suction, antacids, *etc.*
Renal H^+ Loss
Diuretics, excess mineralocorticoids, *etc.*
K^+ depletion ($\Rightarrow$ ECF alkalosis):
H^+-K^+ exchange $\Rightarrow\uparrow [H^+]_i \Rightarrow$ □H^+ secretion$\Rightarrow\uparrow[HCO_3^-]_p$

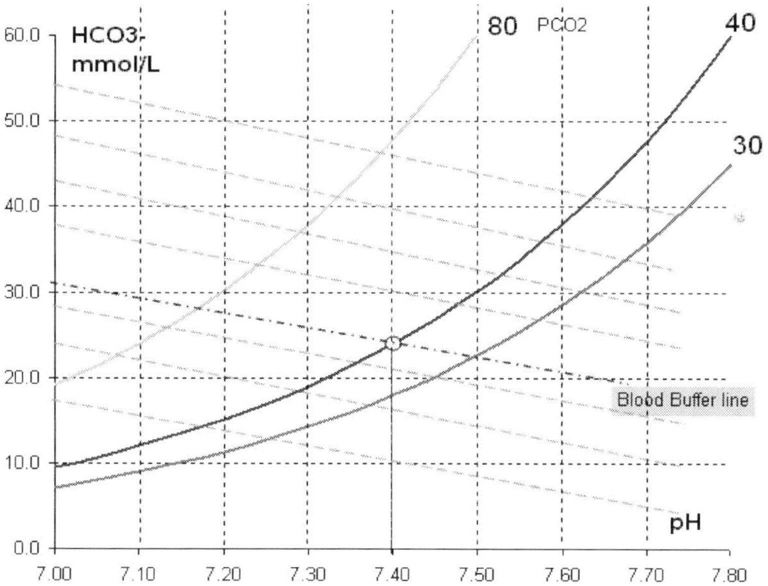

Figure 7: The Davenport diagram showing multiple buffer lines reflecting different levels of base excess (BE = the vertical distance between a given buffer line and the normal one).

EVALUATION OF THE ACID-BASE STATUS

For using the Davenport diagram to evaluate the acid base status one needs to consider both the respiratory status (*which isobar we on*) and the metabolic status (*which blood buffer line we are on*). With a *pure, uncompensated* metabolic disturbance one operated along the normal $PaCO_2 = 40$ isobar, but can develop either a negative or a positive BE by moving away from the normal point along this isobar. With a pure, uncompensated, respiratory disturbance one remains on, and moves along, the normal blood-buffer line from one CO_2-isobar to another. However, acid-base disorders are almost never pure. They are almost always partially compensated. A simple acid-base disturbance consists of the primary disturbance plus its attendant secondary response. A primary non-respiratory disorder is often accompanied by a respiratory compensation and *vice versa* (Fig. **8**).

However, it is not uncommon for two primary disorders to coexist in the same patient at the same time, in which case we speak of **mixed** acid-base disorder. The 3-point method of evaluating ABDs will further clarify how such mixed disorders are easily identified.

Let's look at two simple examples.

In a patient with chronic obstructive pulmonary disease (COPD) and **respiratory acidosis**, we might observe an elevated arterial $PaCO_2$ of 60 mmHg, a $[HCO_3^-]$ of 32 mEq/l and an arterial pH of 7.35. Under these conditions and assuming a normal blood buffering capacity (BC'=10, Eqs. 20 and 21):

$$[HCO_3^-]_{predicted} = 24 + 10(7.40 - 7.35) = 24.5 \text{ mEq/l} \ldots \quad \textbf{(20)}$$

$$BE = 32 - 24.5 = +7.5 \text{ mEq/l} \ldots \quad \textbf{(21)}$$

This base excess results from renal compensation. To represent this graphically we consider two components: *(a)* a respiratory acidosis (Fig. **8A**), moving along the normal blood buffer line from 40 to 60 mmHg isobars; and *(b)* a metabolic (renal) compensatory increase in $[HCO_3^-]$, moving along the 60 mmHg isobar to an arterial pH value of 7.35, and producing a BE of +7.5 mEq/l (Fig. **8A**). In reality, these processes occur simultaneously and incrementally as the disorder develops. Analogous changes take place in metabolic ABDs (Fig. **8B**).

While respiratory compensation for primary metabolic disturbances is relatively rapid, renal compensatory mechanisms are slow. For instance, the renal compensation for the acute respiratory alkalosis associated with high altitude-induced hyperventilation requires 2-3 days.

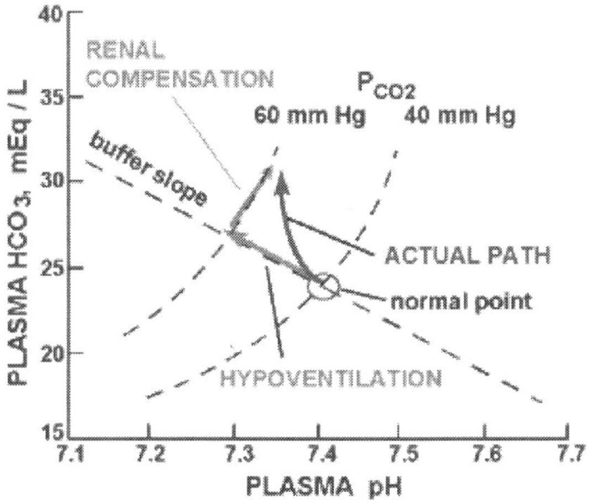

A: Respiratory Acidosis

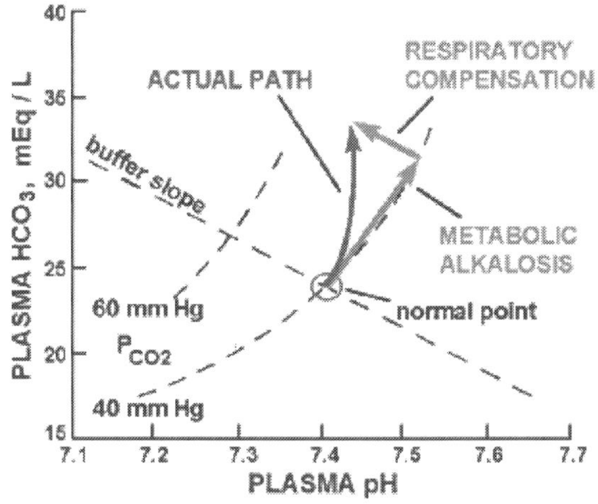

B: Metabolic Alkalosis

Figure 8: Use of the Davenport diagram to follow changes in acid-base parameters brought about by secondary compensations to primary acid-base disorders. Panel A shows the renal compensation for a primary respiratory acidosis. Panel B illustrates the respiratory compensation for a metabolic alkalosis.

The acid-base values alone may be used to make an educated *initial* guess as to the type of acid-base disorder (ABD), as illustrated in Fig. **9**. It is important to bear in mind that we cannot determine what the underlying problem is based on the *acid-base values alone*. Additional information is usually available to help us deduce the nature of an acid-base disorder.

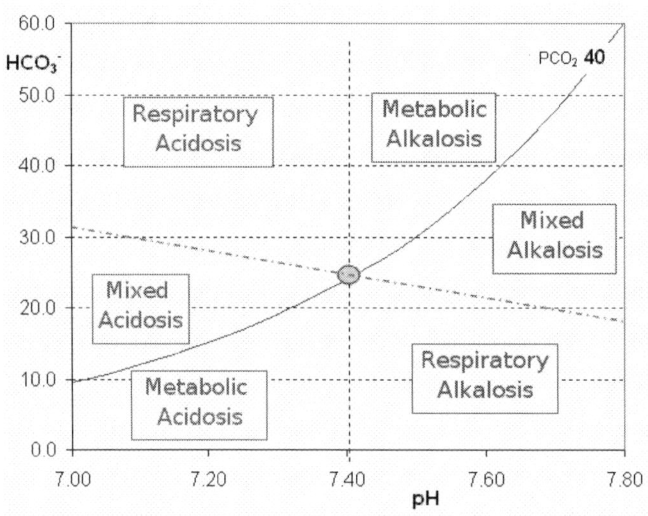

Figure 9: The canvas of the Davenport diagram is divided into 6 distinct areas by the 3 main lines: the 40 isobar, the normal blood buffering line, and the perpendicular line through the normal point. Each area indicates a specific ABD.

CLINICAL (PRACTICAL) METHODS FOR THE EVALUATION OF ACID-BASE DISORDERS

Acid-base disorders (ABDs) are seldom simple and often complicated by multiple comorbidities including organ failure, especially in critically ill patients. Management of serious ABDs requires deliberate diagnosis and treatment of the underlying pathology and may also require measures to hasten restoration of normal acid-base balance. It is essential that one develops a consistent, systematic, approach for the evaluation of ABDs.

Over the past sixty years or so, many approaches for analyzing and quantifying ABDs have been developed. As a result, there are many ways to graphically visualize the acid-base status and countless nomograms and equations, and more recently interactive computer programs and mobile "apps". All of these analytical tools are aimed at facilitating the diagnosis and treatment of ABDs.

Each of these methods has its own terminology and focuses on a particular aspect of the acid-base picture. Therefore, it is not surprising that in general this subject is surrounded by controversy and confusion and that much of the literature deals with conflicting claims of superiority of one method over another. It appears that each medical specialty (*e.g.*, anesthesiology, critical care medicine, nephrology, and so on) has adopted its favorite approach.

Some of these methods are briefly described below. The approach advocated here is a nomogram-free, straightforward, conceptual and practical method that is based on a large volume of experimental data and clinical observations accumulated over decades. Nomogram-based methods are still in use and are described here mostly for their didactic and historical interest. There is in addition a relatively new approach (the **Stewart** method) [4] advocated mainly by some critical care physicians who believe it to be quantitatively (and scientifically) more accurate and diagnostically more useful. However, its use remains very limited because its practical value in a clinical setting is yet to be proven.

SINGER-HASTINGS METHOD

This approach, introduced by Singer and Hastings in 1948, relies on the *in vitro* measurement of "**whole-blood buffer base concentration**" ([BB]), *i.e.*, the sum of the concentrations of all buffer anions in whole blood. These consist mainly of bicarbonate, with a smaller but significant contribution by hemoglobin [5]. The contributions by plasma albumin and inorganic phosphate are negligible. Under normal acid-base balance, [BB] = 48±2 mEq/l. Changes in $PaCO_2$ do not affect the total [BB] value and only affect the redistribution of protons between bicarbonate and non-bicarbonate buffers. Therefore, abnormalities in [BB] are indicative of non-respiratory (metabolic) acid-base processes. After the introduction of this approach, a nomogram was published [6] which enables one to determine the value of [BB] from blood pH and $PaCO_2$, or from $[HCO_3^-]$ and the hematocrit (Hct), or hemoglobin concentration ([Hb]).

STANDARD BICARBONATE/ BASE EXCESS METHOD

This approach was first introduced by Astrup and Siggaard-Anderson in 1960. It utilizes the concepts of standard bicarbonate ($[HCO_3]_{40}$) and base excess (BE) discussed above. To reiterate, the standard bicarbonate is defined as the plasma bicarbonate concentration in fully oxygenated blood in equilibrium *in vitro* with $PaCO_2 = 40$ mmHg at 37° C. The idea is that equilibrating the blood *in vitro* with normal $PaCO_2$ eliminates the effect of the deviations in $PaCO_2$ on the levels of blood buffers ($[HCO_3^-]$ and [BB]). Therefore, any deviation from normal in the level of standard bicarbonate ($[HCO_3]_{40}$) can be attributed to a non-respiratory (metabolic) event. The normal value of $[HCO_3]_{40}$ is 24 mEq/l. The $[HCO_3^-]_{40}$ value can be read off the Siggaard-Anderson nomogram which is based on a linear plot of $PaCO_2$ (on a log scale) *versus* pH (Fig. **10**).

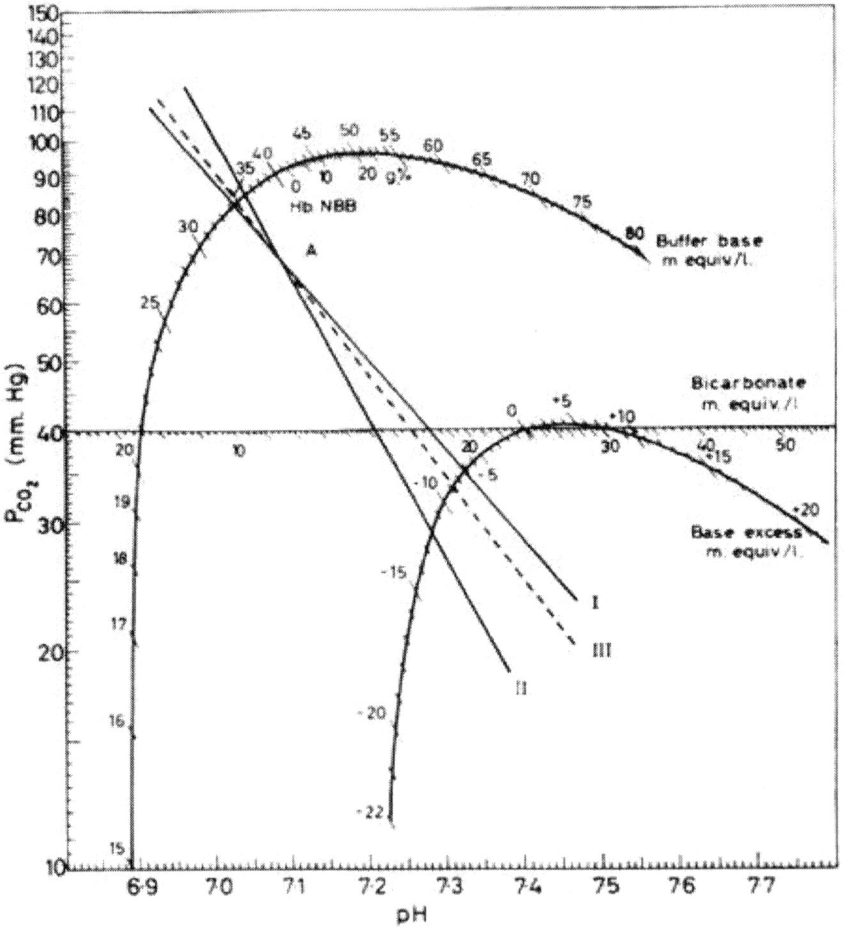

Figure 10: Siggaard-Anderson nomogram / PCO_2-pH plot. Lines I and II represent plots for two samples with pHa = 7.08 and $PaCO_2 = 70$ mmHg. Line I represents plasma and line II represents

whole blood. Line III represents a similar plot for a blood sample diluted with plasma to a hemoglobin concentration of 5 g/100 ml blood. The PCO_2-pH plot is obtained by altering $PaCO_2$ and recording the resulting steady-state pH. The intersection of this line with the $PaCO_2 = 40$ mmHg line gives the actual $[HCO_3]_{40.}$ This value represents what the $[HCO_3^-]$ would be without respiratory compensation. As mentioned earlier, base excess (BE) is the $\Delta[HCO_3^-]_{40}$ multiplied by an empirical factor (1.2) related to the buffer capacity of hemoglobin: BE = 1.2 ($[HCO_3]_{40}$ - 24), BE may be defined as the amount of acid or base (mEq) required to restore normal pH (7.40) to one liter of whole blood *in vitro* at 37° C., Because *in vivo* the buffering effect of hemoglobin is "felt" (diluted) throughout the extracellular compartment, another quantity has been introduced- standard BE which is defined in the same way except that the hypothetical blood sample is assumed to have a [Hb] of 5 g/100 ml blood (roughly 1/3 normal)., In addition to being confusing and mechanical, these methods have at least one serious flaw - they rely on data derived from *in vitro* titration of whole blood and the assumption that the CO_2 titration curve in whole-blood *in vitro* is the same as its titration curve in the whole organism *in vivo*. Laboratory experiments and careful clinical observations clearly indicate that this assumption is at least inaccurate if not outright wrong.

CONCEPTUAL (NOMOGRAM-FREE) APPROACH TO ACID-BASE DISORDERS [7]

Step 1 ("Blink") [8]

Look at the arterial blood acid-base values and identify the apparent, most obvious disturbance. Table **5** shows the tentative diagnosis based on "first look" at the acid-base picture. The arrows signify direction of change relative to normal arterial blood values. Double arrows indicate primary (more pronounced) change and a single arrow indicates secondary (compensatory) response. Note that in each of the four primary acid-base disturbances both $[HCO_3^-]$ and $PaCO_2$ change in the same direction; this is what you would expect from an appropriate physiological response aimed at keeping $[HCO_3^-]/PaCO_2$ ratio close to normal.

Step 2 (Compensation Formula)

Table 5: Blink Diagnosis of ABDs

pH	$[HCO_3^-]$	$PaCO_2$	Primary Acid-Base Disturbance
Lower than 7.35	↓↓	↓	**Metabolic acidosis (non-respiratory)**
Lower than 7.35	↑	↑↑	**Respiratory acidosis**
Higher than 7.45	↑↑	↑	**Metabolic alkalosis (non-respiratory)**
Higher than 7.45	↓	↓↓	**Respiratory alkalosis**

Table 6: Formulas for Expected Secondary Response (Compensation) (metabolic means non-respiratory)

Metabolic Acidosis	**↓↓ $[HCO_3^-]$**	**$PaCO_2 = 1.5\ [HCO_3^-]_p + 8$ or $PaCO_2 = 40 - 1.1\ \Delta[HCO_3^-] \pm 3$**
Metabolic Alkalosis	**↑↑ $[HCO_3^-]$**	**$PaCO_2 = 0.9\ [HCO_3^-]_p + 15$ or $PaCO_2 = 40 + 0.7\ \Delta[HCO_3^-]$ or $PaCO_2 = 40 + 0.6\ \Delta[HCO_3^-] \pm 3$**
Acute Respiratory Acidosis	**↑↑ $PaCO_2$**	**$[HCO_3^-] = 24 + 0.1\ \Delta PaCO_2 \pm 2$**
Chronic Respiratory Acidosis	**↑↑ $PaCO_2$**	**$[HCO_3^-] = 24 + 0.35\ \Delta PaCO_2 \pm 3$**
Acute Respiratory Alkalosis	**↓↓ $PaCO_2$**	**$[HCO_3^-] = 24 - 0.25\ \Delta PaCO_2 \pm 3$**
Chronic Respiratory Alkalosis	**↓↓ $PaCO_2$**	**$[HCO_3^-]_p = 24 - 0.5\ \Delta PaCO_2 \pm 2$**

Determine whether the apparent compensation is consistent (both direction and magnitude) with the expected secondary response according to the well-established formulas derived from clinical observations and *in vivo* whole-body titration experiments (Table **6**).

- In **metabolic acidosis**, the respiratory compensation (hyperventilation) causes $PaCO_2$ to drop approximately 1.2 mmHg for each mEq/l drop in $[HCO_3^-]$. Alternatively, $PaCO_2 = 1.5[HCO_3^-] + 8$. It has also been noted that within certain limits, the $PaCO_2$ in metabolic acidosis is usually numerically close to the last two digits of the arterial pH value (*e.g.*, if pHa = 7.29, $PaCO_2 \simeq 29$ mmHg).

- In **metabolic alkalosis**, the respiratory compensation (hypoventilation) causes $PaCO_2$ to rise by approximately 0.7 mmHg for each mEq/l increase in $[HCO_3^-]$. In the case of respiratory acid-base disturbances, it is important to distinguish between acute and chronic situations.

- In **acute respiratory acidosis**, the apparent secondary compensation (mostly due to the buffering effect) increases $[HCO_3^-]$ by 0.1 – 0.15 mEq/l for each mmHg rise in $PaCO_2$.

- In **chronic respiratory acidosis**, the renal compensation increases $[HCO_3^-]$ by approximately 0.35 mEq/l for each mmHg rise in $PaCO_2$.

- In **acute respiratory alkalosis**, the apparent secondary compensation reduces $[HCO_3^-]$ by approximately 0.2 mEq/l for each mmHg drop in $PaCO_2$.

- In **chronic respiratory alkalosis**, the renal compensation reduces $[HCO_3^-]$ by approximately 0.4 mEq/l for each mmHg drop in $PaCO_2$.

If the apparent compensation is not consistent with the standard formulas, it is likely that we are dealing with a mixed ABD (*e.g.*, lactic acidosis + metabolic alkalosis, two primary metabolic acidosis, or a respiratory plus a non-respiratory ABD, as often occurs in adult patients as a result of salicylate (aspirin) toxicity (respiratory alkalosis plus metabolic acidosis).

Step 3 (Anion Gap):

Determine the anion gap (Eq. 22):

$$AG = [Na^+] - ([HCO_3^-] + [Cl^-]) \ldots \qquad \textbf{(22)}$$

Normally the AG ranges between 9 and 16 mEq/l (average = 12 mEq/l). The normal anion gap reflects, and is accounted for, by the negative changes on protein molecules, mainly albumin. When the plasma albumin level falls, so does the anion gap. An AG > 20 indicates the presence of an "anion gap metabolic acidosis" (*e.g.*, diabetic ketoacidosis, alcoholic ketoacidosis, L-lactic acidosis, D-lactic acidosis, and so on).

If one is dealing with a lactic acidosis or a ketoacidosis, it is useful to compare the rise in AG to the drop in $[HCO_3^-]$:

$ In ketoacidosis: $\Delta[HCO_3^-] = \Delta AG$.

$ In lactic acidosis the drop in $[HCO_3^-]$ is roughly equal to 2/3 ΔAG.

Significant deviations from these expected changes suggest the presence of an additional primary acid base disturbance (ABD).

In each of the following examples the patient starts off with normal acid-base values including a normal anion gap of 12.

Example 1:

A patient develops lactic acidosis and at simultaneously emesis for 2 days; his [HCO_3^-], pH, and $PaCO_2$ remain essentially normal, but his AG increases from 12 to 30 mEq/l. Thus $\Delta AG = 18$. Here we expected a drop in [HCO_3^-] of approximately (2/3)18 = 12 mEq/l, but there is no apparent drop in [HCO_3^-], suggesting the existence of a primary metabolic alkalosis. This is consistent with the effect of emesis [9].

Example 2:

A patient develops severe ketoacidosis and the acid-base picture changes to: pH = 7.08, [HCO_3^-] = 4 mEq/l, $PaCO_2$= 14 mmHg, AG = 22 mEq/l, and ΔAG=10. With ketoacidosis we expect a drop in [HCO_3^-] roughly equal to a rise in AG; in this case the [HCO_3^-] should have been approximately14 mEq/l. The fact that the actual [HCO_3^-] is much lower than expected indicates the presence of a second metabolic acidosis (of the normal anion gap type) [10].

ACID-BASE CASES (N.H.A.)

(Adapted from acidbasedisorders.com with permission of Dr. John Doyle).

Case 1: Morphine Overdose

In the recovery room following surgery, a 23-year-old man was found apneic (not breathing), cyanotic, and unresponsive. About an hour earlier he had received 25 mg of intravenous (IV) morphine for pain relief.

While he was being resuscitated, an arterial blood gas sample was taken and the results came as follows:

$$pHa = 7.12 \; PaCO_2 = 82 \text{ mmHg} \; [HCO_3^-] = 26 \text{ mEq/l}$$

- The patient is clearly acidemic as indicated by the very low pH.
- Since the HCO_3 level is practically normal and the $PaCO_2$ is severely elevated (normal is around 40 mmHg), the primary disturbance is clearly respiratory, that is respiratory acidosis.

- Since we are dealing with a respiratory disturbance, we have to decide whether it is acute or chronic. Here we can make use of the equation of the expected secondary compensation. In this case the measured $[HCO_3^-]$ is close to the level expected for acute respiratory acidosis:

$$[HCO_3^-] = 24 + 0.1\ (82 - 40) \pm 2 = 28.2 \pm 2\ \text{mEq/l}$$

If it were chronic:

$$[HCO_3^-] = 24 + 0.35\ (82 - 40) \pm 3 = 38.7 \pm 3\ \text{mEq/l}$$

Thus the diagnosis is Acute Respiratory Acidosis.

Morphine and other opiate analgesics are respiratory depressants and in large doses will stop breathing. This effect is mediated *via* the μ (mu) opioid receptors in the medulla, the part of the brainstem that regulates breathing and other autonomic functions. When examined, the patient was cyanotic (blue), with pinpoint pupils, but he still had a pulse. He was given 100% oxygen by positive-pressure ventilation and 0.4 mg of IV naloxone (Narcan), an opiate antagonist. The patient quickly improved. Upon review of the incident it was noted that the analgesic order was actually for 25 mg of IV meperidine (Demerol), an amount roughly equal to 2.5 mg of morphine. Drug errors of this kind are frightfully common. The Institute of Medicine estimates that as many as 44,000 to 98,000 people die in U.S. hospitals each year as the result of medical errors. This means that more people die from medical errors than from motor vehicle accidents, breast cancer, or AIDS.

Case 2: Pyloric Stenosis

A 4-week-old baby boy is admitted to hospital with history of projectile vomiting of several days duration. The following blood gases are obtained:

$$pHa = 7.50\ \ PaCO_2 = 49\ \text{mmHg}\ \ [HCO_3^-] = 37\ \text{mEq/l}$$

- The arterial pH is alkalemic (compared to the normal range: 7.35 to 7.45).

- Is the primary disturbance respiratory or metabolic? Since all three parameters are elevated above normal, the primary disturbance is most likely metabolic alkalosis.

- The rise in $PaCO_2$ in the face of alkalemia indicates respiratory compensation rather than a primary respiratory disturbance.

- The expected $PaCO_2$ in metabolic alkalosis may be calculated as follows:

$$0.9 \times [HCO_3^-] + 15 \text{ mmHg} = [0.9 \times 37] + 15 = 48 \text{ mmHg}$$

Since the actual $PaCO_2$ (49) and the expected $PaCO_2$ (48) are approximately the same, this suggests that respiratory compensation is appropriate.

DIAGNOSIS

Metabolic Alkalosis from due to persistent vomiting induced by pyloric stenosis.

Pyloric stenosis is a narrowing of the pylorus, the terminal segment of the stomach that leads to the small intestines. This occurs when the muscle around the pylorus has hypertrophied. Most babies with pyloric stenosis begin to vomit during the second to third week of life. These babies begin with "spitting up" that later becomes projectile vomiting after feeding. The loss of gastric acid is accompanied by the addition of bicarbonate to the blood, hence the metabolic alkalosis in this case. The diagnosis of pyloric stenosis is often suspected on clinical grounds and confirmed by ultrasonic imaging or a barium swallow study.

Also known as infantile hypertrophic pyloric stenosis or gastric outlet obstruction, pyloric stenosis is relatively common, especially in firstborn male infants. Pyloric stenosis is fixed with an operation called a pyloromyotomy, where the surgeon spreads open the muscle around the pyloric valve. Some scientists believe that babies with pyloric stenosis lack receptors in the pyloric muscle to detect nitric oxide (NO), an important chemical messenger that relaxes smooth muscle. As a result, the muscle is in a state of almost continual contraction, which causes it to hypertrophy over time. This process may take some time, which is why pyloric stenosis usually appears in babies a few weeks after birth rather than immediately. Incidentally, do not confuse nitric oxide (NO) with nitrous oxide (N_2O), the "laughing gas" often used in anesthesia.

Case 3: – Woman with Panic Attacks

A 26-year-old woman is undergoing treatment for frequent panic attacks. The attacks are accompanied by hyperventilation, a racing heartbeat (tachycardia), dizziness, feelings of "unreality" and tingling in the hands. In one particularly severe attack, when taken to the emergency department, an arterial blood-gas sample was taken, which revealed the following:

$$pH= 7.52 \ PaCO_2= 26 \text{ mmHg } [HCO_3^-]= 22 \text{ mEq/l}$$

- The pH of the arterial blood is clearly alkalemic (normal range for arterial blood pH is 7.35 to 7.45).
- Since the $PaCO_2$ is markedly reduced and the $[HCO_3^-]$ is also on the low side, the alkalosis in this case is the result of a primary respiratory disturbance.
- Since $[HCO_3^-]$ is only slightly below normal we are dealing with an acute respiratory alkalosis. We can corroborate this conclusion by calculating the level of $[HCO_3^-]$ expected as the result of the secondary (renal) compensation for acute respiratory alkalosis:
- $[HCO_3^-] = 24 - 0.25 (PaCO_2) \pm 3 = 24 - 0.25 (40\text{-}26) \pm 3 = 20 \pm 3$ mEq/l
- Q: If this were a chronic condition, would the $[HCO_3^-]$ have been higher or lower and why?

DIAGNOSIS

Acute Respiratory Alkalosis from Hyperventilation due to Panic Attack

For further reading on panic attack see:
http://www.nimh.nih.gov/anxiety/getpd.cfm

Case 4: – Man with a Flail Chest

A 22-year-old man was severely injured in the chest from a motor vehicle accident. A large flail rib segment in his thorax is compromising his breathing. Flail chest is the paradoxical movement of a segment of chest wall caused by anterior and posterior fractures of 3 or more ribs. A blood gas sample was taken, revealing the following:

$$pH = 7.21 \; PaCO_2 = 65 \text{ mmHg} \; [HCO_3^-] = 25 \text{ mEq/l}$$

- The pH of the arterial blood is clearly acidemic.

- Since $PaCO_2$ is markedly elevated (65 *vs.* 40 mmHg) while the $[HCO_3^-]$ is practically normal, the primary disturbance is respiratory acidosis. We also can immediately see that it is acute because the $[HCO_3^-]$ has not yet risen above normal because the kidneys require time to effect a significant degree of compensation in response to hypercapnia. You may want to confirm that by applying the appropriate formula for the expected $[HCO_3^-]$ level. Therefore, we are dealing with a case of Acute Respiratory Acidosis due to hypoventilation because of Flail Chest Injury.

REFERENCES

[1] $PaCO_2 = (863 \times \dot{V}CO_2)/\dot{V}Ai$; where $\dot{V}CO_2$ is the rate of the CO_2 production (l/min at STPD) and $\dot{V}Ai$ is the ideal alveolar ventilation (l/min at BTPS).

[2] *True plasma* is plasma in whole blood so that it is subject to the buffering effect of hemoglobin. ***Separated** plasma* is plasma without the benefit of the buffering effect of hemoglobin.

[3] CO_2 is hydrated to H_2CO_3, which partially dissociates to HCO_3^- and H^+. Some of the generated H^+ are bound to hemoglobin leaving behind HCO_3^-.

[4] http://www.anaesthesiamcq.com/AcidBaseBook/ab10_1.php
http://www.nature.com/ki/journal/v64/n3/full/4493953a.html

[5] Singer RB. A new diagram for the visualization and interpretation of acid-base changes. Am J Med Sci 1951;221:199-210.

[6] Hemoglobin owes its buffering capacity to the imidazole groups of its histidine residues of which each hemoglobin molecule contains 38. Deoxyhemoglobin (Hb) is a better buffer base (weaker acid; higher pKa) than oxyhemoglobin (HbO_2).

[7] Preston RA. Acid-base, fluids, and electrolytes made ridiculously simple. Miami: MedMaster, Inc; 1997.

[8] This is a reference to: Gladwell M. BLINK. The power of thinking without thinking. New York: Little Brown & Co; 2005. A highly recommend book, particularly to young doctors and cops.

[9] Vomiting means loss of gastric acid and gain in blood $[HCO_3^-]$. It may also mean loss of body fluids, leading to ECF contraction and secondary rise in $[HCO_3^-]$.

[10] These include mild-moderate renal failure, diarrhea (loss of $[HCO_3^-]$), all types of renal tubular acidosis, and so on.

CHAPTER 7

Ventilation-Perfusion Distribution, Blood Shunts and Alveolar Dead Space

Camillo Peracchia

Abstract: This chapter focuses on the relationship between alveolar ventilation and blood perfusion in normal and diseased states. In particular, it explains the reasons for different ventilation-perfusion ratios among lung regions. It explains the functional consequences of pulmonary diseases that alter the ventilation-perfusion ratio, and demonstrates how ventilation-perfusion abnormalities can be quantified. It describes in more detail the "three compartment model" (equivalent of the real lung), the methods used to quantify the fraction of pulmonary blood that does not undergo gas exchange (right-to-left blood shunt or venous admixture) and those used for differentiating between the two major components of venous admixture: maldistribution shunt-like effect and conductive (anatomical) shunt. The various normal and abnormal conditions that result in venous admixture (right-to-left blood shunt) are schematically represented, and the method for quantifying the fraction of alveolar ventilation wasted in alveolar dead space is described. Finally, pros and cons of oxygen therapy and potential complications of prolonged lung exposure to high O_2 fractions, leading to oxygen toxicity, are detailed.

Keywords: Alveolar Dead-Space, Alveolar Gas-Equation, Alveolar-Arterial PO_2-Gradient, Alveolar-Effective Gas, Alveolar-Ideal Gas, Blood R-lines, Conductive-Shunt-Fraction, Gas R-lines, Hyperbaric-Oxygen Therapy, Hypocapnic Bronchoconstriction, Hypoxic Vasoconstriction, Inert-Gas-Method, Maldistribution-Shunt-Like-Effect, Oxygen Therapy, Oxygen Toxicity, Physiological-Shunt-Fraction, Pulmonary Circulation, Shunt-Fraction Equation, Three-Compartment-Model, Ventilation-Perfusion Distribution.

SYMBOLS, ACRONYMS AND NORMAL VALUES: See Appendix 3

Pulmonary *Versus* Systemic Circulation

Pulmonary and systemic circulations differ in many respects due to different functional requirements. While right and left ventricles eject the same amount of blood per minute, the blood ejected by the left ventricle perfuses all of the organs (including ~2% to the lungs *via* bronchial arteries), some of which are at great distance from the heart and others (brain *etc.*) significantly above the heart when the one is standing. In contrast, blood ejected by the right ventricle only perfuses the lungs. The differences between the two systems are reflected by differences in vessel diameter and wall thickness, as well as in blood flow-resistance and pressure (Table **1**).

Table 1: Average Blood Pressure Values

	Arterial (systolic/diastolic)	Arterial Mean	Capillary	Venous	Left Atrial (same as P_{CWP}*)	Right Atrial
Systemic (mmHg)	120/80	100	30→10	10	5	2
Pulmonary (mmHg)	25/8	15	12→8	8		

* P_{CWP} = capillary wedge pressure - also be symbolized as "Pw" (pulmonary wedge pressure) – a catheter is wedged into a pulmonary capillary and the measured pressure reflects that of the left atrium.

The left ventricle needs to maintain a mean pressure approximately six times as high as that of the right ventricle in order to perfuse the brain and deliver blood to organs quite far from the heart. Furthermore, the systemic circulation needs a higher pressure to meet the blood flow requirements of different organs under various functional states, such as skeletal muscles at rest *versus* exercise and digestive system before and after food intake. Therefore, work load and metabolic requirements of the left ventricle are much greater than those of the right ventricle.

Redistribution of blood flow to different organs is regulated by regional vascular resistances, which also calls for sufficiently high systemic blood pressure. The right ventricle on the other hand only needs to generate enough pressure to lift the blood a few centimeters above the heart for perfusing the lungs' apex, and does not need to redistribute its output because all lung units perform the same gas exchange function - so it does not need to be as powerful as the left. Indeed, the thickness of the right ventricle is about a third of that of the left, and the wall of pulmonary arteries is thinner than that of systemic arteries of similar diameter, as it contains fewer smooth muscle cells.

Pulmonary Vascular Resistance

Role of Lung Volume

The pulmonary artery branches into 17 generations of smaller arteries, each generation creating 3.6 smaller branches. This vast vascular tree expands the equivalent cross-sectional area of pulmonary blood flow from ~9 cm^2 at the pulmonary artery to ~45,000 cm^2 at the alveolar level, as there are ~100 billion alveolar capillaries, each 7-8 μm wide and ~12 μm long. This astronomical increase in equivalent diameter results in a large drop of flow velocity, as velocity is inversely related to cross-sectional area, providing ample time for gas exchange – a red blood cells spends approximately ¾ of a second flowing through an alveolar capillary, which gives ample time to gas exchange; indeed, partial pressure equilibration across the blood-gas barrier at rest occurs within ~ ¼ of a second.

Vascular resistance of pulmonary vessels, and so flow rate, vary depending on lung volume and both alveolar and intra-pleural pressures. As the lungs expand, the intra-pleural pressure assumes more negative values - this has opposite effects on alveolar capillaries and extra-alveolar vessels. As the alveoli enlarge, their capillaries are stretched lengthwise, becoming narrower (Fig. **1**). This increases their flow resistance, as resistance is inversely related to the fourth power of capillary radius and directly proportional to capillary length; obviously, the opposite takes place as the lung volume decreases in expiration. In contrast, extra-alveolar vessels are stretch more open at large lung volumes (Fig. **1**), such

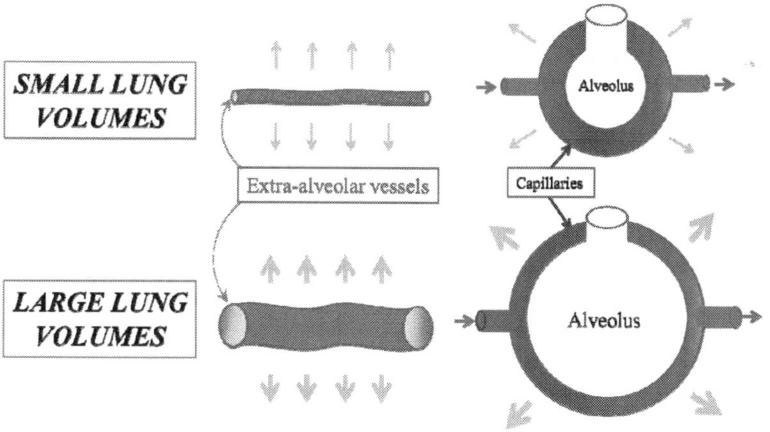

Figure 1: Lung volumes affect differently alveolar and extra-alveolar vessels. As the lungs expand, the intra-pleural pressure becomes more negative. This stretches more open the extra-alveolar vessels (arteries and veins), but narrows and lengthens the alveolar capillaries. The result is that flow resistance decreases in the former and increases in the latter.

that their flow resistance drops. In a sense we are dealing here with two resistors in series, whose lung-volume dependent changes are opposite to each other. The result of these opposing forces is that the total vascular resistance is greatest at both smallest (RV) and largest (TLC) lung volumes, and minimal at the end of a normal expiration (FRC). At RV the narrowed extra-alveolar vessels play a major role in determining the total vascular resistance, whereas at TLC the major role is played by the narrowed and elongated alveolar capillaries.

Since at rest the lungs expand during inspiration by only 250-300 ml (VT), vascular resistance changes only minimally as one breathes from FRC to FRC+VT and *vice versa*. Based on this, one would think that vascular resistance should increase during exercise, as one reaches larger lung volumes in inspiration; this is not the case, however, because in exercise the large increase in capillary recruitment, needed to accommodate for the increased pulmonary blood flow, actually causes a drop in vascular resistance.

Role of Alveolar Pressure

The pressure in the alveolar gas compartment (alveolar pressure) also plays a role in pulmonary vascular resistance. Alveolar pressure changes only slightly during normal breathing at rest, as it shifts from mildly negative during inspiration to mildly positive during expiration, but it might change dramatically as a consequence of certain lung diseases. In patients with obstructive pulmonary diseases such as COPD type A the increase in expiratory airway resistance greatly increases the alveolar pressure, and so the vascular resistance, in expiration because a larger pressure gradient between alveoli and ambient needs to be generated to create adequate gas flow. In patients suffering from asthma, chronic bronchitis or extra-thoracic airway obstruction (laryngeal cancer, for example) airway resistance is increased during both inspiration and expiration; therefore, alveolar pressure, and so vascular resistance, abnormally increases in expiration and decreases in inspiration. Other factors that play a role in determining pulmonary blood flow in these and other diseases will be discussed in Chapter 10.

Alveolar pressure is positive during both inspiration and expiration in patients ventilated by Positive End Expiratory Pressure (PEEP) ventilators. While this method is very useful in many cases to prevent alveolar collapse and consequential conductive blood shunt at small lung volumes, one should be aware that PEEP may increase pulmonary vascular resistance, and so right ventricular work-load, due to compression of alveolar capillaries.

Role of Blood Flow

Other factors that play a role in pulmonary vascular resistance are blood flow and pulmonary venous pressure. As blood flow increases, for example during exercise, pulmonary vascular resistance drops because capillaries un-perfused at rest, especially those at upper lung regions (due to gravity, see below), become perfused. This significantly increases the size of the vascular bed and decreases capillary flow resistance.

Similar increase in vascular bed occurs with mild increase in left atrial pressure. Left atrial pressure can be estimated by measuring the Pulmonary Capillary Wedge Pressure (PCWP; Table **1**), which is accomplished by inserting a small catheter into the pulmonary artery and wedging it with an inflatable balloon into a small arteriole. It is believed that pulmonary edema develops when PCWP reaches values greater than ~20 mmHg.

With a large increase in vascular resistance the right heart may become overloaded. If this results in increased right atrial pressure the foramen ovale may open, causing a right-to-left blood shunt (venous admixture). The foramen ovale is actually patent in ~27% of the normal population in the absence of increased right atrial pressure, but venous admixture rarely occurs because the normal inter-atrial pressure gradient favors a small left-to-right blood shunt.

Distribution of Ventilation and Blood-Perfusion

Due to gravity, alveolar ventilation and blood perfusion vary significantly among lung units. In addition to gravity, several pulmonary diseases such as emphysema, asthma, pulmonary embolism, lung collapse, pneumonia, and so on, may cause large changes in regional alveolar ventilation and/or perfusion, greatly affecting the ventilation-perfusion ratio ($\dot{V}/\dot{Q}$) and significantly altering PO_2 and PCO_2 values in blood and alveolar gas. To facilitate the understanding of the functional consequences of $\dot{V}/\dot{Q}$ abnormalities we will first describe the effects of gravity on lung perfusion and ventilation.

Effect of Gravity on Blood-Flow Distribution

Since the branches of the pulmonary vascular tree are all interconnected, lung perfusion can be equated to a column of blood (30-40 cm high) flowing through the lungs from pulmonary artery to pulmonary veins. Due to gravity, the weight of this column of blood in the erect lung considerably reduces blood pressure and perfusion rate at apical lung regions.

The gradual drop in blood perfusion from base to apex was demonstrated by John West and coworkers [1] through experiments in which radioactive xenon (^{133}Xe) was injected into the superior vena cava through a catheter. As the labeled blood perfuses the lungs, ^{133}Xe diffuses into the alveolar compartment and remains there during breath-hold. The radioactivity of different regions was measured with a scintillation counter and compared to that measured a few seconds later after the subject was asked to re-breathe in order to achieve a uniform distribution of ^{133}Xe among the alveoli. By evaluating the two scans, West and coworkers succeeded in quantifying the blood flow per unit of alveolar volume; their study demonstrated that blood flow progressively decreases from lung's base to apex (Fig. **2**).

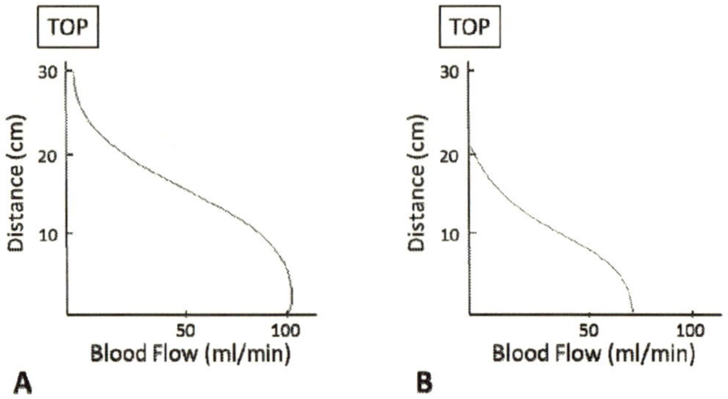

Figure 2: Gradual increase in lung perfusion from apex to base, demonstrated by perfusing isolated lungs with ^{133}Xe at normal (A) or reduced (B) pressure.

Since blood flow is affected by gravity, its distribution depends on posture. When a subject lies supine, blood flow decreases from posterior to anterior lung regions, rather than from base to apex, but the distribution is more homogeneous because the distance is shorter. However, gravity is not the only factor that affects differences in blood flow among lung regions. Another factor is the slight mismatch between the shape of the lungs and that of the chest wall - at the apex lung volume is smaller than chest volume, while at the base lung volume is greater than chest volume. The result is that alveoli are slightly stretched out at the apex and slightly compressed at the base, regardless of the subject's posture.

With mild exercise, blood flow increases in both upper and lower regions, but more so in upper regions, so that flow is more evenly distributed. In diseases that increase blood flow through the lungs (ex. left-to-right blood shunts) flow is distributed more homogeneously than in normal. With pulmonary hypertension due to increased vascular resistance, pulmonary flow is also more homogeneously distributed among lung regions. In patients with increased pulmonary venous pressure, for example in case of mitral valve stenosis, blood flow is more evenly distributed, but in later stages, when severe pulmonary hypertension develops, blood flow distribution may become inverted - flow at apex greater than at base.

The reason for the uneven blood-flow distribution was understood by analyzing data from perfusion experiments on isolated lungs [2]. The lungs were perfused with ^{133}Xe at either normal or reduced pressure. With normal pressure (~32 cm H_2O) blood flow decreased fairly linearly from base to apex, being almost zero at the apex (Fig. **2A**). With reduced pressure (~16 cm H_2O), blood flow also decreased fairly linearly, but fell to zero about 2/3 of the way up the lungs (Fig. **2B**). To account for these data, a "three-zone" model was drawn (Fig. **3**). In zone #1 arterial pressure is lower than alveolar (atmospheric) pressure, so that there is no blood flow and capillaries are collapsed (bloodless). In zone #2 arterial pressure is greater than alveolar (atmospheric) pressure, but the latter exceeds venous pressure, so that capillaries are constricted at the end, where pressure in their lumen is lowest. In zone #3 venous pressure is greater than alveolar (atmospheric), so that capillaries are open and flow is determined by the gradient between arterial and venous pressures. The three-zone model is generally attributed to John West [2], but actually it was published two year earlier by Solbert Permutt and coworkers [3].

In most subjects, a zone #4 is also observed when the subject stands in upright position. In zone #4, which is in the lower lung regions circulation is reduced because the weight of the lungs compresses small vessels.

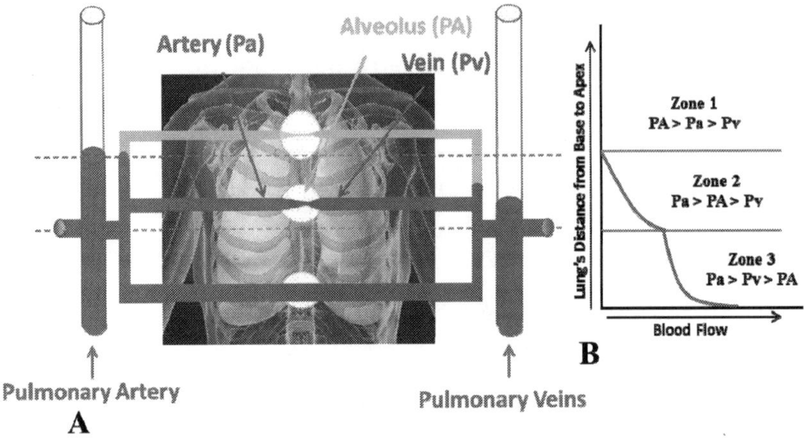

Figure 3: Pressure gradients among alveolar (PA, same as atmospheric), arterial (Pa) and venous (Pv) compartments (A) determine the extent of alveolar blood perfusion. In lungs perfused with ^{133}Xe at half-normal pressure (A), flow is absent at apex, reduced at mid-lung and normal at base (B). Lungs image from Microsoft PowerPoint's Clip Art.

Effect of Gravity on Ventilation Distribution

Ventilation is also uneven in the erect subject due to gravity. Because of the weight of the lungs, the intra-pleural pressure is more negative at the apex than at the base. This causes the upper alveoli to be more expanded (Fig. **4A**) than the lower ones (Fig. **4B**). Consequently, the two operate in different regions of their compliance curve (Fig. **4C**), such that upper alveoli are less compliant that lower ones and expand less during inspiration. This is due to the non-linearity of the compliance curve (Fig. **4C**) - with the same pressure gradient the alveoli at the base expand more than those at the apex because they operate along a more compliant (steeper) region of the compliance curve. The result of this is that at the bottom of upright lungs there is more ventilation per unit alveolar volume than at the apex.

The difference in ventilation among lung regions was demonstrated by West and coworkers through experiments with ^{133}Xe re-breathing (reviewed in [1]). A subject was asked to breathe in and out of a bag that contained ^{133}Xe, while the radioactivity was simultaneously monitored in different lung regions. After a few breaths the count rate achieved steady state as ^{133}Xe equilibrated throughout the lungs-bag-system. The difference between apex and base in terms of first VT, rate of ^{133}Xe equilibration and volumes at FRC, TLC and RV is shown in Fig. **5** and Table **2**.

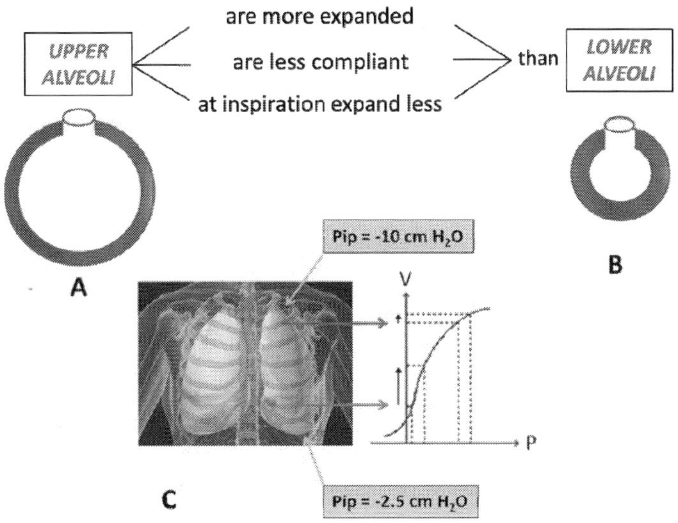

Figure 4: The weight of the lungs causes apical (A) and basal (B) alveoli to differ in size, compliance and expandability. They operate at different levels of the compliance curve (C, right) as they are subjected to different intra-pleural pressures (Pip) – with the same pressure increments, upper alveoli expand less than lower alveoli (C). Lungs image from Microsoft PowerPoint's Clip Art.

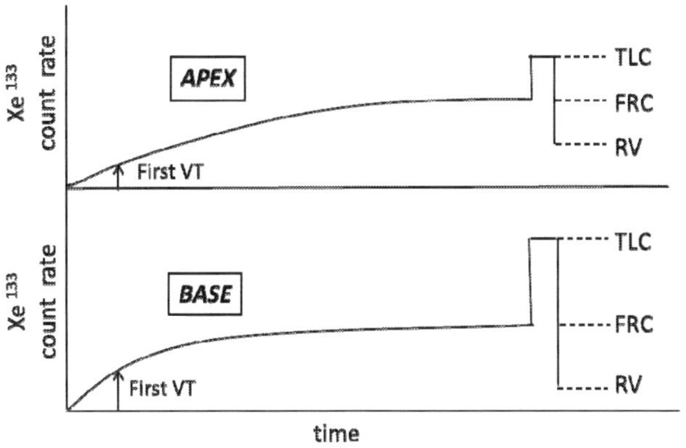

Figure 5: Differences in lung volume between apex and base measured in ^{133}Xe re-breathing experiments. The first VT and the volume increment from FRC to TLC are greater in basal alveoli, whereas FRC and RV are greater in apical alveoli, as apical alveoli are less compliant (more stretched out) than basal alveoli.

Table 2: Volume differences between lung apex and base

	First VT	Vol. at FRC	Vol. at RV	Vol. at TLC - Vol. at FRC
Apex	Small	Big	Big	Small
Base	Big	Small	Small	Big

Effect of Gravity on Regional Ventilation-Perfusion Ratios

Both blood flow and ventilation decrease approximately linearly with distance from base to apex (Fig. **6**), but the drop in blood flow is considerably greater than that of ventilation, such that alveoli at the base are **much more perfused** and more ventilated than those of the apex. Conversely, the alveoli at the apex are **much less perfused** and less ventilated than those of the base. Therefore, regional $\dot{V}/\dot{Q}$ ratios increase from base to apex, ranging from ~0.6 at the base to ~3 at the apex (Fig. **6**). In other words, the alveoli at the base of the lungs are excessively perfused with respect to the amount of ventilation they receive, so that in effect they are hypoventilated (low $\dot{V}/\dot{Q}$ regions). Conversely, the alveoli at the apex are excessively ventilated for the amount of blood perfusion they receive, so that in effect they are hyperventilated (high $\dot{V}/\dot{Q}$ regions).

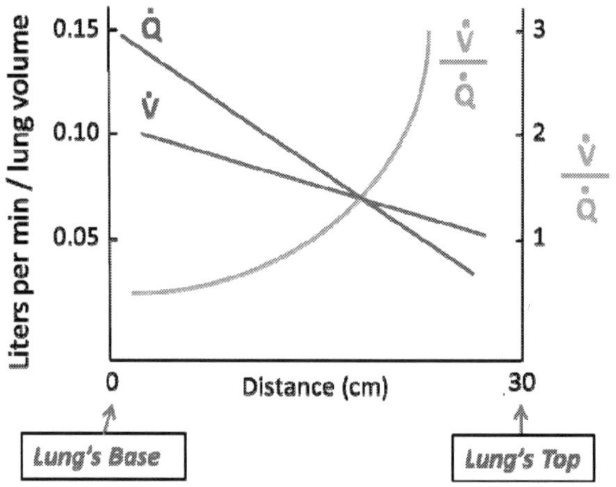

Figure 6: Both perfusion ($\dot{Q}$) and ventilation ($\dot{V}$) decrease from the base to the top of the lung, but $\dot{Q}$ drops more steeply, such that $\dot{V}/\dot{Q}$ progressively increases from base to top.

As a result of this $\dot{V}/\dot{Q}$ maldistribution (Table **3**):

Table 3: Effect of $\dot{V}/\dot{Q}$ maldistribution on regional PO_2 and PCO_2

In Upper Lung Regions	In Lower Lung Regions
High $\dot{V}/\dot{Q}$	Low $\dot{V}/\dot{Q}$
Low PCO_2	High PCO_2
High PO_2	Low PO_2

These differences in regional PCO_2 and PO_2 (Fig. **7C and D**) affect the O_2- and CO_2-contents of corresponding end-capillary blood, as well as regional O_2 uptake, CO_2 release and R values.

Thus, with respect to well matched (ideal) $\dot{V}/\dot{Q}$ units (Table **4**):

Table 4: Effect of maldistribution on high and low $\dot{V}/\dot{Q}$ units as compared to ideal units.

In High $\dot{V}/\dot{Q}$ Units	In Low $\dot{V}/\dot{Q}$ Units
Small increase in O_2 uptake/unit blood	Small decrease in O_2 uptake/unit blood
Large increase in CO_2 release/unit blood	Large decrease in CO_2 release/unit blood
High exchange ratio (R)	Low exchange ratio (R)
pH > 7.4	pH < 7.4
$PCO_2 < 40$, $PO_2 > 100$	$PCO_2 > 40$, $PO_2 < 100$

The reason for different O_2 uptake and CO_2 release in high *versus* low $\dot{V}/\dot{Q}$ units can be understood by examining the curves that plot O_2 and CO_2 partial pressures against O_2 and CO_2 blood contents (O_2 and CO_2 pressure-content curves; Fig. **7A** and **B**). Due to the progressive decrease in steepness of the slope of the O_2 dissociation curve, as Hb approaches saturation, relatively large PO_2 increments have relatively small effects on O_2 uptake per unit blood - they increase only slightly the O_2 content at $PO_2 > 50$ mmHg. In contrast, due to the steeper and more linear (total) CO_2 dissociation curve (Fig. **7A** and **B**), changes in PCO_2 have a great effect on the volume of CO_2 released per unit blood.

By plotting regional PO_2 and PCO_2 values on the O_2-CO_2 diagram (Fig. **8**) one sees that the alveolar gas composition of high $\dot{V}/\dot{Q}$ regions approaches that of inspired air (I), while the composition of low $\dot{V}/\dot{Q}$ regions approaches that of mixed venous blood ($\bar{v}$). The curved line that joins $\bar{v}$ to I (Fig. **8A**) is known as the "ventilation-perfusion ratio line" ($\dot{V}/\dot{Q}$ line). Its path is determined by the large spectrum of regional PO_2 and PCO_2 values, which range from those of mixed venous blood ($\bar{v}$) to those of inspired air (I) - its curved shape is due to the different shapes of O_2 and CO_2 dissociation curves (Fig. **7**).

From the inspired gas point (I), a family of straight lines of different steepness originate (Fig. **8B**).

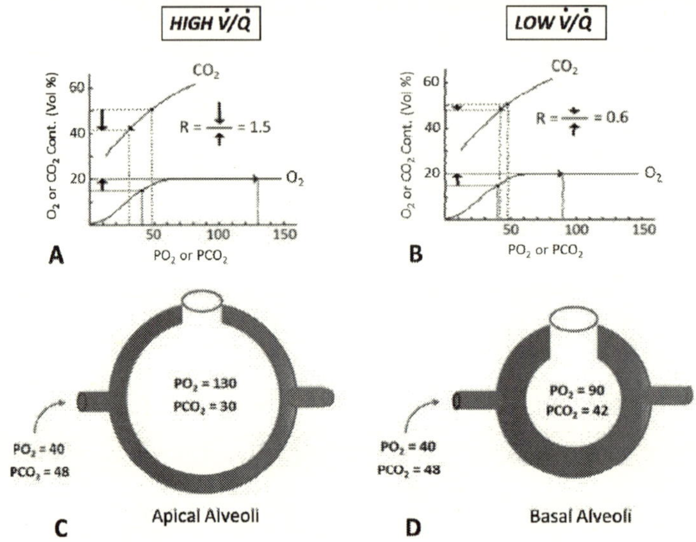

Figure 7: The difference in shape between the O_2 and CO_2 curves that plot partial pressures *versus* blood contents (A and B) causes R and PO_2 to be significantly higher (and PCO_2 lower) in apical (A and C) than basal (B and D) alveoli.

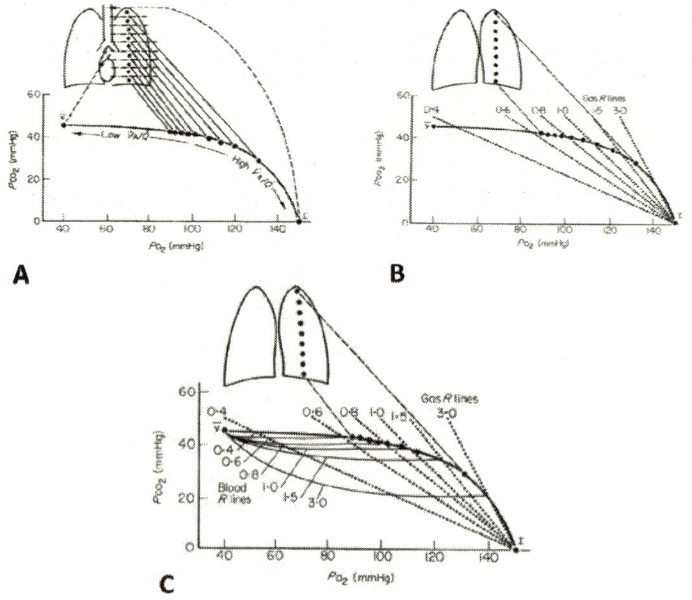

Figure 8: A. $\dot{V}/\dot{Q}$ line plotting gradual changes in PO_2 and PCO_2 from lung's base to apex. B. Gas R-lines; note the gradual increase in exchange ratios from lung's base to apex. C. Blood R-lines; unlike gas R-lines, blood R-lines are curved because of the "S" shape of the O_2 dissociation curve –

due to hemoglobin, in blood pressures and contents are not linearly related. From: West, J.B., Ventilation/blood flow and gas exchange. 3rd Edition, Blackwell Scientific Publications, Osney Mead, Oxford, UK, 1977. Reproduced with permission granted by John Wiley & sons, Inc.

They are the **gas R-lines**, which correspond to exchange ratios of regional alveolar gas compartments (low and high R values correspond to low and high $\dot{V}/\dot{Q}$ regions, respectively). Note that the alveoli of the base operate at low exchange ratios ($R < 0.8$), whereas those of the apex operate at high ratios ($R > 0.8$; Fig. **8B**).

Another family of lines (Fig. **8C**) originates from the mixed venous point ($\bar{v}$); these are the **blood R-lines**. They correspond to the exchange ratios of regional alveolar compartments viewed from the blood side of the alveolar wall. Each line corresponds to a group of alveoli in which the ratio between the volume of CO_2 diffusing out of blood and the volume of O_2 diffusing into blood is as indicated. Note that, as we have seen for the gas R-lines, alveoli with low $\dot{V}/\dot{Q}$ operate along blood R-lines with low R values, whereas alveoli with high $\dot{V}/\dot{Q}$ operate along blood R-lines with high R values (Fig. **8B** and **C**).

In each group of alveoli, both blood and gas R values are the same – each gas R-line meets its corresponding blood R-line at the $\dot{V}/\dot{Q}$ ratio line (Fig. **8C**). The reason for it is that in any particular lung unit the ratio between the volume of CO_2 that enters the alveoli and the volume of O_2 that exits the alveoli (gas R) is obviously the same as the ratio between the volume of CO_2 that exits from the capillary blood and the volume of O_2 that enters the capillary blood (blood R).

Hemoglobin is an Oxygen Buffer

One may ask: why are the gas R-lines straight and the blood R-lines curved? The gas R-lines are straight because in the gas compartment O_2 and CO_2 contents (fractional concentrations) are linearly related to PO_2 and PCO_2 (partial pressures) – at any point in the R line a pressure increment always results in the same content increment. The blood R-lines are curved because in the blood compartment O_2 contents and pressures are not linearly related due to the presence of hemoglobin, whose O_2 dissociation curve is not linear but S-shaped, like buffers; indeed, hemoglobin is an O_2 buffer (Fig. **9A**, bottom).

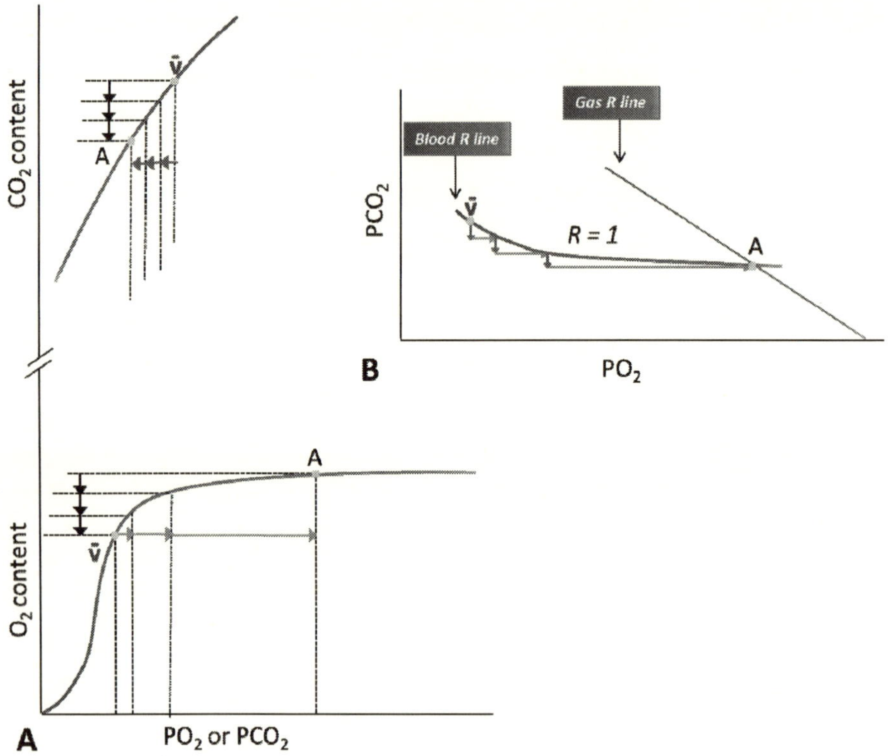

Figure 9: The blood R-line (B) is curved because of the S-shape of the O_2-dissociation curve (A, bottom). In this example, which deals with alveoli with R = 1, one sees that equal changes in O_2 and CO_2 content (A, black arrows) are not matched by equal changes in PO_2 and PCO_2 (A and B, green and blue arrows, respectively) such that the blood R-line becomes progressively flatter as PO_2 increases (B). Note that while the O_2 content is mostly Hb-associated O_2 (A, bottom) the CO_2 content (A, top) represents the total CO_2.

To visualize the phenomenon, imagine that you are navigating along an alveolar capillary on board of a red blood cell. The gradual changes in PO_2 and PCO_2 that you would experience as a result of gas exchange would correspond to those plotted along the blood R-line, as the red blood cell flows from point $\bar{v}$ to point A (Fig. 9B). If in that alveolus the exchange ratio is one (R = 1, Fig. **9B**), the volume of O_2 diffusing into the blood per unit time will be the same as the volume of CO_2 exiting from it - PO_2 will increase and PCO_2 will decrease following the line with R = 1 ($\dot{V}CO_2/\dot{V}O_2 = 1$). Note that the R-line is steep at first and becomes flatter and almost parallel to the X-axis as PO_2 increases and PCO_2 decreases (Fig. **9B**). The steep portion of the R-line corresponds to a region in which the O_2- and

CO_2-dissociation curves have similar steepness (Fig. **9A**), whereas the flatter portion of the R-line corresponds to a region in which the O_2- and CO_2-dissociation curves differ drastically in steepness (Fig. **9A**) - while the CO_2 curve is still steep (Fig. **9A** top) the O_2-dissociation curve is almost flat (Fig. **9A** bottom), as hemoglobin is almost fully saturated with O_2. Therefore, in this region an increment in O_2 content corresponds to a relatively large increase in PO_2, whereas a drop in CO_2 content by the same amount corresponds to a much smaller drop in PCO_2 (Fig. **9A**).

Ventilation-Perfusion Distribution – Effect on Gas Exchange

In the absence of ventilation-perfusion maldistribution (mismatch), average alveolar gas ($\bar{A}$) and arterial blood (a) would have almost the same PO_2 and PCO_2 values - PaO_2 would only be slightly lower than $P\bar{A}O_2$ due to the normal 2-4% anatomical (conductive) right-to-left blood shunt. Because of gravity, however, even in normal subjects there is a small amount of $\dot{V}/\dot{Q}$ maldistribution that generates small fractions of alveolar dead space ventilation and shunt-like effect - the former causes $P\bar{A}O_2$ to be slightly higher than $PAiO_2$ (and $P\bar{A}CO_2$ slightly lower than $PaCO_2$), and the latter causes a further drop in PaO_2 from $PAiO_2$.

The effect of gravity on $\dot{V}/\dot{Q}$ maldistribution in normal people is exemplified in Fig. **10**, which demonstrates how maldistribution generates small amounts of shunt-like effect and alveolar dead space even in the absence of alveoli with $\dot{V}/\dot{Q} = 0$ (conductive shunt) or $\dot{V}/\dot{Q} = \infty$ (alveolar dead space). In the example of Fig. **10**, the lungs are divided into three regions with different $\dot{V}/\dot{Q}$ ratios, simulating lung's base, mid-portion and apex. The base has a relatively low $\dot{V}/\dot{Q}$ (0.83); in the mid-portion $\dot{V}$ and $\dot{Q}$ are well matched ($\dot{V}/\dot{Q} = 1$); the apex has a relatively high $\dot{V}/\dot{Q}$ (1.5). Note, however, that in spite of regional maldistributions, the whole system has $\dot{V}/\dot{Q} = 1$, as both $\dot{V}\bar{A}$ and $\dot{Q}$ are 6 l/min. This is important to realize, because it shows that the total $\dot{V}/\dot{Q}$ ratio has little meaning, as it could be normal even in cases of severe regional $\dot{V}/\dot{Q}$ maldistribution. What really counts in terms gas exchange is not the total $\dot{V}/\dot{Q}$ ratio but rather the extent of regional $\dot{V}/\dot{Q}$ aberrations. To illustrate how irrelevant is the total $\dot{V}/\dot{Q}$ ratio, consider an absurd condition in which the right lung is perfused ($\dot{Q} = 5$ l/min) but unventilated $\left(\dot{V}/\dot{Q} = 0\right)$ and the left lung is ventilated

($\dot{V}$ = 5 l/min) but unperfused ($\dot{V}/\dot{Q} = \infty$). This "impossible lung" with perfect ratio ($\dot{V}/\dot{Q} = 1$) would result in 100% alveolar dead space and 100% shunt, which is obviously incompatible with life.

In Fig. **10**, blood coming from the base has an O_2 content of 19.57 vol%; that from the mid-portion: 19.83 vol%; and that from the apex: 20.22 vol% (see **Appendix 2, A** for calculations). The weighted average of the O_2 content of the three regions is the content of the mixed arterial blood (19.77 vol%), which corresponds to a PaO_2 of ~98 mmHg. The weighted average of the alveolar PO_2 ($P\bar{A}O_2$) is 103 mmHg (see **Appendix 2, A**). Thus, in spite of the absence of true shunt $(\dot{V}/\dot{Q} = 0)$ and true alveolar dead space $(\dot{V}/\dot{Q} = \infty)$ there is a gradient between mixed alveolar and arterial PO_2 values: $(\bar{A} - a)PO_2$= 103 – 98 = 5 mmHg, which is due to the heterogeneity of $\dot{V}/\dot{Q}$ ratios throughout the system. The $(\bar{A} - a)PO_2$ gradient results from to two separate effects of the heterogeneous $\dot{V}/\dot{Q}$ distribution: a dead-space-like effect, caused by the high $\dot{V}/\dot{Q}$ regions, which increases PO_2 and decrease PCO_2 of mixed alveolar ($\bar{A}$) gas with respect to that of ideal (Ai) gas, and a shunt-like effect, caused by the low $\dot{V}/\dot{Q}$ regions, which decreases PaO_2 with respect to that of ideal gas ($PAiO_2$).

Note that both O_2-content (19.77 vol%) and PO_2 (98 mmHg) of arterial blood are closer to those of the low $\dot{V}/\dot{Q}$ region (19.57 vol% and 90 mmHg, respectively) than to those of the high $\dot{V}/\dot{Q}$ regions (20.22 vol% and 130 mmHg, respectively). The reason for this is that 50% of the blood (3/6 of $\dot{Q}$) perfuses low $\dot{V}/\dot{Q}$ regions, whereas only ~17% (1/6 of $\dot{Q}$) perfuses high $\dot{V}/\dot{Q}$ regions. Therefore, high $\dot{V}/\dot{Q}$ regions do not effectively compensate for low $\dot{V}/\dot{Q}$ regions. In other words, high $\dot{V}/\dot{Q}$ regions have only a minimal effect in reducing the shunt fraction caused by the low $\dot{V}/\dot{Q}$ regions.

In this example, the $\dot{V}/\dot{Q}$ maldistribution results in a maldistribution shunt-like effect of only 1.6% of the total $\dot{Q}$ and an alveolar dead space fraction $(\dot{V}Ad/\dot{V}\bar{A})$ of only 1% of the total alveolar ventilation (Fig. **10**; for calculations see Appendix **2, A**). Note that these are equivalent values of shunt and alveolar dead space fractions, because in this example there is no true blood shunt (alveoli perfused but unventilated) and no true alveolar dead space (alveoli ventilated but unperfused).

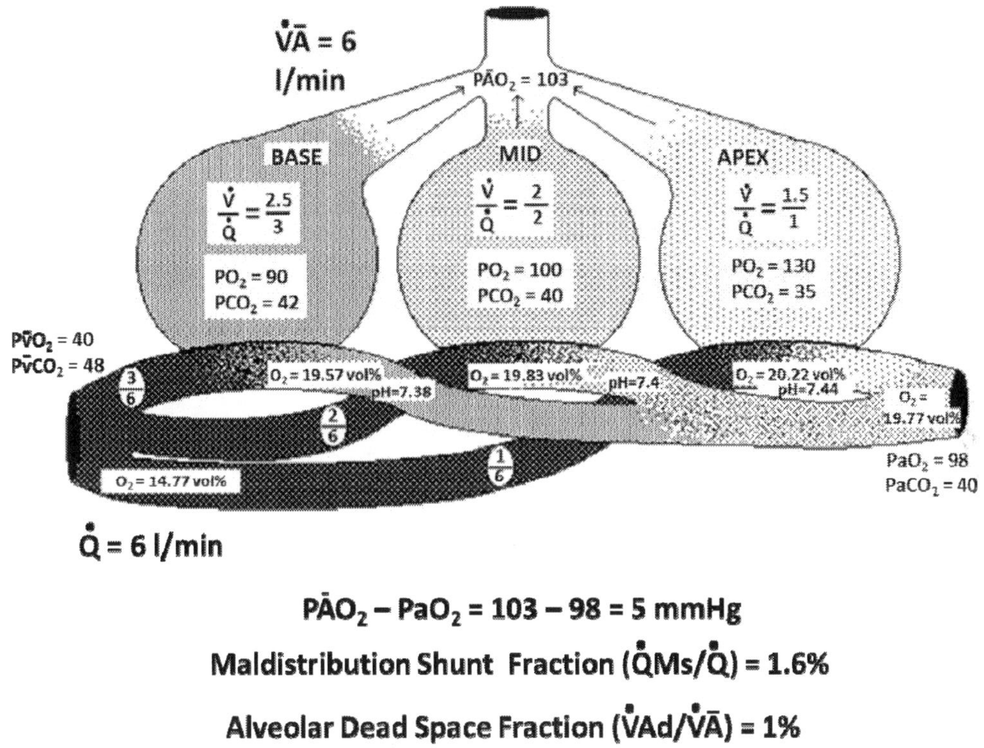

Figure 10: Example of the effect of $\dot{V}/\dot{Q}$ maldistribution on blood shunt and alveolar dead space in a normal subject standing erect - effect of gravity on regional pulmonary ventilation and perfusion.

Functional Equivalent of the Real Lung

In the example described above (Fig. **10**) we were able to estimate the fraction of both maldistribution shunt-like effect and alveolar dead space because we knew the gas and blood values in the three lung regions. This, of course, is not the case in real life, because for evaluating patients suspected of $\dot{V}/\dot{Q}$ maldistribution, all we have available are data from arterial blood (a), mixed alveolar gas ($\bar{A}$) and mixed venous blood ($\bar{v}$)**.** So, how can we evaluate a patient in terms of blood shunt, maldistribution shunt-like effect, diffusion impairment, and alveolar dead space if we don't know regional values of blood and gas compositions? We can do so by simplifying the real lung into a "functional equivalent lung", known as the "three-compartment-model" (see below).

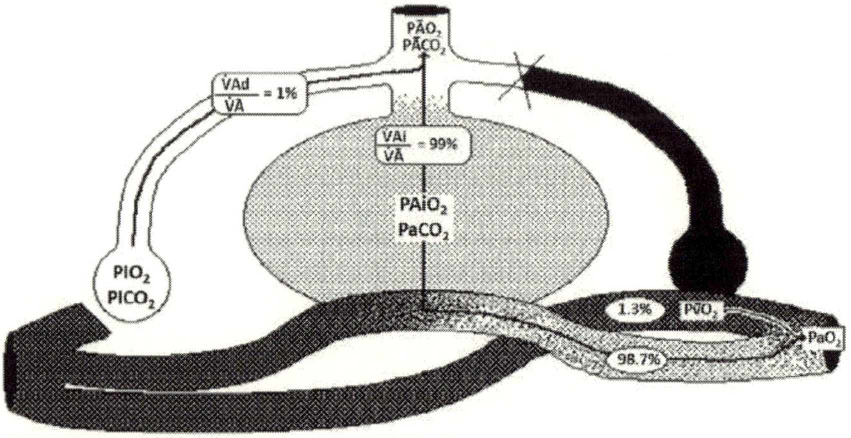

$$PAiCO_2 = PaCO_2$$

$$PAiO_2 = PIO_2 - \frac{1 - FIO_2(1 - R)}{R}\,PaCO_2$$

Figure 11: "Three-compartment-model". The regional $\dot{V}/\dot{Q}$ maldistribution shown in Figs. **7-10** is here simplified into a functionally equivalent three-compartment-model, which contains: an ideal (center), a shunt (right; $\dot{V}/\dot{Q} = 0$) and an alveolar dead space (left; $\dot{V}/\dot{Q} = \infty$) compartment.

The lungs contain as many as half a billion alveoli, each with its particular $\dot{V}/\dot{Q}$ ratio, such that most of them contribute differently to blood shunt or alveolar dead space. In normal people the vast majority of the alveoli have $\dot{V}/\dot{Q}$ ratios very close to ideal values, so that regional $\dot{V}/\dot{Q}$ aberrations minimally contribute to shunt and alveolar dead space, such that the fractions of maldistribution shunt-like effect and alveolar dead space ventilation are only 1-2% of $\dot{Q}$ and $V\overline{A}$, respectively. In contrast, in patients with lung diseases there might be large $\dot{V}/\dot{Q}$ mismatches, causing significant amounts of shunted blood and/or alveolar dead space ventilation.

In the late sixties, John West and coworkers [4] developed a clever method for determining regional distributions of ventilation and perfusion which involves the intravenous injection of a number of inert gases. This powerful method, however, is not easily applicable to patients on a routine basis; but, in most cases one does not need to have a detailed knowledge of regional $\dot{V}/\dot{Q}$ ratios for evaluating a patient's gas exchange efficiency, because what counts is the functional equivalent of the real-lung's $\dot{V}/\dot{Q}$ aberrations.

The "Three-Compartment-Model"

Riley and Cournand [5] have developed a way of simplifying the real lung, with its large range of $\dot{V}/\dot{Q}$ ratios, into a model that divides the lungs into three compartments: alveolar ideal, shunt, and alveolar dead space (Figs. **11** and **12**).

The alveolar ideal compartment (Ai) is defined as the lung region whose alveoli have an exchange ratio (R) identical to the cellular respiratory quotient (R = RQ), and whose PCO_2 is virtually the same as the arterial PCO_2 ($PAiCO_2 \approx PaCO_2$); in this compartment ventilation and perfusion are perfectly matched ($\dot{V}/\dot{Q} = 0.85-1$; Fig. **11**, center), such that gas exchange occurs at maximal efficiency.

The shunt compartment is a region where gas partial pressures and contents are identical to those of mixed venous blood ($\bar{v}$), as if alveoli were perfused but unventilated ($\dot{V}/\dot{Q} = 0$; Fig. **11**, right).

The alveolar dead space compartment is a region where partial pressures are identical to ambient air (at BTPS), as if alveoli were ventilated but unperfused ($\dot{V}/\dot{Q} = \infty$; Fig. **11**, left).

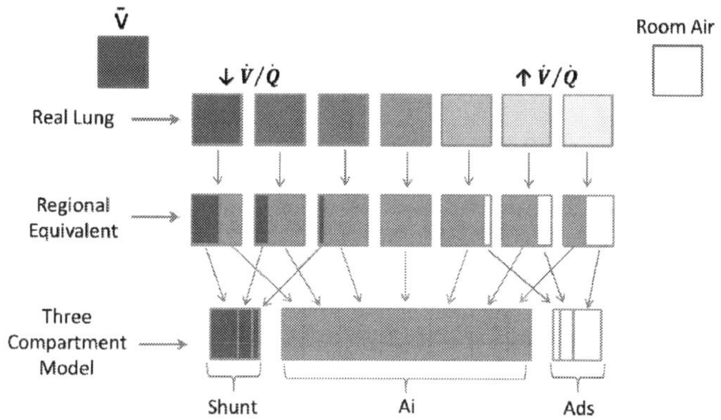

Figure 12: Schematic representation of how the real lung is converted into an equivalent "three-compartment-model. Regional $\dot{V}/\dot{Q}$ maldistributions ($\downarrow \dot{V}/\dot{Q}$, left, and $\uparrow \dot{V}/\dot{Q}$, right) contribute by different fractions to alveolar ideal (Ai), shunt, and alveolar dead space (Ads) compartments.

In a sense, the model simplifies the complexity of the real lung by lumping together the partial contributions of regional $\dot{V}/\dot{Q}$ mismatches to shunt, alveolar dead space and ideal gas exchange, into three virtual compartments: shunt, dead space, and alveolar ideal (Fig. **11**). Fig. **12** schematically describes how the real lung is converted into its functional equivalent three-compartment model. Note that in the equivalent model (Fig. **11** and **12**) any difference between $PAiO_2$ and PaO_2 is due to the mixing of shunted blood ($P\bar{v}O_2$) with blood from the ideal exchanger ($PAiO_2$). Similarly, any difference between $PaCO_2$ and $P\bar{A}CO_2$ (or $PAiO_2$ and $P\bar{A}O_2$) is due to the mixing of gases from the dead space compartment (room air, with $PICO_2 = 0$) with gases from the ideal alveolar exchanger (with $PAiO_2$ and $PaCO_2$). Thus, one can see that the $(Ai - a)PO_2$ gradient reflects the magnitude of shunted blood, the $(Ai - \bar{A})PO_2$ or PCO_2 gradient reflects the magnitude of alveolar dead space ventilation, and the total $(\bar{A} - a)PO_2$ or PCO_2 gradient reflects the combined effect of shunt and alveolar dead space (Figs. **11** and **13**).

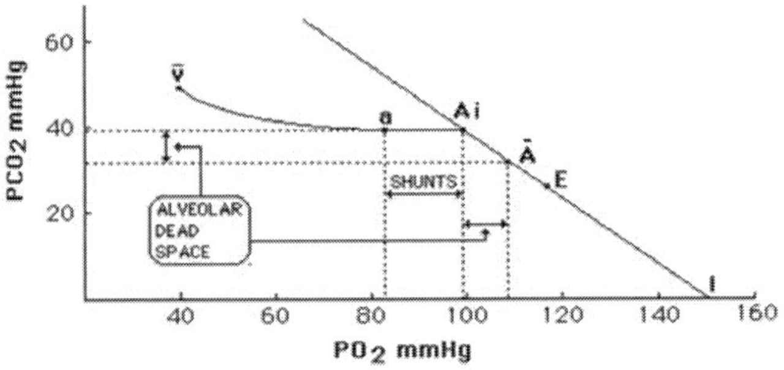

Figure 13: The effect of right-to-left blood shunts and alveolar dead space ventilation on arterial (a) and mixed alveolar ($\bar{A}$) PO_2 and PCO_2 are shown on the PO_2-PCO_2 diagram. Shunts cause a drop in PO_2 from ideal (Ai) to arterial (a) blood, but affect minimally PCO_2 ($PaO_2 \neq PAiO_2$, $PaCO_2 \approx PAiCO_2$). The (Ai-a)PO_2 gradient is entirely due to shunts, whereas the (Ai-$\bar{A}$)PO_2 and (Ai-$\bar{A}$)PCO_2 gradients are entirely due to alveolar dead space ventilation.

How is the Three-Compartment-Model Used for Evaluating Gas-Exchange Efficiency?

To evaluate a patient by means of the three compartment model it is not sufficient to have data from arterial blood (a) and mixed alveolar gas ($\bar{A}$, end tidal) samples, one also needs to know the blood and gas composition of the alveolar ideal compartment (Ai). Obviously, this compartment cannot be sampled, but fortunately its composition can be estimated by capitalizing on the fact that, in spite of blood shunts, alveolar ideal (Ai) and arterial (a) PCO_2 are virtually the same ($PAiCO_2 \approx PaCO_2$), due to the fact that the blood R-line becomes progressively flatter (horizontal) as PO_2 increases (Fig. **13**). In contrast, this is not true for PO_2, as PaO_2 is always lower than $PAiO_2$ ($PAiO_2 \neq PaO_2$, Fig. **13**) due to blood shunts, present even in normal subjects, which affect PO_2 much more than O_2-content when the system operates along the flatter region of the O_2 dissociation curve (Fig. **9A**).

The fact that $PAiCO_2 \approx PaCO_2$ is a **cardinal element** of respiratory physiology because it enables one to quantify PO_2 and O_2-content of the alveolar ideal compartment ($PAiO_2$ and $CAiO_2$, respectively). In turn, this enables us to evaluate individually and quite precisely the "equivalent" magnitudes of right-to-left blood shunt and alveolar dead space ventilation (see below).

Thus, by means of the alveolar gas equation (Eqs. 1 and 2; see Chapter 3) one can calculate $PAiO_2$ and with that the O_2 content of the alveolar ideal compartment:

$$PAiO_2 = PIO_2 - \frac{1-FIO_2(1-R)}{R} - PaCO_2 \ldots \quad \textbf{(1)}$$

In the example of Fig. **10**, using the following values: PB = 760 mmHg; PH_2O = 47 (37°C), FIO_2 = 0.2094, R = 0.8 and $PaCO_2$ = 40 mmHg, $PAiO_2$ is:

$$PAiO_2 = (760 - 47)0.2094 - \frac{1-0.2094(1-0.8)}{0.8} - 40 = 101 \text{ mmHg} \ldots \quad \textbf{(2)}$$

By comparing $PAiO_2$ to PaO_2 (Eq. 3) one notices a difference of:

$$(Ai - a)PO_2 = 101 - 98 = 3 \text{ mmHg} \ldots \quad \textbf{(3)}$$

This $(Ai\text{-}a)PO_2$ gradient is entirely due to maldistribution shunt-like effect (low $\dot{V}/\dot{Q}$ regions), and is completely unaffected by the presence of alveolar dead space (Figs. **11** and **12**).

By comparing $P\bar{A}O_2$ to $PAiO_2$ (Eq. 4) one notices a difference of:

$$(\bar{A} - Ai)PO_2 = 103 - 101 = 2 \text{ mmHg} \ldots \quad \textbf{(4)}$$

This difference is entirely due to alveolar dead space and is completely unaffected by the presence of shunts (Fig. **11**).

The total PO_2 gradient (Eq. 5)

$$(\bar{A} - a)PO_2 = 103 - 98 = 5 \text{ mmHg} \ldots \tag{5}$$

results from both alveolar dead space ventilation and maldistribution shunt-like effect.

CALCULATION OF SHUNT FRACTION

Assume that you are in the intensive care unit (ICU) and have been asked to evaluate a patient with a respiratory problem. The questions you need to answer are: is there an abnormal physiological (total) right-to-left blood shunt fraction ($\dot{Q}Ps/\dot{Q}$)? If so, how much of it is due to $\dot{V}/\dot{Q}$ maldistribution ($\dot{Q}Ms/\dot{Q}$)? How much is due to conductive (anatomical) shunt ($\dot{Q}Cs/\dot{Q}$)? Is there alveolar dead space ventilation? *For shunt calculation see **Appendix 2, B and C**.*

The following data are available (**Table 5**):

Table 5: Laboratory blood and gas data (***PB*** 760 mmHg, ***Hb*** 15g/100 ml blood)

PaO_2, mmHg	80	pHa	7.42
$PaCO_2$, mmHg	35	R	0.8
$P\bar{A}CO_2$, mmHg	30	$(Ca - C\bar{v})O_2$, vol%	5

Just looking at the data what can you tell?

- There is moderate hypoxemia (PaO_2 = 80 mmHg), which is not due to hypoventilation because $PaCO_2$ = 35 mmHg.
- The $PaCO_2$ value indicates mild hyperventilation, which is compensatory to hypoxemia.
- The presence of hypoxemia in spite of hyperventilation indicates that there is abnormal shunt, maldistribution shunt-like effect and/or diffusion impairment - however, note that it would be normal if the

subject were breathing a low PIO_2 gas mixture, for example breathing at high altitude. This, however, is not the case because PB = 760 mmHg.

- $P\bar{A}CO_2$ differs from $PaCO_2$; this proves that there is alveolar dead space ventilation - in normal subjects $P\bar{A}CO_2$ is virtually the same as $PaCO_2$ because there is minimal alveolar dead space ventilation.

- Hb is normal - no anemia.

- pHa is normal

- R is normal, indicating that respiration is at pace with metabolic rate (steady state condition).

- O_2 extraction, $(Ca - C\bar{v})O_2$, is normal (normal $\dot{V}O_2/\dot{Q}$ ratio).

Calculation of Physiological Shunt Fraction

As discussed above, for calculating the shunt fraction we use the "three-compartment-model" (Fig. **14**) of the real lung, in which the cardiac output ($\dot{Q}$), the total volume of blood flowing through the lung per minute (Eq. 6), is assumed to come from two sources: the alveolar ideal compartment ($\dot{Q}Ai$) and the shunt compartment ($\dot{Q}Ps$), which comprises all types of shunt: alveolar (alveoli with low $\dot{V}A/\dot{Q}$, alveoli with $\dot{V}A/\dot{Q} = 0$, and alveoli with diffusion impairment) and extra alveolar shunts:

$$\dot{Q} = \dot{Q}Ai + \dot{Q}Ps \ ... \qquad \textbf{(6)}$$

Similarly, the total volume of O_2 flowing per minute ($\dot{Q} \times CaO_2$; Eq. 7) is the sum of the O_2 content of the two components of $\dot{Q}$:

$$\dot{Q} \times CaO_2 = \dot{Q}Ai \times CAiO_2 + \dot{Q}Ps \times C\bar{v}O_2 \ ... \qquad \textbf{(7)}$$

Since $\dot{Q}Ai$ is cardiac output ($\dot{Q}$) minus physiological shut ($\dot{Q}Ps$; Eq. 8)

$$\dot{Q}Ai = \dot{Q} - \dot{Q}Ps \ ... \qquad \textbf{(8)}$$

by substituting and solving for the physiological shunt fraction ($\dot{Q}Ps/\dot{Q}$) one obtains Equation 9:

$$\frac{\dot{Q}Ps}{\dot{Q}} = \frac{CAiO_2 - CaO_2}{CAiO_2 - C\bar{v}O_2} \ldots \quad \textbf{(9)}$$

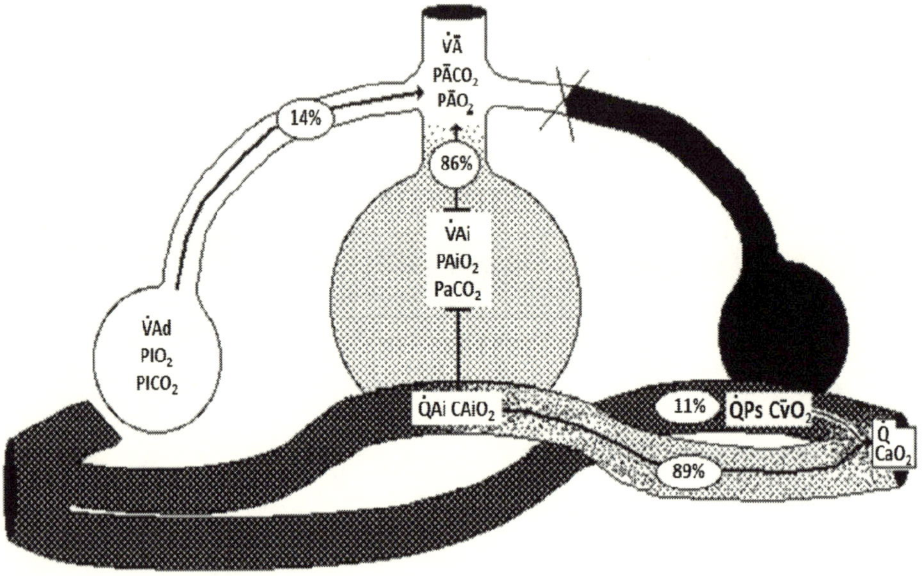

Figure 14: Three Compartment Model. Functional equivalent of diseased lungs that cause 11% physiological shunt ($\dot{\mathbf{Q}}\mathbf{Ps}/\dot{\mathbf{Q}}$) and 14% alveolar dead space ($\dot{\mathbf{V}}\mathbf{Ad}/\dot{\mathbf{V}}\bar{\mathbf{A}}$) fractions in the patient described in the text.

This important equation (Eq. 9) is known as the "***Shunted Blood-Flow Fraction Equation***".

In this patient, the physiological shunt fraction (Eq. 10) is:

$$\frac{\dot{Q}Ps}{\dot{Q}} = \sim 11\% \text{ (normal} = 2 - 4\%) \ldots \quad \textbf{(10)}$$

Since $PAiO_2 = \sim 107$ mmHg (calculated with the alveolar gas equation, see **Appendix 2, B**), the $(Ai\text{-}a)PO_2$ gradient (Eq. 11) is:

$$(Ai - a)PO_2 = 107 - 80 = 27 \text{ mmHg} \ldots \quad \textbf{(11)}$$

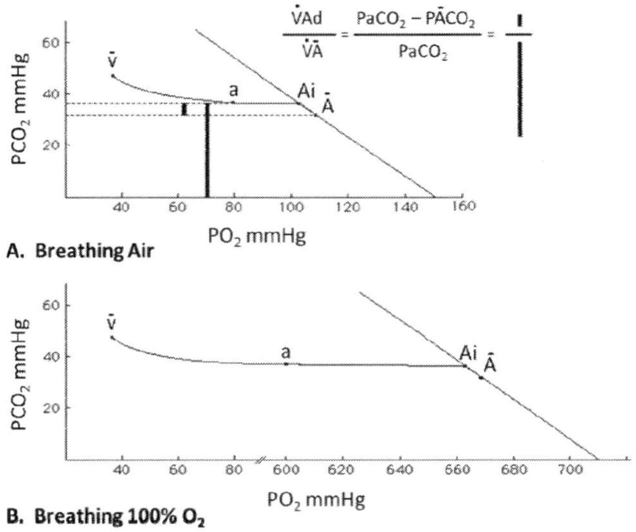

Figure 15: The (Ai-a)PO_2 gradient is a reasonable indicator of shunt magnitude only if a subject is breathing room air. In the case of the patient described in the text, with 100% FIO_2 breathing (Ai-a)PO_2 increased from 27 (A) to 73 (B) mmHg, even though the shunt fraction dropped from 11% to 4.4%. A graphic representation of $\mathbf{\dot{V}Ad/\dot{V}\bar{A}}$ is shown in A.

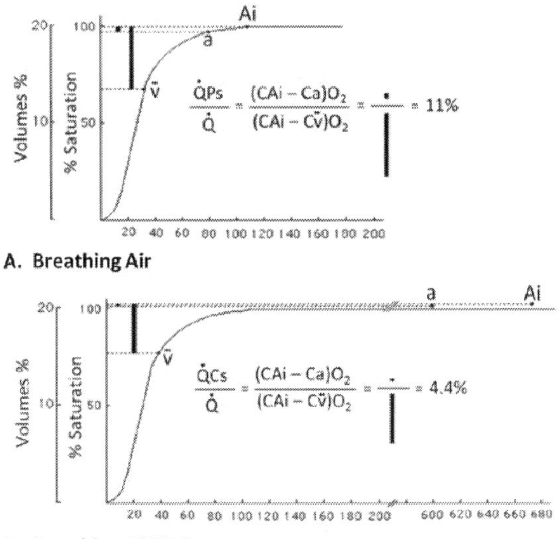

Figure 16: With 100% FIO_2 breathing (B) the system operates along the flat region of the O_2-dissociation curve. In the case of the patient described in the text, while the shunt dropped from 11% (A) to 4.4% (B), (Ai-a)PO_2 increased from 27 (A) to 73 (B) mmHg. $\mathbf{\dot{Q}Ps/\dot{Q}}$ and $\mathbf{\dot{Q}Cs/\dot{Q}}$ are shown graphically in A and B, respectively.

The normal $(Ai - a)PO_2$ gradient ranges from 2 to 6 mmHg, although in older people gradients as high as 10 mmHg are still considered within the normal range. An estimate of the normal $(Ai\text{-}a)PO_2$ can be obtained by calculating the following: (Age+10)/4.

The $(Ai - a)PO_2$ gradient is used as a reasonable indicator of the magnitude of shunt, but one must exercise some caution in interpreting its meaning in patients breathing abnormally high FIO_2 (Figs. **15** and **16**), under hypoxic environmental conditions (high altitude), or severely hypoventilating (see below).

Maldistribution-Diffusion and Anatomical (Conductive) Components of Physiological Shunt

The physiological shunt ($\dot{Q}Ps$) is the sum of several components: anatomical (conductive) shunt ($\dot{Q}Cs$), maldistribution shunt-like effect ($\dot{Q}Ms$), and venous admixture due to gas diffusion impairment (Fig. **17**). In this patient's case (Fig. **14**) we have calculated a physiological shunt fraction of 11%. But, is this shunt fraction mostly due to maldistribution and/or diffusion impairment? Is it mostly conductive shunt? Is it a combination of both?

A simple procedure allows us to differentiate between maldistribution-diffusion and conductive shunt. It involves asking the same patient to breathe 100% FIO_2 for a few minutes, sampling arterial blood during the O_2-breathing period and recalculating the shunt fraction (see Appendix **2, B and C**). This calculation gives the value of just the conductive (anatomical) shunt fraction ($\dot{Q}Cs/\dot{Q}$), because 100% FIO_2-breathing completely eliminates the effect of maldistribution and/or diffusion impairment (Fig. **17**). The reason for it is that by replacing N_2 (almost 80% of inspired air) with O_2 even alveoli with very low $\dot{V}/\dot{Q}$ ratios and/or diffusion impairment will achieve PO_2 values sufficiently high to fully saturate hemoglobin. Even though the PO_2 gradient between low $\dot{V}/\dot{Q}$ alveoli which cause maldistribution shunt-like effect and ideal alveoli will be now much greater than with air breathing (Figs. **15** and **16**), the shunt fraction will decrease because what counts in terms of shunt is not the difference in PO_2, but rather the difference in O_2-content. With 100% O_2-breathing alveoli with low $\dot{V}/\dot{Q}$ and ideal alveoli will have virtually the same O_2 content, because hemoglobin will be fully saturated in both compartments, the only difference being the content of dissolved O_2, which is negligible as the O_2 solubility in water is very low. Since shunt reflects the difference in O_2-content rather that in PO_2, a negligible content difference between low $\dot{V}/\dot{Q}$ and ideal alveoli translates into a negligible shunt fraction.

In contrast, anatomical (conductive) shunts are not affected at all by 100% FIO_2-breathing, because they occur in regions unexposed to 100% FIO_2. Obviously, this is also the case in completely unventilated alveoli ($\dot{V}/\dot{Q} = 0$) - alveoli completely filled with liquid (ex. pneumonia, pulmonary edema, hemorrhagic alveolar flooding, and so on) or collapsed alveoli. Breathing 100% FIO_2 will also virtually eliminate the venous admixture caused by diffusion impairment, because the much greater PO_2 gradient across the alveolar wall will easily succeed in overcoming the larger blood-gas barrier, allowing hemoglobin to achieve saturation.

In our patient, with 100% FIO_2-breathing, the conductive shunt fraction (Eq. 12) and the (Ai-a)PO_2 gradient (Eq. 13) are:

$$\frac{\dot{Q}Cs}{\dot{Q}} = 4.4\% \ldots \qquad \textbf{(12)}$$

$$(Ai\text{-}a)PO_2 = 73 \text{ mmHg}. \qquad \textbf{(13)}$$

Since the physiological shunt fraction (Eq. 14) is:

$$\frac{\dot{Q}Ps}{\dot{Q}} = 10.8\% \ldots \qquad \textbf{(14)}$$

and the maldistribution-diffusion shunt-like fraction is the difference between physiological and conductive shut fractions (Eq. 15)

$$\frac{\dot{Q}Ms}{\dot{Q}} = \frac{\dot{Q}Ps}{\dot{Q}} - \frac{\dot{Q}Cs}{\dot{Q}} \ldots \qquad \textbf{(15)}$$

in this patient, the maldistribution-diffusion shunt fraction (Eq. 16) is:

$$\frac{\dot{Q}Ms}{\dot{Q}} = 10.8 - 4.4 = 6.4\% \ldots \qquad \textbf{(16)}$$

This fraction of maldistribution-diffusion shut (Eq. 16) accounts for ~60% of the total (physiological) shunt. A conductive shunt fraction of 4.4% is just slightly above the normal range (2-4%); therefore, the major problem of this patient in terms of venous admixture (right-to-left shunt) is $\dot{V}/\dot{Q}$ maldistribution and/or diffusion impairment; diffusion impairment, however, is not very common. Therefore, most of the shunts eliminated by 100% FIO_2-breathing are likely to result from $\dot{V}/\dot{Q}$ maldistribution (alveoli with abnormally low $\dot{V}/\dot{Q}$ ratios).

Caveat! The (Ai-a)PO_2 Gradient Not Always is a Reliable Index of Shunt Magnitude

In most cases the (Ai-a)PO_2 gradient increases proportionally to shunt magnitude, but there are conditions in which it is not a reliable indicator of shunt magnitude. In the case presented above, for example, with 100% FIO_2 breathing the shunt fraction decreased from 10.8% to 4.4%, while, paradoxically, the (Ai-a)PO_2 gradient increased from 27 to 73 mmHg (Figs. **14** and **15**). As mentioned above, the reason for it is that at high PO_2 hemoglobin is 100% saturated, and so we now operate along the flat (horizontal) portion of the O_2-dissociation curve where relatively large changes in PO_2 result in very small changes in O_2 content (mostly as dissolved O_2). A rule of thumb is that in normal subjects the (Ai-a)PO_2 gradient increases by 5-7 mmHg for each 10% increase in FIO_2. In clinical practice, a more accurate estimate of the shunt magnitude in patients breathing high FIO_2 can be obtained by calculating the (Ai/a)PO_2 gradient which, in contrast to the (Ai-a)PO_2 gradient, is not affected by changes in FIO_2. The changes in the (Ai-a)PO_2 gradient and the magnitude of shunt can be readily appreciated in the O_2-CO_2 diagram (Figs. **13** and **15**) and the O_2-dissociation curve (Fig. **16**).

The disconnect between shunt fraction and (Ai-a)PO_2 gradient does not occur only with high FIO_2 breathing. While with abnormally high FIO_2 the gradient increases in spite of a drop in shunt fraction, the opposite occurs when one breathes under hypoxic conditions - low in PIO_2 due to low barometric pressure at high altitude, for example. With hypoxic breathing both $PAiO_2$ and PaO_2 are lower than normal, and so that they shift to steeper regions of the O_2 dissociation curve where changes in O_2-content due to shunt correspond to relatively small changes in PO_2 (see Chapter 9).

Lower than expected (Ai-a)PO_2 gradients also occur in hypoxemic patients; this is more pronounced when hypoxemia is caused by hypoventilation, because in this case both $PAiO_2$ and PaO_2 shift to steeper regions of the O_2 dissociation curve. In contrast, if hypoxemia is caused by shunt, the disconnect between (Ai-a)PO_2 gradient and shunt magnitude is not as obvious because while PaO_2 shifts to steeper regions of the O_2 dissociation curve, the compensatory hyperventilation maintains $PAiO_2$ in the flat regions of the O_2 dissociation curve.

Types of Right-to-Left Blood Shunt

There are several physiological and pathological conditions that cause an influx of venous blood into well oxygenated blood, causing the arterial blood entering the aorta to be less oxygenated than blood exiting from the ideal alveolar compartment (Fig. **17**). In normal subjects, virtually all of the shunted blood comes from two sources: "venae cordis minimae" and broncho-pulmonary anastomoses.

The "venae minimae", also known as Thebesian veins, were discovered in 1708 by the German anatomist Adam Christian Thebesius (1686-1732). These tiny veins, that carry deoxygenated blood form the myocardium, are located in the inner surfaces of the cardiac walls and empty their blood directly into the atria and ventricles; those that empty into the left atrium and ventricle cause a small amount of conductive right-to-left shunt.

The other source of normal conductive shunt is from broncho-pulmonary anastomoses, small passageways that allow blood exchange between bronchial and pulmonary veins. Due to the pressure gradient between bronchial and pulmonary circulation, these anastomoses cause a small amount of venous blood to flow into pulmonary veins, which contain well oxygenated blood.

Since in normal subjects the maldistribution shunt-like effect is minimal, virtually all of the shunt is conductive and it amounts to only 2-4% of the cardiac output.

Several pathological conditions cause additional blood shunts that result in further de-oxygenation of arterial blood (Fig. **17**). Pathological shunts can be divided into alveolar and non-alveolar. Alveolar-based venous admixtures may result from alveoli with abnormally low $\dot{V}/\dot{Q}$ (maldistribution), alveoli with $\dot{V}/\dot{Q} = 0$, and/or alveoli with diffusion impairment. Non-alveolar shunts are mostly intra-cardiac shunts, resulting from atrial or ventricular septal defects. In these cases, venous admixture only occurs when the blood pressure of the right cardiac chambers exceed that of the left chambers, an obvious example being diseases that result in pulmonary hypertension.

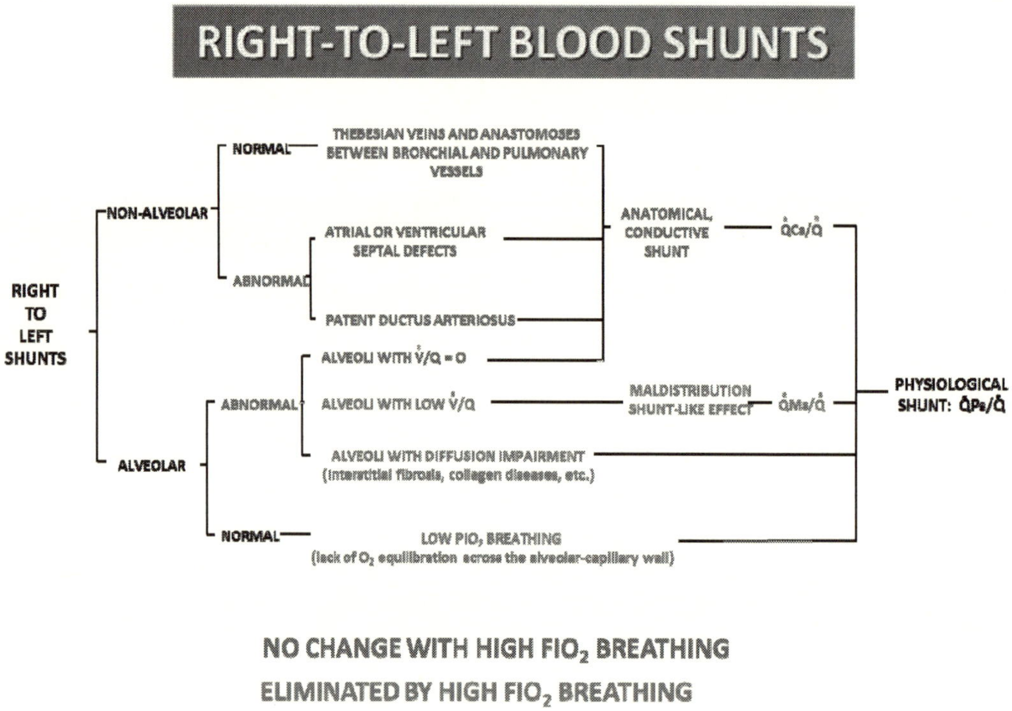

Figure 17: Components of physiological right-to-left blood shunt. Hypoxemia caused by conductive (anatomical) shut is insensitive to increased FIO_2. In contrast, hypoxemia caused by maldistribution shunt like effect, diffusion impairment or low PIO_2 is eliminated by ventilation with high FIO_2.

Non-alveolar shunt also results from patent "ductus arteriosus" in newborn children. Before birth, this arterial duct that joins the aorta to the pulmonary artery allows blood from the right ventricle to bypass the compressed lungs. Soon after birth the expansion and oxygenation of the lungs rapidly reduces the pulmonary vascular resistance and artery pressure, causing the duct to close. If the duct remains open, the pressure gradient between aorta and pulmonary artery causes blood to diffuse into the pulmonary artery, resulting in a left-to-right shunt; blood flow, however, can reverse course, resulting in right-to-left shunt, when pulmonary arterial pressure exceeds aortic pressure, for example during crying spells, which increase pulmonary vascular resistance, or in cases of pathological pulmonary hypertension.

Calculation of Alveolar Dead Space and Ideal Alveolar Ventilation

For determining the magnitude of alveolar dead space ventilation we simplify the real lung, as we did for the shunt calculation, into the lung equivalent "three compartment model" (Fig. **14**), in which mixed alveolar ($\dot{V}\bar{A}$) gas is assumed to come from two compartments: ideal exchanger ($\dot{V}Ai$) and alveolar dead space ($\dot{V}Ad$, alveoli with $\dot{V}/\dot{Q} = \infty$). Therefore, the total alveolar ventilation ($\dot{V}\bar{A}$) is the sum of ideal ($\dot{V}Ai$) and dead space ($\dot{V}Ad$) ventilations (Eq. 17):

$$\dot{V}\bar{A} = \dot{V}Ai + \dot{V}Ad \ ... \qquad \textbf{(17)}$$

Similarly, the total flow of CO_2 per minute is the sum of CO_2 exiting from the ideal compartment and CO_2 exiting from the alveolar dead space compartment (Eqs. 18-20):

$$\dot{V}\bar{A} \text{ x } F\bar{A}CO_2 = \dot{V}Ai \text{ x } FAiCO_2 + \dot{V}Ad \text{ x } FICO_2 \ ... \qquad \textbf{(18)}$$

since:

$$\dot{V}Ai = \dot{V}\bar{A} - \dot{V}Ad \ ... \qquad \textbf{(19)}$$

and $FICO_2 = 0$,

by solving for the alveolar dead space fraction and converting fractions to partial pressures one obtains Equation 20:

$$\frac{\dot{V}Ad}{\dot{V}\bar{A}} = \frac{PaCO_2 - P\bar{A}CO_2}{PaCO_2} \ ... \qquad \textbf{(20)}$$

This equation (Eq. 20) represents the fraction of the total alveolar ventilation ($\dot{V}\bar{A}$) wasted in alveolar dead space ($\dot{V}\bar{A}d$; Fig. **14**A). If the value of $P\bar{A}CO_2$ is not available, the alveolar dead space fraction can be calculated by measuring $\dot{V}\bar{A}$ and

$\dot{V}Ai$ (**Appendix 4, B2**). In normal subjects this fraction is virtually zero (minimal alveolar dead space ventilation). In our patient $\dot{V}Ad/\dot{V}\bar{A}$ = 14%, meaning that 14% of the alveolar ventilation is wasted into alveolar dead space (for the alveolar dead space calculation see **Appendix 2, B**).

The calculation of the alveolar dead space fraction gives an equivalent value of alveolar dead space ventilation. It shows that the lungs of this subject function as if 14% of the total alveolar ventilation were taking place in alveoli ventilated but not perfused at all ($\dot{V}/\dot{Q} = \infty$). In other words, this idealized calculation lumps together all of the partial contributions of high $\dot{V}/\dot{Q}$ units, in terms of dead space, into two compartment ($\dot{V}Ad$), with $\dot{V}/\dot{Q} = \infty$, and $\dot{V}Ai$, with perfect $\dot{V}/\dot{Q}$ (Fig. **12**). In this patient's lungs it is very unlikely that there are alveoli ventilated but totally unperfused ($\dot{V}/\dot{Q} = \infty$) but rather there are probably lots of alveoli (perhaps 40%, 50%, or more) with different degrees of abnormally high $\dot{V}/\dot{Q}$, whose functional equivalent is that 14% of the alveoli have a $\dot{V}/\dot{Q} = \infty$ and 86% have a perfect $\dot{V}/\dot{Q}$.

Functionally, to have an alveolar dead space fraction greater than normal is like having inside the chest a plastic bag connected to one of the bronchi. With each breath air enters and exits the plastic bag, but this is obviously no use to gas exchange because the bag is not perfused with blood - it only takes up space, so that the patient needs to ventilate more than normal for maintaining sufficiently ventilated the ideal alveolar compartment (Ai). If the patient does not compensate by increasing total ventilation (hyperpnea), the gas exchange will be insufficient (hypoventilation) - $PaCO_2$ will climb (hypercapnia) and PaO_2 will drop (hypoxemia).

Below are the expected fractions of wasted ventilations in conductive (Cd, Eq. 21), physiological (Pd, Eq. 22) and alveolar (Ad, Eq. 23) dead space compartments in a normal subject (no alveolar dead space) breathing with a normal breathing pattern at resting conditions:

$$\frac{\dot{V}Cd}{\dot{V}E} = \frac{P\bar{A}CO_2 - PECO_2}{P\bar{A}CO_2} = \frac{40-27}{40} = 33\% \ldots \quad \textbf{(21)}$$

$$\frac{\dot{V}Pd}{\dot{V}E} = \frac{PaCO_2 - PECO_2}{PaCO_2} = \frac{40-27}{40} = 33\% \ldots \quad \textbf{(22)}$$

$$\frac{\dot{V}Ad}{\dot{V}\bar{A}} = \frac{PaCO_2 - P\bar{A}CO_2}{PaCO_2} = \frac{40-40}{40} = 0\% \ldots \quad \textbf{(23)}$$

Below are the expected fractions of wasted ventilation in conductive (Cd, Eq. 24), physiological (Pd, Eq. 25) and alveolar (Ad, Eq. 26) dead space compartments in a patient with 50% alveolar dead space ventilation at resting conditions:

$$\frac{\dot{V}Cd}{\dot{V}E} = \frac{P\bar{A}CO_2 - PECO_2}{P\bar{A}CO_2} = \frac{20-13.5}{20} = 33\% \ldots \quad \textbf{(24)}$$

$$\frac{\dot{V}Pd}{\dot{V}E} = \frac{PaCO_2 - PECO_2}{PaCO_2} = \frac{40-13.5}{40} = 66\% \ldots \quad \textbf{(25)}$$

$$\frac{\dot{V}Ad}{\dot{V}\bar{A}} = \frac{PaCO_2 - P\bar{A}CO_2}{PaCO_2} = \frac{40-20}{40} = 50\% \ldots \quad \textbf{(26)}$$

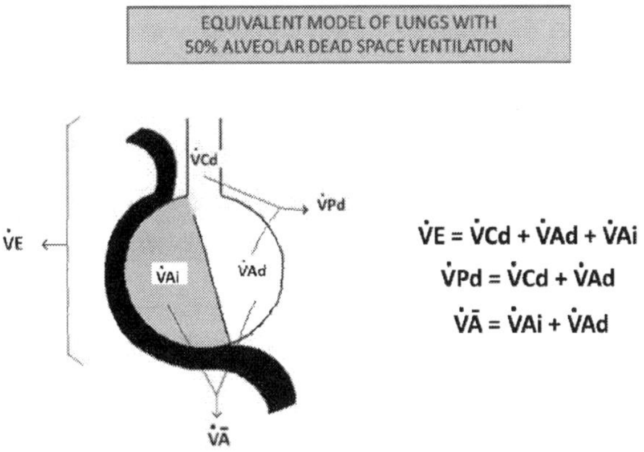

Figure 18: Functional equivalent ventilatory compartments in a patient with 50% alveolar dead space.

Fig. **18**, shows the functional-equivalent ventilatory compartments in a patient with large alveolar dead space ventilation ($\dot{V}Ad/\dot{V}\bar{A} = 50\%$).

"Ideal" *versus* "Effective" PO_2 and PCO_2

In calculations of shunt and alveolar dead space fractions (see above) we have assumed that $PaCO_2 \approx PAiCO_2$. This is a reasonable assumption, because their values are usually very similar since the blood R-line is almost flat (horizontal) as it approaches the ideal point (Figs. **13, 15** and **19**). However, one should realize that in diseases that result in very large blood shunts, PaO_2 and $PaCO_2$ shift farther away from the Ai point, as they move toward slightly steeper regions of the blood R-line (closer to the $\bar{v}$ point). This means that $PaCO_2$ assumes values slightly greater than $PAiCO_2$ (Fig. **19**, points "a" and "Ai", respectively) and, consequently, $PAiO_2$ "*calculated*" by means of the alveolar gas equation from the measured $PaCO_2$ (Fig. **20**, point "Ae"), is slightly lower than the "*actual*" $PAiO_2$ (Fig. **19**, point "Ai") - the point of intersection between gas and blood R-lines which cannot be calculated.

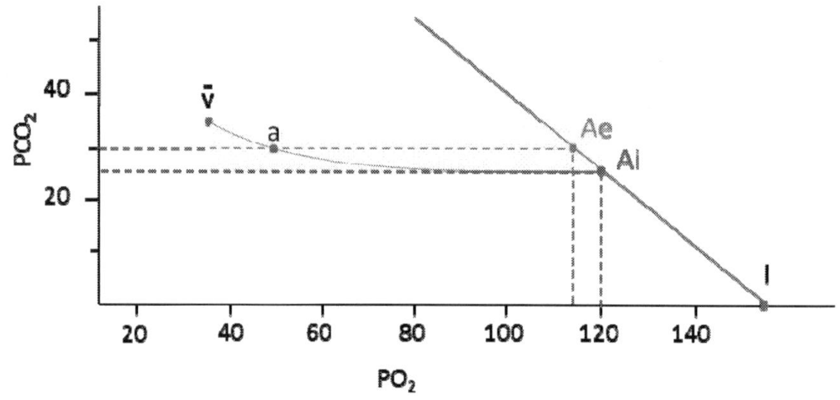

Figure 19: This example shows that even in cases of very large shunts that cause a shift of the arterial (a) point to steeper regions of the blood R-line, effective (Ae) and ideal (Ai) PO_2 values differ by only a few mmHg (~5 mmHg, here).

Riley and coworkers [6] have named this "*calculated*" value "effective" (e), rather than "ideal" (i); based on this, $PaCO_2 = PAeCO_2$, and the "*calculated*" $PAiO_2$ is symbolized as $PAeO_2$ (Fig. **17**, point "Ae"). Therefore, in patients with large shunt fractions, and so large $(Ai\text{-}a)PO_2$ gradients (Fig. **19**), calculations of shunt fractions by means of $PaCO_2$ and $PAeO_2$ values, slightly underestimate the actual shunt fraction, because $PAeCO_2$ is slightly higher that $PAiCO_2$, and $PAeO_2$ is slightly lower than $PAiO_2$ - consequently, $CAeO_2 < CAiO_2$.

Riley and coworkers[36] have worked out a way to correct for this relatively small error. However, even under extreme conditions that result in large shunt fractions this correction makes a relatively small difference. As an example, let's compare "effective" (e) *versus* "ideal" (i) values and shunt fractions (**Table 6**) in the patient with the following lab values (Fig. **19**): $PaO_2 = 50$ mmHg, $PaCO_2 = 30$ mmHg, pHa = 7.45, $CaO_2 = 17.64$ vol%, O_2-extraction = 5 vol%, Hb = 15 g/100 ml blood, R = 0.8, body temperature = 37°C (breathing air at sea level).

Table 6: Comparison between ideal and effective values

pHAe	7.45	**$PAiO_2$ (mmHg)**	**1120**
pHAi	**7.48**	$CAeO_2$ (vol%)	20.1
$PAeCO_2$ (mmHg)	30	**$CAiO_2$ (vol%)**	**20.2**
$PAiCO_2$ (mmHg)	**27**	$\dot{Q}Ps/\dot{Q}$ "e" (%)	33
$PAeO_2$ (mmHg)	113	**$\dot{Q}Ps/\dot{Q}$ "i" (%)**	**33.9**

Indeed, it would hardly be relevant to learn that in this patient a physiological shunt fraction calculated as it is usually done is 33% (Table **6**, $\dot{Q}Ps/\dot{Q}$ "e"), whereas the (correct) shunt fraction calculated by means of "ideal" values is 33.9% (Table **6**, $\dot{Q}Ps/\dot{Q}$ "i"). A 0.9% difference for this shunt fraction, which is more than eight times the normal fraction, is clearly negligible.

Similarly, in calculating $\dot{V}Ad/V\bar{A}$ (see above) we have assumed, as usual, that $PaCO_2 \approx PAiCO_2$. However, as mentioned above, in patients with large shunt fractions $PaCO_2$ is actually higher than $PAiCO_2$ (Fig. **19**). Therefore, in patient with large shunt fractions who also have abnormal alveolar dead space fractions, the calculated $\dot{V}Ad/V\bar{A}$ is greater than the actual fraction (which cannot be calculated). As an example, let's assume that in the patient, whose values are shown in Fig. **19** and Table **6**, $P\bar{A}CO_2$ is 20 mmHg. In this case, $\dot{V}Ad/V\bar{A}$ calculated using $PaCO_2$ (same as $PAeCO_2$) is (Eq. 27):

$$\frac{\dot{V}Ad}{\dot{V}\bar{A}} = \frac{PaCO_2 - P\bar{A}CO_2}{PaCO_2} = \frac{30-20}{30} = 33\% \ldots \quad \textbf{(27)}$$

whereas, if we were able to calculate $\dot{V}Ad/V\bar{A}$ by using $PAiCO_2$, it would be (Eq. 28):

$$\frac{\dot{V}Ad}{\dot{V}\bar{A}} = \frac{PAiCO_2 - P\bar{A}CO_2}{PAiCO_2} = \frac{27-20}{27} = 26\% \ldots \quad \textbf{(28)}$$

This is a significant difference. However, note that in this case we are dealing with an extreme condition, as the shunt fraction is more than eight times the normal value.

Therefore, in this book the term "ideal" is consistently used, with an understanding that under most pathological conditions "ideal" and "effective" values are virtually the same.

Compensatory Mechanisms for Ventilation-Perfusion Maldistribution

As mentioned above, regional $\dot{V}/\dot{Q}$ mismatches result in shunt-like effect and/or alveolar dead space ventilation. However, the effects of $\dot{V}/\dot{Q}$ maldistribution would be greater if there weren't compensatory mechanisms.

One of them is the "pulmonary hypoxic vasoconstriction response". In low $\dot{V}/\dot{Q}$ regions, the alveolar PO_2 is lower than normal. This regional alveolar hypoxia causes vasoconstriction of local pulmonary arterioles and consequentially decreases the regional blood flow. The resulting increase in regional $\dot{V}/\dot{Q}$ and PO_2 translates into a regional increase in O_2-content and reduced shunt fraction. Simultaneously, the increased vascular resistance in these low $\dot{V}/\dot{Q}$ regions causes a shift in pulmonary blood flow toward poorly perfused (high $\dot{V}/\dot{Q}$) regions, partially reducing the fraction of alveolar dead space ventilation.

Hypoxic vasoconstriction starts developing when the local alveolar PO_2 drops below 70-75 mmHg (Fig. **20**) and reaches its maximum (a decrease in blood flow to approximately half normal) at PO_2 values ranging from 20 to 50 mmHg. Hypoxic vasoconstriction is further potentiated by higher regional PCO_2 and lower than normal regional blood pH. A pH drop of 0.1-0.2 units triples the effect of hypoxic vasoconstriction. This is very important because hypoxia, hypercapnia and acidemia often occur altogether in low $\dot{V}/\dot{Q}$ regions. Another compensatory mechanism for $\dot{V}/\dot{Q}$ maldistribution is the "hypocapnic bronchoconstriction". The lower than normal PCO_2 in high $\dot{V}/\dot{Q}$ regions causes the smooth muscle of regional bronchioles to contract. This reduces the regional ventilation, decreasing the regional $\dot{V}/\dot{Q}$ ratio and so the fraction of alveolar dead space ventilation.

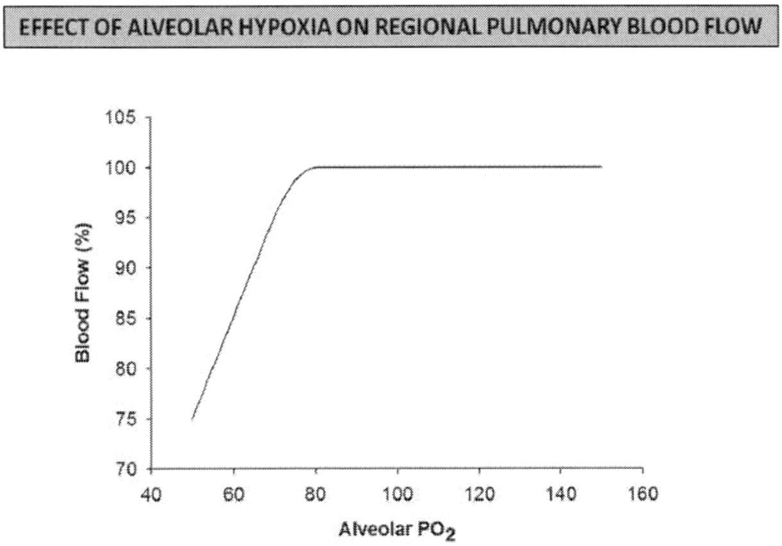

Figure 20: Regional drops in PAO_2 to values lower than ~70-80 mmHg, activate a local hypoxic vasoconstriction response, which decreases regional blood flow and shifts it to better oxygenated regions.

The hypoxic vasoconstriction response is a useful mechanism for reducing the effects of $\dot{V}/\dot{Q}$ maldistribution, but it can cause problems for cardiac patients breathing under hypoxic conditions, such as at high altitudes. Hypoxic breathing causes generalized pulmonary vasoconstriction, leading to pulmonary hypertension and possibly right heart failure. In these patients, O_2 therapy will obviously help by lowering the pulmonary blood pressure.

In pulmonary patients with $\dot{V}/\dot{Q}$ maldistribution, O_2 therapy increases the ventilation-perfusion mismatch and may result in CO_2 retention (hypercapnia). While it is true that administration of high fractions of O_2 eliminates the fraction of shunt caused by maldistribution-diffusion (see above) and reduces pulmonary hypertension, the higher alveolar PO_2 worsens the $\dot{V}/\dot{Q}$ maldistribution, because it eliminates the compensatory hypoxic vasoconstriction (see below: "Oxygen Therapy").

Inert-Gas-Method for Quantifying Ventilation-Perfusion Distribution

As mentioned above, the $\dot{V}/\dot{Q}$ distribution can be evaluated by a clever method devised in 1974 by the group of John B. West [7]. In this method, a series of six inert gases, dissolved in saline, are infused intravenously. When a steady state elimination of the gases is reached at the lungs, their concentrations are measured by gas chromatography in samples of arterial blood and expired gas. Since the gases have different solubility characteristics, they partition between blood and gas according to the $\dot{V}/\dot{Q}$ ratio of different lung units; this enables one to plot a continuous distribution of $\dot{V}/\dot{Q}$ ratios.

Fig. **21** exemplifies the distribution of $\dot{V}/\dot{Q}$ ratios in a normal young subject (**A**), where most of the ventilation and blood flow occur in units with a $\dot{V}/\dot{Q}$ ratio close to 1, and in a patient with chronic obstructive pulmonary disease (COPD) of type A (emphysema; **B**), where large areas with $\dot{V}/\dot{Q}$ ratios much greater than 1 are present.

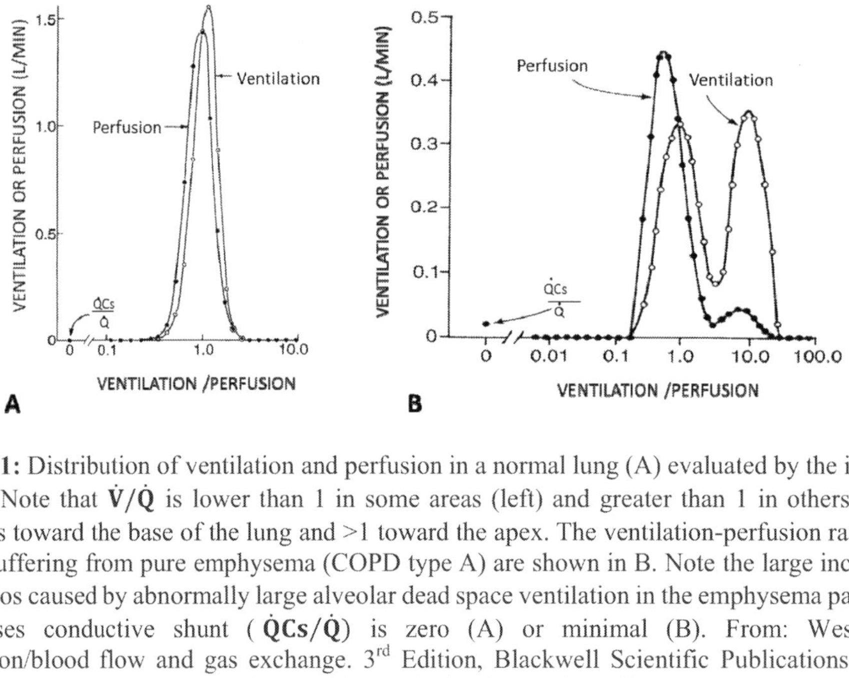

Figure 21: Distribution of ventilation and perfusion in a normal lung (A) evaluated by the inert gas method. Note that $\dot{V}/\dot{Q}$ is lower than 1 in some areas (left) and greater than 1 in others (right). $\dot{V}/\dot{Q}<1$ is toward the base of the lung and >1 toward the apex. The ventilation-perfusion ratios of a patient suffering from pure emphysema (COPD type A) are shown in B. Note the large increase in $\dot{V}/\dot{Q}$ ratios caused by abnormally large alveolar dead space ventilation in the emphysema patient. In both cases conductive shunt ($\dot{Q}Cs/\dot{Q}$) is zero (A) or minimal (B). From: West, J.B., Ventilation/blood flow and gas exchange. 3rd Edition, Blackwell Scientific Publications, Osney Mead, Oxford, UK, 1977. Reproduced with permission from John Wiley & sons, Inc.

Causes of Hypoxemia

There are four major conditions that result in hypoxemia (low PaO_2, Table 7). By and large the most important of them are **shunt** and **hypoventilation**. Any type of venous admixture (right-to-left blood shunt), whether it is conductive shunt, maldistribution shunt-like effect, diffusion impairment, or a mixture of them, results in hypoxemia because O_2-desaturated blood (mixed venous) mixing with oxigenated blood causes a drop in arterial PO_2; the most common causes of shunt-induced hypoxemia are schematized in Fig. **17**. If PaO_2 drops significantly below normal (< 70-75 mmHg) the hypoxic stumulus results in a compensatory increase in ventilation, which reduces the hypoxemia and causes hypocapnia. Therefore, in patients with abnormal right-to-left blood shunts both PaO_2 and $PaCO_2$ will be lower than normal (hypoxemia with compensatory hypocapnia), as long as the patients are able to compensate for hypoxemia by hyperventilation.

Note that for the same shunt fraction hypoxemia is more severe if $P\bar{v}O_2$ is lower than normal (for example, when O_2 extraction is greatly increased due to a drop in $\dot{Q}$) because the same fraction of venus admixture containing more desaturated blood will cause a greater drop in CaO_2 and PaO_2. For example, with a shunt fraction of 10% and a normal O_2 extraction of 5 vol%, PaO_2 would be about 80 mmHg, whereas with the same shunt fraction an increase in O_2 extraction to 10 vol% will cause PaO_2 to drop to ~68 mmHg.

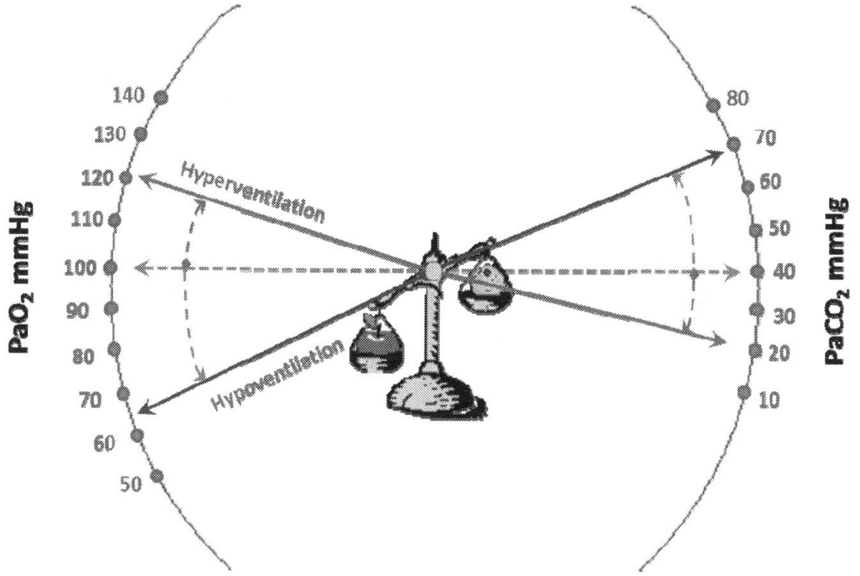

Figure 22: In normal subjects breathing room air at sea level and at steady state (R = RQ), hypoventilation and hyperventilation cause PaO_2 and $PaCO_2$ to change in a balanced fashion - as $PaCO_2$ rises or drops, PaO_2 drops or rises, respectively, by approximately the same amount.

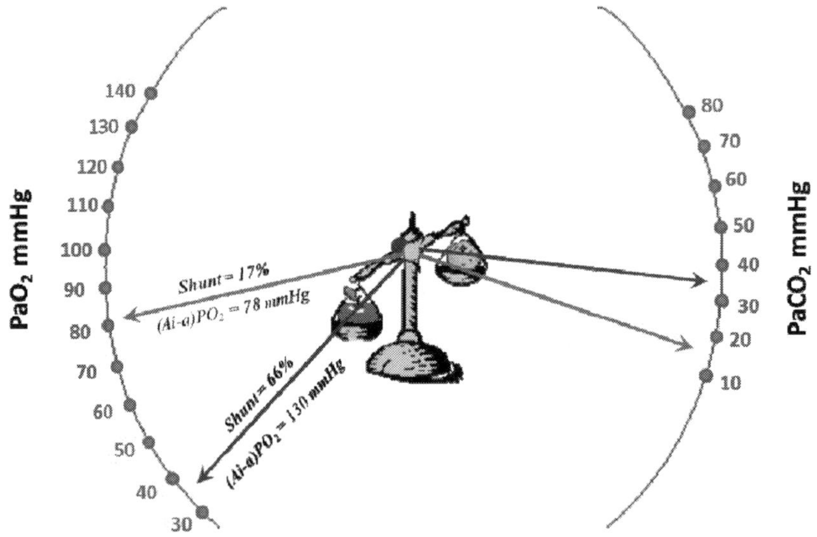

Figure 23: In cases of hypoxemia caused by abnormal shunt fractions, diffusion impairment, or exposure to low FIO_2, the PaO_2-$PaCO_2$ balance is broken. In this example, the hypoxemia (PaO_2 = 82 mmHg) caused by a shunt fraction of 17% is reasonably well compensated by a $PaCO_2$ drop to 16 mmHg. In contrast, the severe hypoxemia (PaO_2 = 36 mmHg) caused by a 66% shunt fraction is only minimally compensated by a $PaCO_2$ drop to 36 mmHg.

Table 7: Pathological and physiological conditions that result in hypoxemia (lower than normal arterial PO_2)

CAUSES OF HYPOXEMIA (LOW PaO_2)
• SHUNT
• HYPOVENTILATION
• DIFFUSION IMPAIRMENT
• LOW PIO_2

Hypoxemia caused by hypoventilation can easily be differenciated from that caused by abnormal right-to-left shunts because with hypoventilation the low PaO_2 is associated with high $PaCO_2$ (hypoxemia and hypercapnia). With pure hypoventilation the magnitude of PaO_2-drop matches reasonably well that of $PaCO_2$-increase (Fig. **22**). This is because at steady state the changes in PaO_2 and $PaCO_2$ follow the gas R-line of the O_2-CO_2 diagram (Fig. **13**). For example, if the exchange ratio (R) has a value of "1", an increase in $PaCO_2$ by 20 mmHg (from 40 to 60) would cause PaO_2 to drop by ~20 mmHg (from 95 to ~75 mmHg); since the R value is usually ~0.85, a 20 mmHg increase in $PaCO_2$ would cause PaO_2 to drop by ~23.5 mmHg. In a normal subject with minimal shunt fraction ($\dot{Q}Ps/\dot{Q}$ = 2-4%), breathing room air at sea level and steady state (R=RQ), hypoxemia due entirely to hypoventilation causes PaO_2 and $PaCO_2$ to change in a balanced fashion - as $PaCO_2$ rises PaO_2 drops by approximately the same amount, and *vice versa* (Fig. **22**).

In contrast, when hypoxemia is caused by abnormally high shunt fractions (conductive shunt and/or maldistribution shunt-like effect), diffusion impairment, or exposure to low FIO_2 (hypoxia at high altitude, for instance), the PaO_2-$PaCO_2$ balance is broken - in the examples shown in Fig. **23**, one sees that with shunt both PaO_2 and $PaCO_2$ dropped below normal values - with a 17% shunt the hypoxemia was reasonably well compensated by a drop in $PaCO_2$ to 16 mmHg, whereas with a 66% shunt the hypoxemia was only minimally compensated as $PaCO_2$ only dropped to 36 mmHg.

Hypoxemia due to alveolar diffusion-impairment is fairly rare in clinical setting because under normal conditions a red blood cell entering an alveolar capillary achieves the same PO_2 value of the alveolar gas as early as in the first third of its transit time through the capillary. This represents a significant reserve of diffusing capacity, such that even in heavy exercise there is virtually complete equilibration of oxygen pressure across the alveolar-capillary barrier in spite of the increase in perfusion velocity (albeit, moderated by increased capillary recruitment). Even in pathological conditions such pulmonary fibrosis or pulmonary edema, diffusion impairment appears to play a minor role in hypoxemia, most important being the role of $\dot{V}/\dot{Q}$ maldistribution (shunt-like effect). Hypoxemia due to diffusion impairment is accompanied by hypocapnia, as in the case of shunt, so also in this case the PaO_2-$PaCO_2$ balance is broken (Fig. **23**).

Hypoxemia due to low PIO_2 occurs at high altitude, where hypoxia is the consequence of reduced barometric pressure. In this case, as with shunt, the reduced PaO_2 causes hyperventilation and consequential hypocapnia due to the hypoxic stimulus.

Oxygen Therapy

Oxygen therapy is a treatment for hypoxemia that involves delivery of oxygen to the lungs at fractions higher than normal atmospheric values (FIO_2 >21%). High oxygen fractions can be delivered by nasal cannulas, mask, trans-tracheal micro-catheters, tents, or endotracheal tube (mechanical ventilation). Oxygen therapy is used widely in patients suffering from respiratory failure, a conditions in which the respiratory system is unable to efficiently delivering oxygen to pulmonary capillaries and removing from them carbon dioxide.

Hypoxemia caused by respiratory failure can be acute or chronic, and is usually classified into two major categories: Hypoxic Respiratory Failure (HRF) and Hypercapnic Hypoxic Respiratory Failure (HHRF). In HRF the drop in PaO_2 is associated with normal or lower than normal $PaCO_2$ (Fig. **23**), whereas in HHRF the drop in PaO_2 is associated with an increase in $PaCO_2$ (Fig. **22**).

Not all forms of hypoxemia can be improved with oxygen therapy. In HRF, O_2 therapy is beneficial in most but not all of the cases. As mentioned above, high FIO_2 does not significantly increase PaO_2 if the hypoxemia is entirely due to abnormally high conductive shunt fractions, because obviously PO_2 does not increase if blood is not exposed to high FIO_2, as in the case of alveoli perfused but unventilated, collapsed (atelectasis), or flooded with edema, exudate or blood ($\dot{V}/\dot{Q} = 0$). This is also true in patients suffering from extra-pulmonary shunts caused, for example, by atrial or ventricular septal defects or patent ductus arteriosus, when the blood pressure gradient favors venous admixture.

Although it is true that by increasing FIO_2 from 21% to 100%, for example, the content of dissolved O_2 in blood of ventilated alveoli increases from ~0.3 vol% to ~2.1 vol%, this only negligibly increases PaO_2 in arterial blood, which is a mixture of shunted and oxygenated blood, because in the latter hemoglobin was already virtually saturated with O_2, and the addition of a minute amount of dissolved O_2 increase only minimally CaO_2 and PaO_2. For example, the data given in Table **8** show that in a pneumonia patient with a large conductive shunt fraction an increase in FIO_2 from 21% to 100% would only increase CaO_2 and PaO_2 by ~2.5 vol% and ~7 mmHg, respectively.

In contrast, an increase in FIO_2 significantly reduces or totally eliminates hypoxemia when HRF results from maldistribution shunt-like effect and/or diffusion impairment, because in both cases the large increase in alveolar PO_2 will allow the hemoglobin of blood flowing through diseased alveoli to reach

O_2-saturation. As mentioned above, if FIO_2 is increased to 100%, for example, all of the alveolar N_2 is replaced by O_2 such that in alveoli with low $\dot{V}/\dot{Q}$ ratios and/or diffusion impairment PO_2 will become high enough to fully saturate hemoglobin. There will still be a PO_2 gradient between diseased and normal alveolar end-capillary blood but the difference in O_2-content will be minimal, because hemoglobin will be O_2-saturated in both compartments. Similarly, hypoxemia due to low FIO_2 (breathing at high altitude, for example) will be eliminated by high FIO_2 breathing.

Table 8: Laboratory data from a pneumonia patient breathing either air or 100 FIO_2

	Air	**O_2**
pHa	7.3	7.3
$PaCO_2$ (mmHg)	36	36
PaO_2 (mmHg)	**36**	**43**
Hb (g/ml blood)	14	14
PB (mmHg)	747	747
R	0.8	0.8
FIO_2 (%)	21	100
$\dot{V}O_2$ (liters/min, STPD)	0.32	0.32
O_2 extraction (vol%)	4	4
Body Temperature (°C)	39	39
$\dot{Q}Cs/\dot{Q}$ (%)	66	66
CaO_2 (vol%)	**10.43**	**12.9**

In the case of HHRF the supply of high FIO_2 is very effective in correcting the hypoxemia because it is primarily caused by hypoventilation (low $\dot{V}/\dot{Q}$) of the ideal alveolar compartment ($\dot{V}Ai$), rather than by unventilated (yet perfused) alveoli ($\dot{V}/\dot{Q} = 0$) or extra-alveolar shunts. Hypoventilation in HHRF is caused by a reduction of minute ventilation due to patients' inability to provide sufficient respiratory work for maintaining the metabolic needs. This may occur during respiratory failure in asthmatic patients suffering from prolonged, severe, asthma attacks (status asthmaticus), in patients suffering from large alveolar dead space ventilation (COPD type A) who have reached a state of exhaustion, or in patients with COPD type B, who have adapted to chronic hypercapnic conditions (chronic, partially compensated, respiratory acidosis).

High FIO_2 in HHRF patients is certainly beneficial, but has some important caveats, the most relevant being the worsening of hypercapnia and respiratory acidosis. The mechanism behind this type of hypercapnia (CO_2 retention) involves the elimination of both hypoxic vasoconstriction and hypoxic drive. Before O_2 therapy, the hypoxia present in severely hypoventilated regions caused vasoconstriction and consequential reduction in blood perfusion. This had some benefits as it reduced the maldistribution shunt-like effect and shifted some blood to poorly perfused alveoli, partially reducing alveolar dead space, if present. The elimination of hypoxic vasoconstriction by high FIO_2 significantly increases the perfusion of hypoventilated alveoli, causing a significant drop in regional $\dot{V}/\dot{Q}$ and consequentially increasing PCO_2. Somewhat less relevant is the elimination of the hypoxic drive which was present before O_2 therapy if PaO_2 was lower than ~70 mmHg - the elimination of the oxygen drive worsens the hypoventilation, causing a further increase in $PaCO_2$. So, in HHRF the benefits of eliminating the maldistribution shunt-like effect, and the consequential hypoxemia, may be complicated by increased hypercapnia and worsened respiratory acidosis. The obvious way of preventing these complications is to supply FIO_2 not greater than ~50%, which is usually sufficient to correct the hypoxemia, and, if needed, to assist ventilation to prevent CO_2 retention.

Another potential complication of O_2 therapy is alveolar collapse, a phenomenon known as "absorption atelectasis". This phenomenon, however, may only occur with supply of very high FIO_2 (80-100%) and in very poorly ventilated areas; in this case, the reduction of the maldistribution shunt-like effect is counterbalanced by an increase in conductive shunt ($\dot{V}/\dot{Q} = 0$). The reason for absorption atelectasis is that with high FIO_2 the reduction, or complete removal, of alveolar N_2 causes the O_2 diffusion into alveolar capillaries to exceed the influx of O_2 by ventilation - the increased O_2 diffusion is due to the large increase in PO_2 gradient across the alveolar-capillary barrier. Alveolar atelectasis can be prevented by supplying FIO_2 not greater than ~60% to patients breathing on their own. Higher FIO_2 (80-100%) can be supplied to patients connected to mechanical ventilator that maintains tidal volumes large enough to prevent alveolar collapse; particularly useful in these cases is the use of Positive End Expiratory Pressure (PEEP) ventilation.

Hyperbaric Oxygen Therapy

Administration of oxygen at pressures higher than atmospheric pressure is used for treating a few special cases such as carbon monoxide poisoning, cyanide intoxication severe anaerobic infections and traumas [8, 9]; in carbon monoxide poisoning, exposure to high PO_2 facilitates CO-dissociation from hemoglobin. Hyperbaric oxygen is delivered in specially designed pressure chambers where 100% FIO_2 is supplied at a pressure of three atmospheres. Since under normal atmospheric pressures a PaO_2 = 100 mmHg is sufficient to virtually saturate hemoglobin, any additional increase in PO_2 only results in increased physically dissolved O_2 – for each 1000 mmHg increase in PO_2, dissolved O_2 increases by 3 vol%. This is significant, however, because in a normal subject an increase in PaO_2 from 100 to ~2000 mmHg (at 3 atmospheres) results in ~29% increase in CaO_2 (from ~20.4 to ~26.3 vol%).

Hyperbaric oxygen therapy is usually administered for no longer than five hours, and at pressures not exceeding three atmospheres. Longer exposures result in oxygen toxicity. In experimental animals, prolonged exposures result in retinal damage, characterized by a lesion known as "cytoid body" - a round darkly-stained lesion within swollen nerve fiber layer, caused by segmental degeneration of axons. This lesion is believed to result from O_2-induced retinal vasoconstriction and consequential ischemia. Hyperoxia also causes a drop in heart rate and cardiac output. Oxygen-induced peripheral vasoconstriction results in regional drop in blood flow and increased vascular resistance in the systemic circulation.

Decompression from hyperbaric oxygen therapy needs to follow precise decompression schedules to avoid "decompression sickness". Too rapid decompression may cause gas embolism and neurological deficit, which in extreme cases could result in paralysis, coma, and even death.

Oxygen Toxicity

Oxygen therapy employing high FIO_2 (80-100%) for prolonged periods of time may cause oxygen toxicity resulting in the so called "fibroprolipherative disease". This complication, described in experimental animals, involves damage to the endothelium of alveolar capillaries and the alveolar epithelial cells Type 1 (EP1), development of interstitial edema, and proliferation of epithelial cells Type 2

(EP2). Its mechanism is believed to involve the formation of oxygen free-radicals, which cause peroxidation of unsaturated fatty acids, protein degradation, enzyme inactivation, carbohydrate oxidation, and ultimately cell death. An additional complication is that EP1 cells are incapable of multiplying by mitosis such that, once destroyed, their population can only be rebuilt by mitosis and differentiation of EP2 cells, a process that takes days. Destruction of EP1 cells breaches the alveolar barrier, causing plasma to leak into alveoli (alveolar edema → conductive shunt).

There are several defense mechanisms, however, that the lungs are able to activate. They include the generation of detoxifiers such as superoxide dismutase, catalase, and glutathione peroxidase, in addition to anti-oxidant systems such as hemoglobin, vitamin E and reduced glutathione. In view of these effective defense mechanisms, it is hard to predict which patient may develop oxygen related injury, as factors such as age, nutrition, *etc.* may play a role. Furthermore, in those very serious conditions requiring high FIO_2 treatment, such as in ARDS, it is hard to separate damages caused by oxygen toxicity from those resulting from the disease process. Indeed, some authors [10] believe that lung damage by high FIO_2, described primarily in experimental animals, is hard to compare with what might occur in patients, as the animal tests may have used insufficiently humidified inspired gas. These authors feel that there is insufficient evidence to suggest that the supply of 100% FIO_2 in ARDS patients is dangerous; furthermore, they report that there is worldwide evidence that ARDS patients treated for weeks with 100% O_2 survived without consequences.

In premature infants, extensive exposure to high FIO_2 may cause the so called "retrolental fibroplasia ". The eye damage causes blindness by the formation of fibrous tissue behind the lens. The mechanism involves localized vasoconstriction resulting from exposure to high PO_2 in the incubator. This complication can be avoided by preventing PaO_2 from rising above ~140 mmHg.

REFERENCES

[1] Reviewed in: West JB. Ventilation/blood flow and gas exchange. Oxford, UK: Blackwell Scientific Publications; 1980.

[2] West JB, Dollery CT, Naimark A. Distribution of blood flow in isolated lung: relation to vascular and alveolar pressures. J Appl Physiol 1964;19:713-724.

[3] Permutt S, Bromberger-Barnea B, Bane HN. Alveolar pressure, pulmonary pressure, and vascular waterfall. Med Thorac 1962;19:239-269.

[4] Wagner PD, Saltzman HA, West JB. Measurement of continuous distributions of ventilation-perfusion ratios: theory. J Appl Physiol 1974;36:533–537.

[5] Riley RL, Cournand A. "Ideal" alveolar air and the analysis of ventilation-perfusion relationships in the lungs. J Appl Physiol 1949;1:825–847.

[6] Riley RL, Cournand A, Donald KW. Analysis of factors affecting the partial pressures of oxygen and carbon dioxide in gas and blood of lung: methods. J. Appl Physiol 1951;4:102-120.

[7] Wagner PD, Saltzman HA, West JB. Measurement of continuous distributions of ventilation-perfusion ratios: theory. J Appl Physiol 1974;36:588-599.

[8] Camporesi EM, Moon RE, Grande CM. Hyperbaric medicine: an integral part of trauma care. Crit Care Clin. 1990;6:203-19.

[9] Camporesi EM, Vezzani G, Bosco G, Mangar D. and Bernasek TL. Hyperbaric oxygen therapy in femoral head necrosis. J Arthroplasty. 2011;25(6 Suppl):118-123.

[10] Artigas A. *et al.* American-European Consensus Conference on ARDS, Part II. Ventilatory, pharmacologic, supportive therapy, study designed strategies and issues related to recovery and remodeling. Intensive Care Med 1998;24:378-98.

Send Orders for Reprints to reprints@benthamscience.net

CHAPTER 8

Control of Breathing

Nasr H. Anaizi

Abstract: The automatic rhythm of breathing is generated by specialized neurons of the medulla oblongata: the Dorsal Respiratory Group (DRG) and the Ventral Respiratory Group (VRG). The DRG represents the "inspiratory center" whereas the VRG is mostly expiratory; the caudal portion of VRG, together with the Bötzinger complex in its vicinity, constitutes the "expiratory center". Normally, inspiration occurs actively *via* signals from the inspiratory neurons to the inspiratory muscles (mainly the diaphragm). Expiration occurs passively owing to the elastic recoil of the lungs. Expiratory neurons are activated only under certain conditions such as increased physical activity. The Pontine Respiratory Group (PRG, upper pons) represents the "pneumotaxic center", which acts as an "off" switch controlling the point at which inspiration is terminated and therefore determining the depth and frequency of breathing. Ventilation is also subject to direct voluntary control by the cerebral cortex, as it occurs during such maneuvers as breath holding. The activity of the respiratory centers is constantly modified in response to feedback from a variety of sensors in the periphery as well as within the brain. Both the long term and the moment-to-moment regulation of alveolar ventilation are primarily the task of chemosensitive cells in the ventrolateral aspect of the medulla (central chemoreceptors) and in the carotid and aortic bodies (the peripheral chemoreceptors). These chemical sensors monitor the levels of CO_2, O_2, and H^+ in arterial blood.

Keywords: Apneustic Breathing, Bötzinger Complex, Breuer-Hering, Central Chemoreceptors, Chemical Control, Chemosensory Transduction, Deflation Reflex, Dorsal Respiratory Group (DRG), Inhalation Reflex, Inspiratory Center, J-Receptors, Mechanoreceptors, N. Tractus Solitarius (NTS), Neurogenic Control, Peripheral Chemoreceptors, Pneumotaxic Center, Pontine Respiratory Group (PRG), Pre-Bötzinger Complex, Sleep Apnea, Ventral Respiratory Group (VRG).

INTRODUCTION

The primary function of the respiratory system is to deliver oxygen (O_2) and remove carbon dioxide (CO_2) for sustaining cell metabolism and maintaining normal cellular activity. This task is accomplished by maintaining the arterial partial pressures of oxygen (PO_2) and carbon dioxide (PCO_2) relatively constant. Another vital function of the respiratory system is to maintain the pH of body fluids within the normal range despite fluctuations of metabolic demands (the role of respiration in acid-base homeostasis is discussed in Chapter 6).

In addition to these homeostatic, involuntary functions, the respiratory system plays a role in behavioral (voluntary) functions such as speaking and singing (phonation). The normal breathing pattern may be momentarily interrupted by protective reflexes that result from coughing or sneezing.

CONTROL SYSTEM

The complex control system responsible for the regulation of respiratory functions is essentially a negative feedback system composed of: a ***central controller, sensors***, and ***effectors*** (Figs. **1** and **2,** and Table **1**). In addition to generating the basic automatic respiratory rhythm, the central controller is responsible for adjusting its motor output to the respiratory muscles in order to meet the organism's homeostatic needs. Alterations in the controlled variables (PCO_2, $[H^+]$, and PO_2) from their normal values (or set points) are sensed by specialized receptors or sensors. The information is conveyed *via* neural signals to the central controller, which receives and integrates the information, compares it to set point values, and responds accordingly. The response, or output commands of the central controller modify the output of the effectors (*i.e.*, the respiratory muscles), leading to the changes in alveolar ventilation and gas exchange needed for restoring the controlled variables to their normal level.

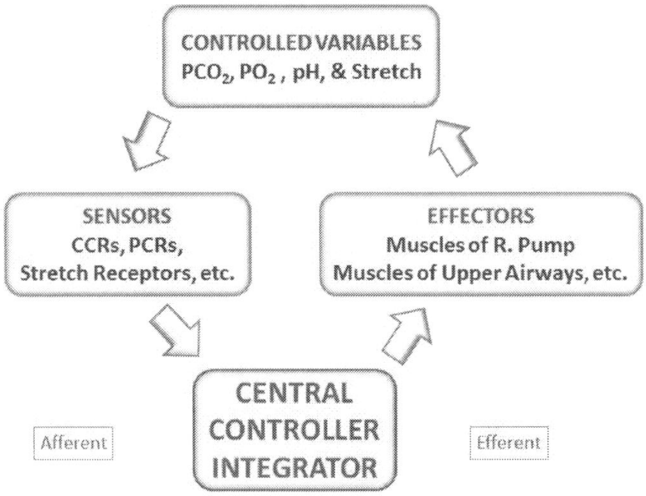

Figure 1: Basic components of a control system: controlled variables, sensors, central integrator/controller, effectors, and afferent and efferent pathways.

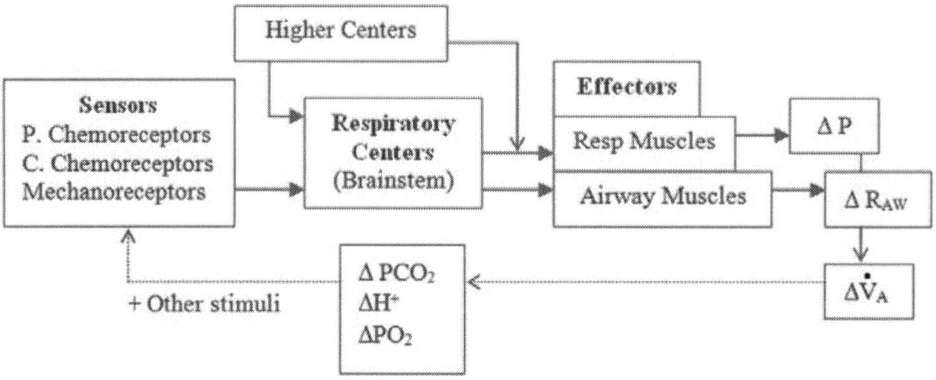

Figure 2: Components of the respiratory control system. Note that the higher centers in the cerebral cortex can modify breathing *via* the brainstem centers as well as through direct projections to the spinal motor neurons. R_{AW} = Airway Resistance. $\Delta\dot{V}A$ = change in alveolar ventilation rate.

NEUROGENIC CONTROL OF BREATHING

The mechanisms that regulate breathing have puzzled and fascinated scientists and physicians since the times of Galen (AD 130-200), the Greek physician who took care of many gladiators with spinal cord injury. A good understanding of respiratory control is essential for the physician because the automaticity of respiration can be altered by numerous conditions such as system immaturity in premature infants, and defects or overstress of the system caused by airway obstruction, obesity, drug overdose, heart failure, injury to the central nervous system (CNS), and so on.

In healthy individuals, breathing is usually involuntary as it is automatically and rhythmically driven by the activity of the CNS. Indeed, the definition of brain death is based on the ability of the CNS to sustain respiration. However, breathing is subject to a complex hierarchy of control mechanisms aimed at dynamically adjusting the ventilatory rate, in terms of both depth (tidal volume, V_T) and frequency of breathing (f), for matching the ever changing metabolic needs, while simultaneously allowing non-homeostatic (behavioral) functions to be carried out normally and seamlessly.

Table 1: Components of the Respiratory Control system

Controlled Variables	**PO_2, PCO_2, pH, Level of Lung Inflation (Distension or Stretch)**
Sensors / Receptors	Within Brain: ***Central chemoreceptors*** (ventral medulla) ***Temperature receptors*** (hypothalamus) ***Pain Receptors*** (through the limbic system) Outside Brain: ***Peripheral Chemoreceptors*** (carotid & aortic bodies) ***Upper Airway Receptors*** (in nose, pharynx, & larynx) ***Lung Receptors***: **Stretch Receptors**: slowly adapting stretch receptors in airways' smooth muscle layer; myelinated vagal fibers stimulated by lung inflation; Breuer-Hering ***inflation*** reflex. (Response: bronchodilation, hyperpnea, and tachycardia) **Irritant receptors**: rapidly adapting receptors among airway epithelial cells; myelinated vagal fibers) (stimulus: cigarette smoke and inflammatory mediators like histamine and prostaglandins; lung hyperinflation) (Breuer-Hering ***deflation*** reflex) (Response: bronchoconstriction; mucous secretion, and cough) **J-Receptors**: Unmyelinated C-fibers endings in the alveolar interstitium closely associated with the capillaries; unmyelinated vagal fibers (stimulus: distension of alveolar interstitial space due to edema or fibrosis) (Response: apnea followed by rapid shallow breathing as seen in patients with pulmonary edema, pneumonia, or embolism; bronchoconstriction; bradycardia; hypotension; mucous secretion) ***Chest Wall Receptors***: proprioceptors in joint, tendon, and muscle spindle receptors (in respiratory muscles and costo-vertebral joints)
Controller Integrator	Medullary Respiratory Groups: **Dorsal Respiratory Group (DRG)** (primarily "Inspiratory Center") **Ventral Respiratory Group (VRG)** (mostly expiratory; rostral portion inspiratory) **Pontine Respiratory Group (PRG)**: a total of four clusters of neurons, two on each side of the brainstem in the upper dorsolateral areas of pons with some neurons firing immediately before inspiration and others immediately before expiration. These neurons function as on-off switches
Effectors	Inspiratory Muscles: diaphragm and external intercostals Expiratory Muscles: internal intercostals and abdominal muscles

At rest, there is a regular cyclic pattern of inspiration and expiration. Inspiration occurs as a result of the contraction of inspiratory muscles (diaphragm and external intercostals), whereas expiration is most often a passive event caused by the elastic recoil of the lung tissue. During each breathing cycle, the frequency of the inspiratory action potentials starts low and accelerates in a ramp-like fashion so that lung inflation occurs smoothly. The rhythmic contractions of the inspiratory muscle fibers are dependent on intact neuronal connections from the brainstem through the motor-neurons in the spinal cord and the phrenic and intercostal nerves.

This automatic rhythm is generated by regular bursts of nerve impulses from specialized neurons of the medulla oblongata and pons located in areas collectively referred to as **respiratory centers**. These include nuclei located in the medulla oblongata (the dorsal and ventral respiratory groups, DRG & VRG, respectively, and the Bötzinger complex), and dorsolateral areas in upper pons (pontine respiratory group or PRG).

The baseline activities of respiratory centers, motor-neurons, and inspiratory muscles are continuously modified to meet the metabolic (homeostatic) needs of the organism as well as to allow for behavioral functions to take place. Breathing is also coordinated with other voluntary activities such eating and drinking (swallowing), as well as with protective reflexes such coughing and sneezing triggered by irritants and allergens.

The central controller/integrator receives afferent (sensory) signals from various sensors, including central and peripheral chemoreceptors (CCR & PCR), lung-inflation (stretch) receptors embedded in lung tissue and airway wall, chest wall proprioceptors, as well as several other sources of protective reflexes (Table **1**). Once the information is analyzed and integrated, the controller issues efferent impulses (output commands) to the effectors to alter their activity. Consequently, the ventilatory rate is altered to meet the demands of the situation. The efferent impulses from the respiratory center in the medulla are carried by fibers that cross below the obex and join the reticulo-spinal tracts, whereas those originating in the cerebral cortex travel in the cortico-spinal tracts and bypass the respiratory centers to transmit voluntary commands directly to the spinal motor neurons that control respiratory muscles. All of the efferent fibers destined to respiratory muscles synapse in the anterior horns of the spinal cord with motor-neurons of phrenic and intercostal nerves. Additional fibers originating in the cerebral premotor and motor cortex descend *via* the cortico-bulbar tracts to innervate the muscles of upper airways.

Respiratory Centers

Over a century ago, Thomas Lumsden (1923), using the crude approach of sectioning the brain of anesthetized cats at different levels, established that the involuntary (automatic) control of breathing is entirely localized in the medulla oblongata and the pons. The complete separation of the brainstem (specifically, medulla oblongata and pons) from the rest of the brain (with a transection at the pons-midbrain junction) had no effect on the normal pattern of breathing. In contrast, a mid-pons transection (immediately above the cerebellar peduncles) resulted in a deep, slow breathing pattern (*i.e.*, increased VT and reduced f). This transection pointed to the presence of the ***"pneumotaxic center"*** in the upper half of the pons whose activity was thought to promote expiration. If in addition to this transection the vagi were cut (to block sensory input from the lungs), a pattern known as ***apneustic breathing*** was produced, which consisted in deep and prolonged inspirations followed by brief expirations. This suggested the presence of inspiration-promoting neurons in lower pons and gave rise to the notion of an "apneustic center" whose activity is normally kept in check by sensory inputs from the lungs and other related sites. Later research proved the assumption of the existence of an apneustic center to be a misinterpretation of the results of the earlier transection experiments. However, the "apneustic center" still appears in many texts. Thus, although apneustic breathing can and does occur in certain disease states, there is no evidence to support the existence an apneustic center.

A transection between the medulla and the pons using the same crude technique resulted in a breathing pattern best described as gasping, consisting of prolonged and deep inspirations separated by short expirations. However, more refined techniques revealed that the medulla alone is capable of generating a regular respiratory rhythm with deep slow pattern. Further electrophysiological experiments revealed that neurons located in several areas of the brainstem fire with each breath, indicating that various neuronal groups or "centers" interact with each other and function in unison to generate the perpetual respiratory rhythm.

There are three paired groups of respiratory nuclei oriented in columns in the tegmentum of the brainstem (Fig. **3**):

1. **Medullary Dorsal Respiratory Group (DRG)**, located in the ventrolateral sub-nucleus of the nucleus tractus solitarius (NTS). Here and in the rostral portions of the VRG (see below) are located most of the inspiratory neurons, some of which directly and monosynaptically connect to motor neurons of the phrenic nucleus (cervical levels C3-C7) that innervate the diaphragm as well as those that innervate the external intercostals (located at thoracic levels T1-T11). Since the DRG is associated primarily with inspiration it is often referred to as "***the inspiratory center***".

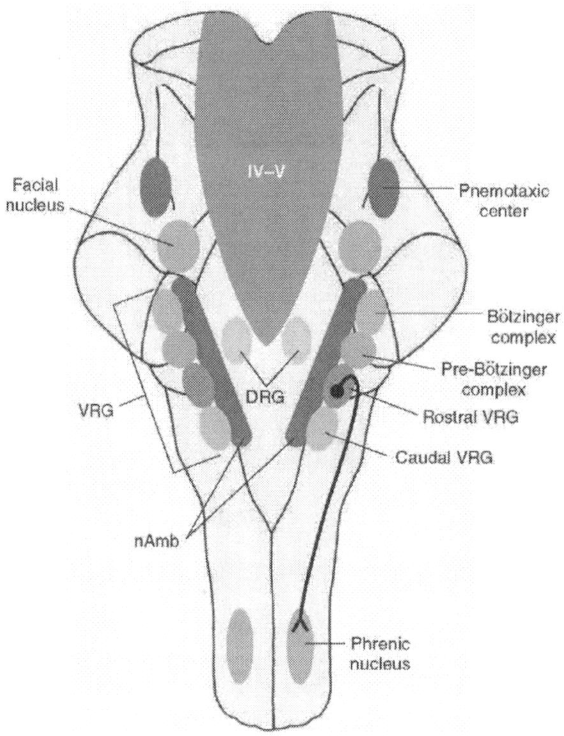

Figure 3: Respiratory neurons in the brainstem. Location of the main centers of respiratory control in the brainstem based on animal experiments and limited human pathology. There are three paired groups of nuclei: (1) The dorsal respiratory group (*DRG*), containing mainly inspiratory neurons, located in the ventrolateral subnucleus of the nucleus of the tractus solitarius; (2) a ventral respiratory group (*VRG*), situated near the nucleus ambiguus (nAmb) and containing in its caudal part neurons that fire predominantly during expiration and in its rostral part neurons that are synchronous with inspiration - the latter structure merges rostrally with the Bötzinger complex, which is located just behind the facial nucleus and contains neurons that are active mostly during expiration; and (3) a pontine pair of nuclei (*PRG*), one of which fires in the transition between inspiration and expiration and the other between expiration and inspiration.

2. **Medullary Ventral Respiratory Group (VRG)**, located along the ventral aspect of the medulla near the nucleus ambiguous, is active during both expiration (caudal region, cVRG) and inspiration (rostral region, rVRG). More rostral to the rVRG and just behind the nucleus of the facial nerve lies the **Bötzinger complex**, which is considered by some to be part of the VRG; it contains neurons that are active mostly during expiration [1]. Thus, the VRG comprises three functionally distinct parts (cVRG, rVRG, and Bötzinger complex). Recently, an area located just caudal to the Bötzinger complex, called pre-Bötzinger complex, has been suggested to play a special role in the genesis of the respiratory rhythm. However, the general consensus is that a regular, controlled respiratory rhythm requires the input and interaction of several clusters of respiratory neurons in both medulla and pons. As pointed out above, at rest expiration occurs passively. However, under certain conditions such as increased metabolic demand, for example, expiratory muscles (mainly internal intercostal and abdominal muscles) may be actively recruited to effect faster and more complete expirations. This recruitment occurs under the control of the expiratory neurons (cVRG + Bötzinger complex) which project to the spinal motor-neurons and at the same time exert an inhibitory influence on the inspiratory neurons.

3. **Pontine Respiratory Group (PRG)**: consists of two clusters of cells of the dorsolateral pons in the region of the nucleus parabrachialis. Experiments involving electrical stimulation indicate that neurons in the dorsal pons may act as "on–off" switches between inspiration and expiration.

Damage to any of the neural components of the respiratory control system can have a profound impact on the patient's capacity to breathe normally. Damage to the fibers arising in the inspiratory neurons and terminating on the phrenic nerve motor-neurons causes the loss of the automatic but not the voluntary movements of the diaphragm ipsilaterally. These fibers lie laterally to the anterior horns of the first three cervical spinal cord segments (C_1-C_3). Damage to the phrenic motor neurons - a thin column in the medial ventral horns extending from the 3rd to the 5th cervical spinal cord segments - prevents both automatic and voluntary breathing.

Chemical Control of Breathing

The chemical composition of the internal environment in terms of PO_2, PCO_2 and protons (H^+) is of paramount importance for the normal functioning of cells and biological systems and is constantly regulated through alterations in the rate of alveolar ventilation ($\dot{V}A$). Although the basic rhythm of breathing is established by the respiratory centers discussed above, both the long term and moment-to-moment control of $\dot{V}A$ are primarily the task of specific chemosensitive cells located in the ventrolateral aspect of the medulla (central chemoreceptors) and in the carotid and aortic bodies (the peripheral chemoreceptors; Figs. **4A** and **4B**). These cells are ultimately responsible for the maintenance of constant levels PO_2, PCO_2 and $[H^+]$ in the arterial blood, protecting the brain from hypoxia and ensuring that the $\dot{V}A$ matches the metabolic rate.

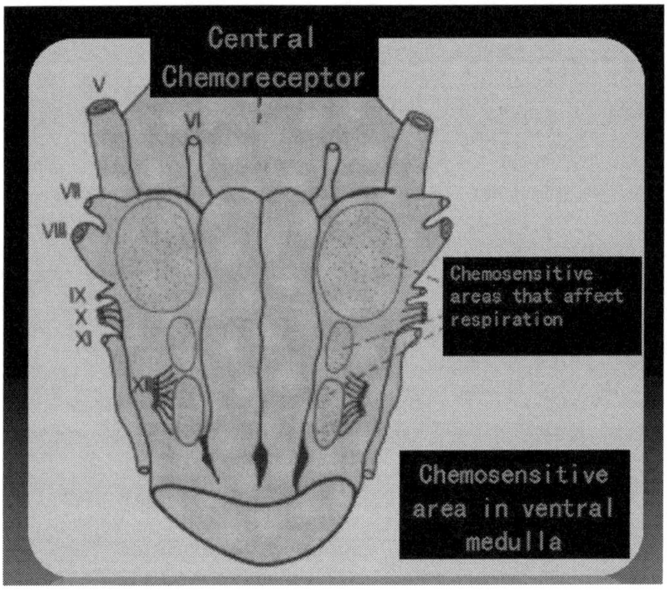

Figure 4A: The central chemoreceptors consist of several clusters of chemosensitive neurons located bilaterally just beneath the surface of the ventrolateral aspect of the medulla oblongata. Note the close association with cranial nerves.

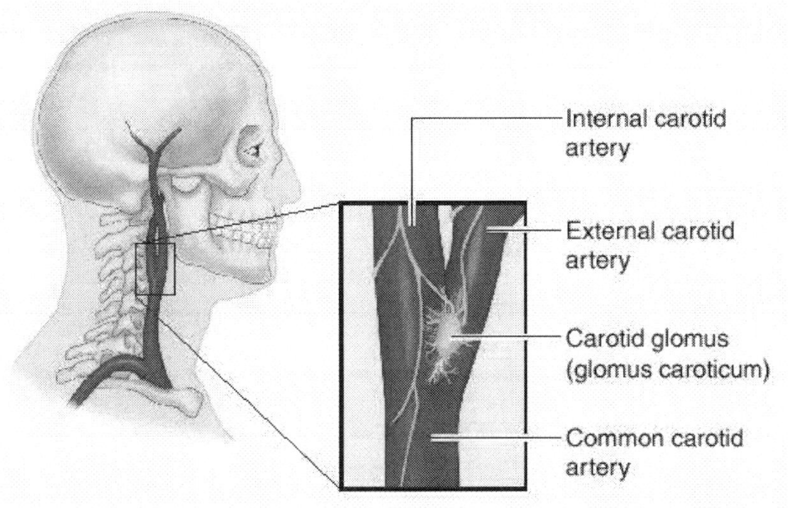

Figure 4B: The carotid body (Glomus caroticum) is a small neurovascular structure lying in the bifurcation of the right and left carotid arteries. It is innervated by a plexus of glossopharyngeal, vagal, and sympathetic fibers. Similar structures are found in the aortic arch. From the Free Dictionary by Farlex http://medical-dictionary.thefreedictionary.com/body

Central Chemoreceptors

The central chemoreceptors are perhaps the most important sensors of the respiratory control system. These specialized, chemosensitive neurons are situated superficially on the ventral aspect of the medulla. They are bathed by the brain's interstitial fluid (ISF) and are in close proximity to the cerebrospinal fluid (CSF; Fig. **5**). The central chemoreceptor cells respond only to $\Delta[H^+]$ in their immediate environment, which is affected by both $\Delta[H^+]_{ISF}$ and $\Delta[H^+]_{CSF}$. Acute increases in arterial PCO_2 elicit marked increases in alveolar ventilation, and the level of this response is markedly influenced by arterial PO_2 (Fig. **6**). It should be noted that while hypoxia directly depresses the respiratory centers it increases ventilation rate by stimulating the peripheral chemoreceptors.

Since CO_2 is highly lipid soluble and diffuses easily through biological membranes, including the blood-brain barrier (BBB), the respiratory response to hypercapnia is relatively rapid. The BBB separates the medullary ISF from the arterial blood. Because of its permeability and transport properties, $\Delta[H^+]$ in arterial blood associated with non-respiratory acid-base disturbances are only partially reflected in the composition of the brain's ISF. By contrast, changes in arterial PCO_2 are transmitted within seconds to both the brain ISF and CSF and have an immediate influence on the activity of the central chemoreceptors and the ventilation rate.

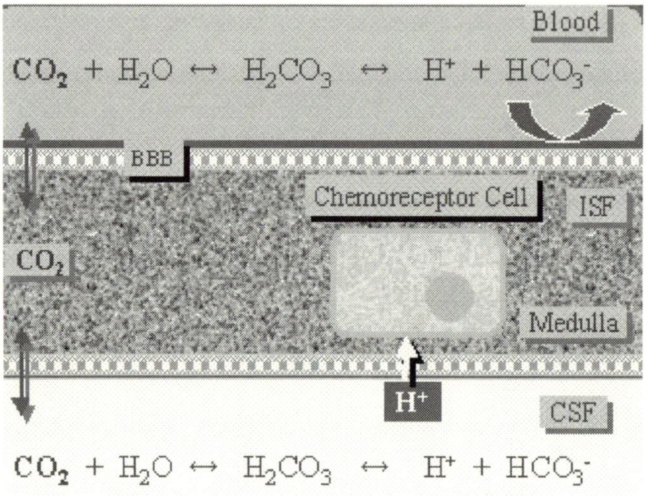

Figure 5: Schematic representation of a chemosensitive cell and its relationship to arterial blood, blood-brain barrier (BBB), interstitial fluid (ISF), and cerebrospinal fluid (CSF). Note that while $\mathbf{HCO_3^-}$ cannot cross the BBB, CO_2 diffuses freely.

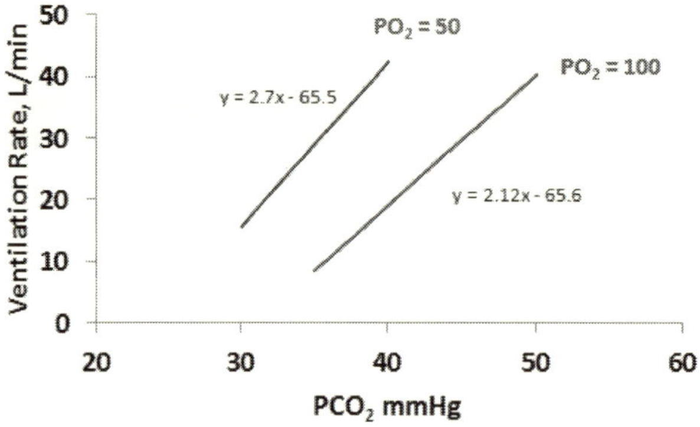

Figure 6: Effect of alveolar PCO_2 on ventilation rate and of hypoxemia on the response to ΔPCO_2. A: normal O_2 tension; B: hypoxemia which directly depresses the respiratory centers, but increases ventilation rate by stimulating the peripheral chemoreceptors.

The CSF is separated from the brain interstitial fluid (ISF) by the brain-CSF barrier and from the blood in the arachnoid plexus by the blood-CSF barrier. The latter consists primarily of ependymal cell lining the CSF cavity. Although the brain's

ISF surrounds the chemosensitive cells, it is the CSF composition that dictates the behavior of the central chemoreceptors (Fig. **5**).

Several characteristics account for the predominant role of the CSF in the regulation of central chemoreceptors' activity:

- The CSF is in intimate contact with a very rich blood supply from the arachnoid plexus, which allows very rapid transmission of any alteration in arterial PCO_2.
- Due to its very low protein concentration, the CSF has very little buffering capacity compared to the medullary ISF, which is surrounded by cells that provide substantial buffering capacity. As a consequence, the same rise in PCO_2 will result in a substantially greater increase in $[H^+]_{CSF}$ than in $[H^+]_{ISF}$.
- The CSF is strategically located immediately underneath the chemosensitive cells. Therefore, the diffusion distances are very short, allowing for the diffusion of H^+ from the CSF toward the chemosensitive neurons.

When exposed to chronic hypercapnia, the central chemoreceptors show a marked degree of adaptation (Fig. **7**).

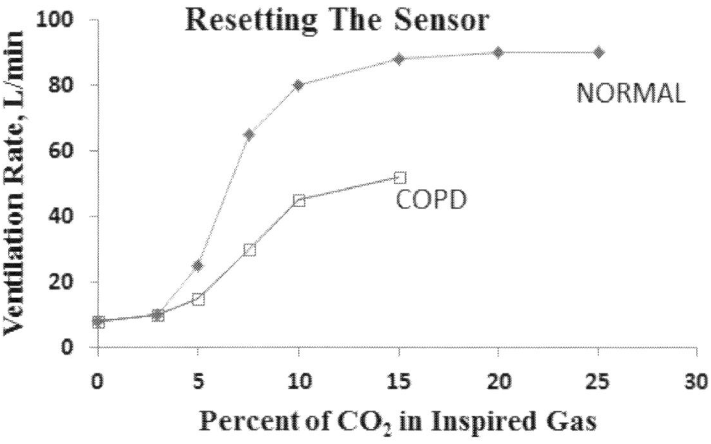

Figure 7: Adaptation of central chemoreceptors to chronic hypercapnia.

A few days after the beginning of hypercapnia, the magnitude of the ventilatory response decreases by about 80%. This is believed to result from the active transport of blood HCO_3^- into CSF across ependymal membranes. As a result, the $[HCO_3^-]_{CSF}$ rises, the $[H^+]_{CSF}$ falls toward its normal value, and the firing activity of the chemosensitive cells drops. This phenomenon accounts for the fact that patients with chronic obstructive pulmonary disease (COPD) and **chronic hypercapnia** become dependent on **hypoxemia** as the primary drive for ventilation. In these patients, aggressive correction of the hypoxemia that would raise the PO_2 above 65 mmHg by administration of O_2-enriched gas eliminates the hypoxia stimulus and leads to CO_2 retention (see Chapter 7). Fig. **8** illustrates the critical importance of the hypoxia drive.

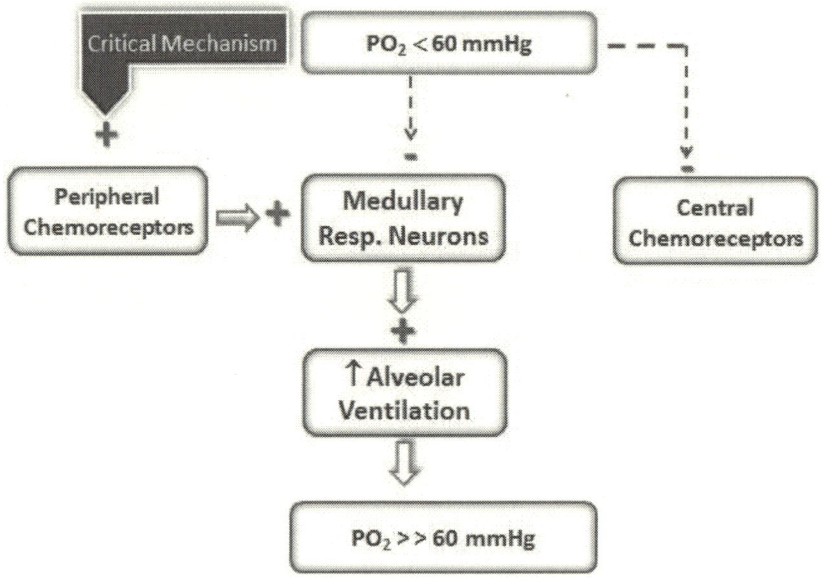

Figure 8: Hypoxia (PO_2 <60 mmHg) is the main stimulus of peripheral chemoreceptors and represents a critical survival mechanism in patients with chronic lung disease.

Peripheral Chemoreceptors

These are clusters of specialized chemosensitive cells capable of chemo-transduction. They are found in the **carotid bodies**, located at the bifurcation of the common carotid arteries, and the aortic body, located in the aortic arch. In humans, the carotid bodies represent the predominant peripheral chemoreceptors; their main function is to maintain an adequate oxygen tension (PO_2) in the arterial blood by stimulating alveolar ventilation. They are responsible for the short-term, moment-to-moment control of alveolar ventilation rate in order to protect brain cells from hypoxia.

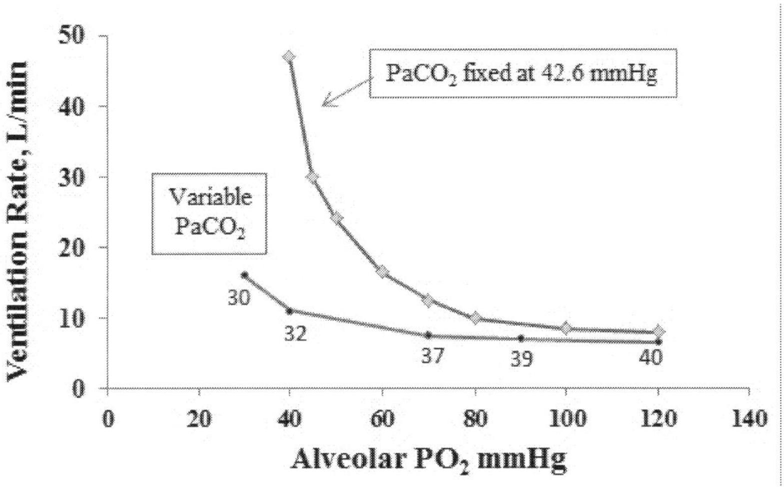

Figure 9: Response of the peripheral chemoreceptors to hypoxemia. Note the greater response when PCO_2 is maintained constant at a nearly normal level.

When in experimental animals carotid and aortic bodies are denervated, hypoxia fails to stimulate ventilation, which highlights their critical importance in maintaining adequate PO_2. Since the carotid bodies possess the highest blood flow (20 ml/g/min) of any tissue in the body and have an extremely low oxygen-extraction, they are well suited for their function, *i.e.*, the constant monitoring of arterial PO_2. The primary *adequate stimulus* for the peripheral chemosensitive cells is **hypoxemia** (⇓PaO_2). However, these cells normally maintain a baseline firing rate even in the presence of hyperoxia ($PO_2 > 400$ mmHg). Under non-isocapnic conditions, their firing rate does not rise significantly until PaO_2 drops well below 60 mmHg. If $PaCO_2$ is kept constant (isocapnia) at its normal level, the peripheral chemoreceptors become more active at higher PO_2 (< 80 mmHg) and the slope of their response curve becomes steeper (Fig. **9**). It should be noted that changes in O_2 content have no effect on the firing rate of the peripheral chemoreceptors. Therefore, neither anemia nor carbon monoxide poisoning stimulates these receptors.

The chemosensitive cells of the carotid bodies can also respond to increases in $[H^+]$ (acidemia), $[K^+]$ (hyperkalemia), and $PaCO_2$ (hypercapnia). The response to hypercapnia appears to be independent of the associated change in $[H^+]$. The effect of hyperkalemia on the peripheral chemoreceptors may play a significant role in the body's response to physical exercise.

Mechanism of Chemosensory Transduction

Adenosine-5'-triphosphate (ATP) is believed to play a key role in the transduction of the chemosensory response of the medullary chemosensitive cells (central chemoreceptors) as well as the glomus cells of the carotid body (peripheral chemoreceptors). Experimental evidence indicates that in response to hypoxia ATP is released by the O_2-sensitive glomus cells of the carotid body. ATP activates the afferent fibers of the carotid sinus nerve, which transmit the information to the brainstem. Similarly, hypercapnia causes the release of ATP from the cells of the central chemoreceptors located in the medulla - ATP acts locally within the medullary respiratory network. The end result in both cases is an adaptive increase in alveolar ventilation ($\dot{V}A$). However, the molecular details of how ATP mediates chemosensory transduction are still unclear [2, 3].

Control of Breathing During Exercise

Metabolic rate is closely linked to alveolar ventilation ($\dot{V}A$). O_2 consumption and CO_2 production increase many folds depending on the intensity of the exercise, up to 20 fold with maximal exertion. Simultaneously, there is a commensurate rise in minute ventilation ($\dot{V}E$), and hence in $\dot{V}A$ with most of the rise occurring at the onset of exercise [4]. The linear relationship between metabolic demand (exercise intensity) and ventilatory response is illustrated in Fig. **10**.

Significantly, all of relevant chemical variables (PO_2, PCO_2, and pH) of arterial blood remain virtually unchanged relative to the normal, resting conditions. In the past, it was believed that the rise in CO_2 production, and hence in PCO_2, is directly responsible for the rise in $\dot{V}A$ that occurs in exercise, but this theory has been proven incorrect. Therefore, the obvious question is: *what triggers the rise in ventilation that occurs within the first few breaths of exercise*?

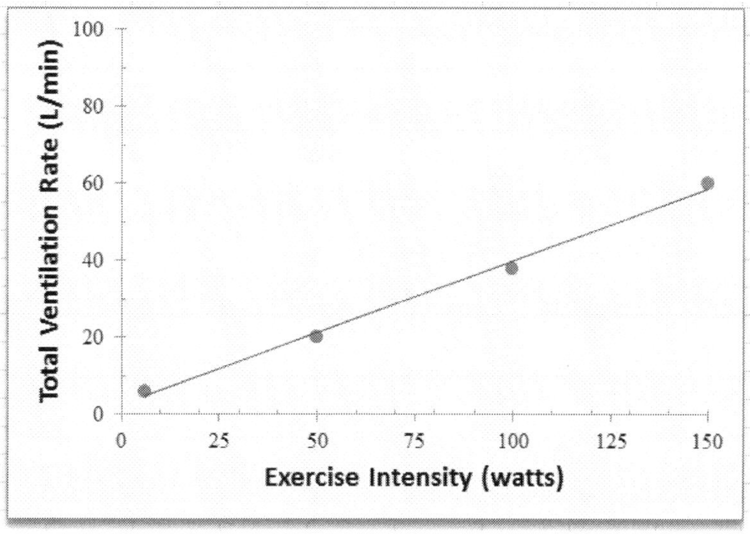

Figure 10: Ventilatory response to exercise intensity. Note the linear relationship.

Evidence indicates that when motor impulses are transmitted to skeletal muscles at the beginning of physical exercise, stimulatory impulses from higher brain centers are also simultaneously transmitted to the respiratory centers of the brainstem, causing an increase in ventilation rate. Afferent impulses from proprioceptors in joints and skeletal muscles are also thought to significantly contribute to stimulating the respiratory centers. Significantly, even with fairly intense exercise the full response of the respiratory system is attained within the first 2-3 minutes. These neurogenic mechanisms account for the initial rise in $\dot{V}E$ but, as exercise continues, chemical stimuli as well as the activity of central and peripheral chemoreceptors play a role in modulating and fine-tuning the respiratory response needed for maintaining adequate tissue oxygenation and acid-base homeostasis. With more intense exercise, the anaerobic threshold is reached. This causes significant lactic acid production, but the compensatory increase in $\dot{V}E$ minimizes the drop in arterial pH.

Control of Breathing During Sleep

The neural control of sleep resides in the supra-chiasmic nuclei of the ventral-anterior region of the hypothalamus. Based on electroencephalographic (EEG) activity, sleep is divided into 4 stages: N1, N2, N3, and R. R stands for rapid-eye movement (REM) and N for non-rapid eye movement (NREM).

In humans, the onset of sleep is associated with a number of physiological changes including a significant reduction in ventilatory rate and ventilatory response to chemical stimuli (reduced chemo-sensitivity). The sleep-related ventilatory depression is accompanied by upper airway atonia and increased upper airway resistance. Some data indicate that the ventilatory depression is centrally mediated, and temporally associated with cessation of activity in the reticular formation and a rise in GABAergic (inhibitory) activity. During REM sleep there is an additional inhibitory activity from cholinergic neurons in the pons that contributes to breathing irregularities and the associated depression of ventilatory rate and response to chemical stimuli.

Sleep Apnea Hypopnea Syndrome (SAHS)

Sleep apnea is a common and potentially serious disorder in which breathing stops and re-starts repeatedly during sleep. Hundreds of such breathing interruptions can occur over the course of a single night with each interruption lasting 10 to 20 seconds. Following each of the long apneic periods the individual is jolted out of the normal sleep phase - the sleep rhythm is disrupted and the individual suffers from fatigue and daytime sleepiness. Other indicative signs of serious sleep apnea include long apneic periods (>15 seconds), loud snoring, choking or gasping during sleep, irritability, headache, depression, nightmares, and so on. If untreated, sleep apnea can lead to serious disorders including obesity, diabetes, hypertension and stroke.

There are three main types of sleep apnea depending on their cause. The most common variety is the Obstructive Sleep Apnea (OSA), which results from upper airway obstruction due to hypotonia and collapse of the posterior pharyngeal muscles. OSA is characterized by cyclic loud snoring - a common problem in obese individuals and patients with endocrine disorders such as hypothyroidism or acromegaly. A common cause of OSA in children is the hypertrophy of tonsils and/or adenoids. Central sleep apnea (CSA) results from reduced central respiratory drive. Complex sleep apnea is a combination of both obstructive and central apneas.

Central sleep apnea occurs when brainstem respiratory neurons fail to stimulate the inspiratory muscles. In some cases, CSA may be a manifestation of cerebrovascular diseases such as lateral medullary infarction. However, many other conditions are associated with CSA, including brainstem encephalitis, anoxic encephalopathy, bulbar poliomyelitis, Creutzfeldt-Jacob ("mad cow") disease, and various brain degenerative diseases. Certain medications may also play a role in CSA. In infants, the cause may be prematurity or congenital diseases. In addition, there is a rare neurological syndrome of idiopathic congenital hypoventilation known as Ondine's Curse [5] which results in total loss of spontaneous breathing, especially during sleep - even in the awake state the "cursed" patients must consciously force themselves to breathe. This disorder is believed to result from the absence of certain respiratory nuclei of the medulla oblongata.

For further reading on the topic of sleep apneas the reader may find these sources helpful [6-8].

REFERENCES

[1] It has been demonstrated that neuronal damage in the area of the Bötzinger complex by neurotoxins or cooling leads to complete loss of respiratory rhythm (Duffin).

[2] Gorine AV. On the peripheral and central chemoreception and control of breathing: an emerging role of ATP. J Physiol 2005;568:715-724.

[3] Ackland GL, Kasymov V, Gourine AV. Physiological and pathophysiological roles of extracellular ATP in chemosensory control of breathing. Biochem Soc Trans 2007;35:1264-1268.

[4] During maximal exercise $\dot{V}E$ may be around 100 l/min whereas the maximum breathing capacity maybe about 150 l/min indicating a substantial physiological reserve.

[5] Nannapaneni, R., Behari S, Todd NV, Mendelow AD. Retracing "Ondine's curse". Neurosurgery 2005;57:354-63.

[6] Callop N, Cassel DK: Snoring and sleep disordered breathing. In: Lee-Chiong T Jr, Sateia M, Carskadon M, Eds: Sleep Medicine. Philadelphia: Hanley & Belfus, 2002;349-355.

[7] Sleep Apnea: Siamak T. Nabili, MD, MPH and Jay W. Marks, MD. http://www.medicinenet.com/sleep_apnea/article.htm

[8] Sleep-Disordered Breathing: Puneet S. Garcha, Loutfi S. Aboussouan, and Omar Minai. http://www.clevelandclinicmeded.com/medicalpubs/diseasemanagement/pulmonary/sleep-disordered-breathing/

CHAPTER 9

Respiration at Rest and During Exercise at Sea Level and High Altitude

Camillo Peracchia

Abstract: This chapter describes the physiological changes that occur when the organism is subjected to physical exercise, from resting state, at sea level and at high altitude. In particular, it focuses on compensatory mechanisms that regulate major respiratory functions, such as: gas exchange, ventilation-perfusion distribution, tissue oxygenation, pulmonary and systemic circulation, and acid-base balance. In addition, mechanisms involved in acclimatization to high altitude, acute and chronic mountain sickness, and adaptation to high altitude are briefly described.

Keywords: Acid-Base Balance, Acute Mountain-Sickness, Alkalosis, Chronic Mountain-Sickness, Exercise, High-Altitude Acclimatization, High-Altitude Adaptation, High-Altitude Oxygen-Pressure, Hypocapnia, Hypoxia, Hypoxic Vasoconstriction, Joint Receptors, Metaboreceptors, Pulmonary Circulation, Pulmonary Edema, Pulmonary Hypertension, Shunt Fraction, Systemic Circulation, Ventilation-Perfusion Distribution, Ventilation-Perfusion Maldistribution.

SYMBOLS, ACRONYMS AND NORMAL VALUES: See Appendix 3

Atmospheric Changes from Sea Level to High Altitude

As one climbs from sea-level to high altitude, composition and physical properties of inspired air gradually change. While the fractional concentration of oxygen (FIO_2) does not change, the inspired pressure of oxygen (PIO_2) progressively drops (Table **1**) as barometric pressure (PB) decreases from 760 mmHg at sea level to values as low as 240 mmHg at the top of Mount Everest (8,848m, 29,029 ft.; 1 m = 3.28084 ft.). In addition, air cools and humidity drops; in spite of that the air that reaches the alveoli is still warmed to body temperature (37°C) and humidified to 100% saturation (47 mmHg).

Since the partial pressure of saturated water vapor in the lungs depends entirely on body temperature regardless of PB, at 37°C PH_2O is still 47 mmHg at any altitude. This significantly contributes to further lowering PIO_2 from atmospheric PO_2, such that while at sea level PO_2 drops from ambient to trachea by ~5%, at 20,000 ft.

(6,096 m) it drops by ~11% (see Table **1**). The combined effect of high altitude hypoxia and pulmonary gas humidification is such that PIO_2 drops by almost 60% going from sea level to 20,000 ft. (see Table **1**). When air reaches the alveoli, PO_2 further drops as some of the alveolar volume is occupied by CO_2. The combined effect is such that even if a subject attempts to compensate by hyperventilating, a reasonable assumption is the alveolar PO_2 at 20,000 ft. will range from 40 to 50 mmHg, which is less than half the sea level value.

Table 1: Oxygen Pressure At Different Altitudes

Altitude (ft.)	Altitude (m)	PB (mmHg)	Atmospheric PO_2 (mmHg, %S 50, 23°C)	PIO_2 (trachea, mmHg, %S 100, 37°C)	%PO_2 drop (Atm.→Trachea)
0	0	760	157	149	5
10,000	3,048	523	107	100	6.5
20,000	6,096	349	71	63	11
30,000	9,144	226	45	37	18

John Climbs from Sea Level to La Rinconada (Peru)

To learn about the effect of high altitude on respiratory physiology, we will follow a fictitious young man (John) whose cardio-respiratory function is tested both at sea level and high altitude (see Table **2**; some of the data were obtained from: Sutton, *et al.*, 1988 [1]).

John, is a healthy, athletic twenty eight year old (180lb weight), who decided to climb from sea-level (PB = 760 mmHg) to the Peruvian town of La Rinconada. This gold-mining town, located at an altitude of 16,732 ft. (5,100m), is one of the world's highest dwellings; its average PB is ~400 mmHg. After being tested at sea level, both at rest and during steady state exercise (12 watts work level, on bicycle exerciser; see Table **2**), John started climbing and reached La Rinconada in a month or so. There, a few days after his arrival John was tested again both at rest and during steady state exercise at the same work load (see Table **2**).

Table 2: Laboratory blood and gas data - comparison between sea level and high altitude conditions

	Sea Level At Rest	Sea Level Exercise	16,732 ft. At Rest	16,732 ft. Exercise
GAS EXCHANGE				
FIO_2 (%)	21	21	21	21
VT (liters, BTPS)	0.75	1.78	1.32	2.6
F (breaths/min)	9	25	11	37
$\dot{V}E$ (l/min, BTPS)	6.75	44.5	14.52	89.5
VCd (liters, BTPS)	0.180	0.180	0.180	0.180
$\dot{V}O_2$ (l/min, STPD)	0.275	1.8	0.329	2.0
$\dot{V}CO_2$ (liters/min, STPD)	0.220	1.75	0.280	1.94
R	0.8	0.97	0.85	0.97
VENTILATION-PERFUSION				
$PAiO_2$ (mmHg)	104	110.8	51.3	54.7
PaO_2 (mmHg)	98	105	48	50
$PaCO_2$ (mmHg)	38	38	20	19
pHa	7.42	7.39	7.5	7.4
Hb (g/100 ml blood)	14	14	16	16
Hematocrit (%)	40	40	50	50
$CAiO_2$ (vol%)	18.95	18.33	19.73	19.43
CaO_2 (vol%)	18.84	18.17	19.23	18.73
$C\bar{v}O_2$ (vol%)	13.84	10.9	13.73	5.03
$CaO_2 - C\bar{v}O_2$ (vol%)	5	11.05	5.5	13.7
$(Ai\text{-}a)PO_2$ (mmHg)	5	5.8	3.3	4.7
$\dot{Q}Ps/\dot{Q}$ (%)	2.2	1.5	8.3	5
$\dot{V}Ad/\dot{V}\bar{A}$ (%)	2.6	0.7	3.7	1.6
$\dot{V}\bar{A}/\dot{Q}$	0.9	2.42	2.1	5.7
CIRCULATION				
$\dot{Q}$ (l/min)	5.5	16.5	6	14.6
Heart Rate	64	120	75	130
Stroke Volume (ml)	86	137	80	112
Mean Pulmonary Artery Pressure (mmHg)	20	25	35	40
TISSUE OXYGENATION				
$P\bar{v}O_2$ (mmHg)	40	23	31	16.2
$pH\bar{v}$	7.38	7.3	7.45	7.31
2,3-DPG (mmol/l)	1.7	1.7	3.8	3.8
ACID-BASE				
$[HCO_3]^-$ (mEq/l plasma)	24	22.6	15.5	11.8
Base Excess (mEq/l plasma)	0.2	-2.4	-7.4	-12.2
$P\bar{v}CO_2$ (mmHg)	50	57	26	30
GENERAL				
Body Temperature (°C)	37	37	37	37
PB (mmHg)	760	760	400	400

Rest *versus* Exercise at Sea Level

Gas Exchange

John's VT and f Increased Rapidly with Exercise. VT More Than Doubled and f Almost Tripled, Such that $\dot{V}E$ Increased 6.6 Times

There is a linear relationship between metabolic rate and ventilation up to exhaustive exercise. When $\dot{V}O_2$ is greater than 2.5 l/min (~63% of $\dot{V}O_2$max), $\dot{V}E$ may actually exceed maximum voluntary ventilation (MVV). This apparent paradox is believed to result from both airway dilatation [2] and a reflex-induced improved balance between respiratory frequency and tidal volume. With vigorous exercise $\dot{V}E$ may increase more rapidly than $\dot{V}O_2$ because some muscle fibers convert to anaerobic metabolism and generate lactic acid, which stimulates the central chemoreceptors.

Surprisingly, ventilation starts increasing immediately with exercise, in spite of the fact that arterial blood gases are at normal level. This phenomenon puzzled physiologists for decades. While its mechanism is still not fully understood, there is evidence that stimuli from muscle metaboreceptors and joint receptors sensitive to limb movement cause virtually instantaneous hyperpnea. Stimuli from joints result in increased ventilation even with passive limb movements, and joint denervation abolishes the effect. Afferent myelinated fibers of group III originating from mechanoreceptors and unmyelinated fibers of group IV are thought to play a role. In addition, receptors known as " nocireceptors" are activated by a variety of chemicals, including metabolites released by working muscles.

Both humoral- and neural-derived stimuli are believed to play a role according to the "neurohumoral theory of ventilator control in exercise". Neural drive is thought to originate in the cortex, hypothalamus, and other sites of the CNS; indeed, stimulation of certain areas of the hypothalamus elicits cardio-respiratory responses comparable to those observed in exercise. Additional stimuli may come from yet unidentified venous receptors sensitive to increased CO_2. These receptors may be located in the venae cavae. Another hypothesis proposes that peripheral chemoreceptors may be stimulated by PO_2 and PCO_2 oscillations that occur during exercise.

With exercise, airway resistance decreases. This facilitates gas flow as its rate is greatly increased. For this reason, the severity of asthma decreases with exercise, but after exercise asthma significantly increases due to a rebound effect.

$\dot{V}O_2$ and $\dot{V}CO_2$ Increased 6.5 and 8 Times, Respectively, and R from 0.8 to 0.97

The large increase in $\dot{V}O_2$ and $\dot{V}CO_2$ does not result in hypoxemia and hypercapnia because the increased ventilation adequately compensates for the increased metabolic demand. The increase in R is not due to acute hyperventilation, as it is stated that John had reached steady state, but rather to metabolic changes. At rest, cells burn a mixture of glucose (RQ = 1) and lipids (RQ = 0.7), resulting in RQ values ranging from 0.8 to 0.85, while during exercise muscle fibers preferentially burn glucose. Tissue hypoxia may develop in vigorous exercise causing muscle fibers to switch to anaerobic metabolism and produce lactic acid; in this case, R values may increase above 1, as protons stimulate the central chemoreceptors causing hyperventilation. In prolonged exercise, for example during a marathon run, R values may progressively decrease toward 0.7 as glycogen reserves become depleted, forcing muscles to burn lipids.

Ventilation-Perfusion Distribution

With Exercise, the Fraction of Alveolar Ventilation Wasted in Alveolar Dead Space Dropped by 73%

The most likely reason for this is that with exercise the effect of gravity on regional pulmonary circulation was minimized. As pulmonary artery pressure and blood flow increase, the lung perfusion becomes more homogeneous. This reduces the regional $\dot{V}/\dot{Q}$ maldistributions and consequently decreases the magnitude of both alveolar dead space and maldistribution shunt-like effect, even though in John's case they were minimal even at rest. Other reasons for the drop in shunt fraction are: the increase in gas diffusion across the blood-gas barrier, due to increased diffusing capacity of the barrier, the large recruitment of blood-filled alveolar capillaries, the increased ventilation in poorly ventilated areas, and the increase in Hb concentration due to sympathetic stimulation.

While the Shunt Fraction Decreased, the (Ai-a)PO_2 Gradient Increased by 16%

This apparent inconsistency is explained by two factors. One is that with an increase in $PAiO_2$ and PaO_2 the relationship between PO_2 and blood O_2 content shifts toward a flatter region of the O_2 dissociation curve. In this region of the curve, greater PO_2 increments are required to produce the same increase in O_2 content. This outweighs the very small right-shift of the O_2 dissociation curve due to a small drop in pHa. The other factor is the metabolic change from mixed to mostly glucose burning. This increases the exchange ratio from 0.8 to 0.97, which raises $PAiO_2$ above the resting value.

Tissue Oxygenation

$P\bar{v}O_2$ Dropped by 42.5% and $pH\bar{v}$ from 7.38 to 7.3

The $P\bar{v}0_2$ drop results from a large increase in O_2 extraction, which almost doubled. Since $P\bar{v}0_2$ represents the average tissue PO_2, it is obvious that the PO_2 of venous blood flowing from working muscles is much lower. However, $P\bar{v}0_2$ would be significantly lower if $pH\bar{v}$ had not dropped to 7.3, which right-shifts the O_2 dissociation curve facilitating the O_2 unloading at tissues, especially in working muscles where pH is even lower. Also beneficial are the higher PCO_2 and temperature at working muscles, which further right-shift the O_2-dissociation curve. The change in base excess to slightly negative indicates that some muscles have switched to anaerobic metabolism and produced lactic acid because of regional tissue hypoxia.

Pulmonary Circulation

Mean Pulmonary Artery Pressure Increased by 25%

Pulmonary artery pressure increases moderately with exercise because in spite of the increased blood flow, due to increased cardiac output, the vascular resistance decreases. The drop in vascular resistance is not caused by a reduction in smooth muscle tone at pulmonary arterioles, but rather it involves two mechanisms: capillary recruitment and capillary distension. While at rest a number of alveolar capillaries are collapsed (un-perfused), in exercise the increased blood flow causes them expand, as the increased hydrostatic pressure outweighs their critical opening pressure. In addition, the increased perfusion pressure increases the trans-mural pressure of the capillary wall causing capillary enlargement; capillaries are easily enlarged because their wall is very distensible (compliant).

Somewhat offsetting this beneficial effect is the increase in tidal volume. At larger lung volumes alveolar capillaries are stretched lengthwise and their diameter decreases, which tends to increase vascular resistance. However, at larger lung volumes the intra-pleural pressure becomes more negative causing extra-alveolar vessels (arteries and veins) to enlarge, as their wall is stretched out, and consequently decreasing their perfusion resistance. In conclusion, the result of these opposing factors is a mild increase in mean pulmonary artery pressure and, minimally, in wedge pressure. The pulmonary wedge pressure is indicative of left atrial pressure and is measured by wedging a catheter with an inflatable balloon into a small branch of the pulmonary artery.

Systemic Circulation

Cardiac Output ($\dot{Q}$) Tripled, as SV and HR Increased by ~60% and 87.5%, Respectively

There is a linear relationship between heart rate and oxygen consumption up to the so called anaerobic threshold, beyond which oxygen consumption increases by greater increments than heart rate. This is caused by the progressive conversion of muscle fibers to anaerobic metabolism with production of lactic acid. John is likely to have just reached the anaerobic threshold, as lactic acid starts accumulating resulting in negative base excess. With exercise, systemic blood pressure usually increases slightly due to increased tension in abdominal and working muscles and increased sympathetic tone. However, the effect of these factors is curbed somewhat by metabolically induced vasodilation in working muscles.

Acid-Base

pHa Dropped from 7.42 to 7.39, BE Became Negative (-2.4) and pH$\bar{v}$ Dropped from 7.38 to 7.3

The negative base excess results from accumulation of small amounts of lactic acid, but pHa is still within the normal range. Due to an increase in $P\bar{v}CO_2$, pH$\bar{v}$ dropped by a greater amount than pHa. As the volume of O_2 taken up by the tissue increases (increased O_2-extraction), causing a drop in $P\bar{v}O_2$, the volume of CO_2 diffusing from tissues into venous blood also increases, causing an increase in $P\bar{v}CO_2$ (greater $P\bar{v}CO_2/PaCO_2$), and consequential drop in $pH\bar{v}$ (greater $pHa/pH\bar{v}$).

Sea Level *versus* High Altitude at Rest

Gas Exchange

VT Increased by 76% and f by Over 20%, Such that $\dot{V}E$ More Than Doubled

The increase in ventilation is not due to a large increase in metabolic rate, as $\dot{V}O_2$ only increases by ~20%, but rather to the hypoxic environment. At 16,732 feet, PIO_2 is only ~74 mmHg; without an increase in ventilation (John's sea level $PaCO_2$ = 38 mmHg), PaO_2 would be less than 30 mmHg, a level likely to cause unconsciousness. The severe hypoxemia strongly stimulates peripheral chemoreceptors, resulting in dramatic increase in ventilation. In John's case, this halves $PaCO_2$ and raises PaO_2 to 48 mmHg, which is hardly tolerable but enough to maintain consciousness.

At High Altitude, $\dot{V}O_2$ and $\dot{V}CO_2$ Increased by 19.6% and 27%, Respectively, and R from 0.8 to 0.85

The increase in metabolic rate results from increased work of breathing ($\dot{V}E$ more than doubled). Elastic work increases because the lungs expand to larger volumes and more frequently. Resistive work increases to a lesser extent because airway resistance drops at high altitude due to decreased air density.

Increased sympathetic discharge and thyroid activity also contribute to increasing metabolic rate. The rise in thyroid activity is likely to be secondary to increased secretion of thyrotropic hormone (TSH) caused by hypoxia and colder temperature. The minimal change in R value indicates that John's ventilation is still at steady state with his metabolic rate, and that no significant change in metabolism from the normal carbohydrate-lipid consumption has occurred.

Ventilation-Perfusion Distribution

At High Altitude, the Alveolar Dead Space Fraction did not Significantly Change, While the Shunt Fraction Almost Quadrupled

The alveolar dead space fraction does not increase at high altitude and in some cases may even decrease slightly due to pulmonary hypertension, which improves perfusion at apical lung regions. In contrast, the hypoxic vasoconstriction increases $\dot{V}/\dot{Q}$ maldistribution in the shunt direction; increased diffusion impairment may also contribute to increasing the physiological shunt fraction.

The $\dot{V}/\dot{Q}$ maldistribution at high altitude results from a number of factors. The non-uniform hypoxic vasoconstriction and consequential pulmonary hypertension results in uneven perfusion that may result in interstitial and perivascular edema. In some alveoli the increase in vascular pressure may cause fluid leakage from capillary walls, resulting in alveolar flooding and consequential conductive shunt (alveoli perfused by unventilated). An additional factor affecting pulmonary perfusion and increasing vascular pressure is the greater blood viscosity due to polycythemia (see below).

Hypoxic vasoconstriction results from contraction of vascular smooth muscles secondary to Ca^{2+}-influx through L-type Ca^{2+}-channels. Among possible reasons for non-uniform hypoxic vasoconstriction are: preexisting regional $\dot{V}/\dot{Q}$ abnormalities, regional variations in nitric oxide (NO) release by endothelial cells, and possibly differences in the number of smooth muscle cells among arterioles. Hyperventilation compensatory to hypoxemia, and consequential alkalosis and increased PAO_2, partially reduce the pulmonary vasoconstriction; this also benefits from greater NO release.

Peribronchial edema and mucous obstruction of small airways may lower regional $\dot{V}/\dot{Q}$ ratios, exaggerating the extent of the maldistribution shunt-like effect. In addition, there might be areas where bronchioles are completely obstructed and alveoli are filled with liquid, which would result in $\dot{V}/\dot{Q} = 0$, adding conductive shunt. Diffusion impairment is also likely to occur at high altitude. Due to hypoxic breathing, the drop in pressure gradient at the alveolar-capillary barrier may cause the end-capillary PO_2 to be lower than alveolar PO_2; this would add to the shunt-like fraction. To determine the fraction of physiological shunt due to maldistribution plus diffusion impairment one needs to ventilate the subject with 100% O_2; this completely eliminates these shunt components, enabling one to determine the conductive shunt fraction (see Chapter 7).

While the Shunt Fraction Almost Quadrupled, the (Ai-a)PO_2 Gradient Decreased to a Value Lower than at Sea Level

The reason for the low (Ai-a)PO_2 gradient is that with hypoxic breathing and hypoxemia - in John's case both $PAiO_2$ and PaO_2 dropped by ~50% - the system operates along the steep portion of the O_2-dissociation curve, where even large changes in O_2 content correspond to relatively small changes in PO_2 - hemoglobin is an O_2-buffer and its O_2 buffering capacity at $PO_2 \approx 50$ mmHg is still pretty large (see Chapter 7).

Tissue Oxygenation

$P\bar{v}O_2$ Dropped by ~23%

The ~23% drop in $P\bar{v}O_2$ (from 40 to 31 mmHg) is relatively small compared to the 51% drop in PaO_2 (from 98 to 48 mmHg). This can be explained by considering several conflicting phenomena taking place here: 1. the increase in pHa to 7.5 shifts the O_2 dissociation curve to the left – this would facilitate O_2-loading at the lungs; 2. the doubling in 2,3-DPG concentration, causes a right-shift – this would facilitate O_2 downloading at the tissue; 3. John's adaptation to high altitude has increased his hemoglobin concentration and hematocrit, greatly enhancing his blood's O_2-carrying capacity. The combined effect of these factors contributes to making John's arterial O_2 content paradoxically ~2% higher than at sea level in spite of the large drop in PaO_2, and contributes to maintaining an adequate O_2 content in venous blood, reflected by a higher than expected $P\bar{v}O_2$; this explains why tissue oxygenation has not deteriorated further.

Pulmonary Circulation

Mean Pulmonary Pressure Increased by 75%

Mean pulmonary artery pressure easily rises above 30 mmHg at high altitude. This is due to hypoxic vasoconstriction, which increases pulmonary vascular resistance, and partially to increased blood viscosity due to polycythemia. Capillary pressure also increases by 2-7 mmHg from ~18 mmHg at sea level; higher capillary pressure may result in pulmonary edema. In contrast, the pulmonary capillary wedge-pressure (P_{pcw}), which monitors the venous side of the pulmonary circulation, does not significantly change from the normal range of 8-10 mmHg. The rise in vascular resistance overloads the right ventricle, with serious consequences in COPD patients (the effect of high altitude on circulation is reviewed in [3]). An increase in right atrial pressure may open the foramen ovale causing additional conductive shunt – note that the foramen ovale is actually open in ~27% of the normal population, although venous admixture rarely occurs in normal people because the inter-atrial pressure gradient favors a small left-to-right shunt.

Systemic Circulation

Cardiac Output ($\dot{Q}$) Increased by 9%, SV Dropped by ~7% and HR Increased by 17%

The drop in stroke volume results in part from a chain of events initiated by the increase in pulmonary vascular resistance and consequential right ventricle overload. As the right ventricle becomes more dilated the inter-ventricular septum shifts to the left sacrificing both volume and filling of the left ventricle. The increase in heart rate caused by sympathetic stimulation compensates for the drop in SV and results in mildly increased cardiac output.

Acid-Base

pHa Increased from 7.42 to 7.50, BE Changed to Negative (-7.4) and pH$\bar{v}$ Increased from 7.38 to 7.45

Since $PaCO_2$ is 20 mmHg (almost half the value at sea level) and BE has a negative value, John's acid-base status is defined as partially compensated respiratory alkalosis. This is obviously brought about by the chain of events caused by hypoxic breathing. As PaO_2 drops, the compensatory increase in ventilation causes hypocapnia with drastic increase in pHa. Hypocapnia then induces the kidneys to release HCO_3^-, causing a drop in pHa. These phenomena initiate a vicious cycle, because as pHa drops, ventilation further increases, causing more HCO_3^- release, and so on. After a week or so, this cycling decreases and pHa starts returning to near normal values.

Rest *versus* Exercise at High Altitude

Gas Exchange

VT Doubled and f Tripled with Exercise, Such that $\dot{V}E$ Increased ~6 Times

Percent-wise, tidal volume, frequency and total ventilation increased as they did at sea level, but $\dot{V}E$ was twice as large because at high altitude ventilation needs to compensate for both the hypoxic environment and the work-related rise in metabolic rate.

$\dot{V}O_2$ and $\dot{V}CO_2$ Increased 6 and ~7 Times, Respectively, and R Increased from 0.85 to 0.97

The increase in ventilation matches the increase in both $\dot{V}O_2$ and $\dot{V}CO_2$, such that PaO_2 is maintained approximately as it was at rest. The increase in R is due to a change in metabolism as working muscle fibers preferentially burn glucose (RQ = 1).

Ventilation-Perfusion Distribution

Alveolar Dead Space and Shunt Dropped by 57% and ~40%, Respectively

As at sea level, the alveolar dead space ventilation, already very low at rest, decreased even further with exercise, due to improved perfusion at apical lung regions (reduced regional $\dot{V}/\dot{Q}$), brought about by an increase in pulmonary artery pressure from 32 to 40 mmHg. The drop in shunt fraction is due to increased ventilation in low $\dot{V}/\dot{Q}$ regions (reduced maldistribution shunt-like effect). In spite of the drop in shunt fraction, the $(Ai\text{-}a)PO_2$ gradient increases slightly. As at sea level this is due to both an increase in $PAiO_2$ and PaO_2 and the increase in R value from 0.85 to 0.97, which increases $PAiO_2$ by greater fractions than at rest.

In some alveoli, diffusion impairment may be enhanced due to increased $\dot{Q}$, which adds to the effect of reduced alveolar PO_2 - the faster flow rate of capillary blood may reduce the available time for PO_2 equilibration across the blood-gas barrier. However, in John's case, the shunt-like effect due to increased diffusion impairment, if any, must have been significantly outweighed by improved $\dot{V}/\dot{Q}$ distribution, because $\dot{Q}Ps/\dot{Q}$ dropped from 8.3% to 5%.

Tissue Oxygenation

$P\bar{v}O_2$ Dropped from 31 to ~16 mmHg and pH$\bar{v}$ from 7.45 to 7.31

The very low $P\bar{v}O_2$ indicates severe tissue hypoxia. Its 58% drop from the resting level results from a large increase in O_2 extraction, which more than doubled. However, $P\bar{v}O_2$ would be even lower if pH$\bar{v}$ had not dropped from 7.45 to 7.3 and $P\bar{v}CO_2$ had not increased - right-shift of the O_2 dissociation curve. The right shift is even greater in working muscles, where PCO_2 is even greater, pH is even lower and temperature is higher. In spite of these favorable factors, however, tissue hypoxia is severe and based on the significantly more negative base excess (see below) it is obvious that many cells have switched to glycolytic metabolism, producing lactic acid.

Pulmonary Circulation

Mean Pulmonary Artery Pressure Increased from 32 to 40 mmHg

Pulmonary artery pressure increased by 25%, as it did at sea level, for reasons explained above. However, the difference at high altitude is that this increase worsens a preexisting, albeit mild, hypertensive status. In John's case, pulmonary hypertension is still relatively mild both at rest and with exercise, but in some people it might increase well over 100 mmHg. In these cases, while wedge pressure usually remains relatively normal, indicating unaltered pulmonary vein pressure, alveolar capillary pressure may increase to 20-25 mmHg, which is above the threshold values of 17-24 mmHg for edema formation [3]. The consequence of increased capillary pressure is the so called High Altitude Pulmonary Edema (HAPE). This is a very serious condition because, by causing large conductive shunt fractions, further complicates the already severe hypoxemia secondary to hypoxic breathing. As HAPE develops, the subject starts experiencing dyspnea and reduced exercise tolerance, and may cough-up pink and foamy expectorate. As HAPE worsens, symptoms of cerebral edema such as ataxia and reduced level of consciousness may develop.

Systemic Circulation

Cardiac Output ($\dot{Q}$) More Than Doubled, as SV and HR Increased by 40% and 73%, Respectively

While with exercise the metabolic rate increased by similar percent values at both sea level and high altitude (555% and 508% increase in $\dot{V}O_2$, respectively), cardiac output had tripled at sea level but only doubled at high altitude. The lower cardiac output increment with exercise at high altitude reflects a drop in work capacity with respect to sea level.

At high altitude HR increased by a smaller percent than at sea level. This seems to result from enhanced parasympathetic activity, because pharmacological vagus inhibition restores HR to sea level values.

Acid-Base

pHa Dropped from 7.5 to 7.4, BE Changed from -7.4 to -12.2, and $pH\bar{v}$ Dropped from 7.45 to 7.31

The significant increase in negative BE is obviously the consequence of lactic acid production in hypoxic working muscles. This base deficit adds to the preexisting negative BE, which resulted from excretion of HCO_3^- compensatory to respiratory alkalosis. The drop in $pH\bar{v}$ is due to a small increase in $P\bar{v}CO_2$ during exercise.

Acclimatization to High Altitude

As mentioned above, with acute exposure to high altitude the hypoxemia-induced hyperventilation, which causes alkalosis and compensatory drop in HCO_3^-, initiates a vicious cycle among these four parameters. This cycling decreases after a week or so and pHa starts returning to near normal values.

After a few days of exposure to high altitude, the ability to respond to CO_2, which was lost due to the large drop in $PaCO_2$ with hypoxia-driven hyperventilation, starts recovering in spite of continuous hyperventilation; this follows the end of the cycling between HCO_3^--excretion and hyperventilation mentioned above. The recovery of CO_2 sensitivity allows the cerebrospinal fluid's pH to progressively recover to a normal value (7.32). Tolerance to hypoxia slowly improves as the organism adapts to hypoxemia and hypocapnia.

Adaptation to high altitude also involves blood changes that significantly improve its O_2 carrying capacity. The hematocrit rises acutely, possibly by transfer of fluid out of the vascular compartment, and chronically by an increase in the erythrocyte population (polycythemia). The latter is due to an increase in erythropoiesis caused by hypoxia-driven stimulation of erythropoietin synthesis. In John's case, the limited amount of time spent at high altitude was sufficient to increase the hematocrit by 25% and the hemoglobin concentration by ~14%.

An additional change is the increase in 2,3-diphosphoglycerate (2,3-DPG) in erythrocytes, due mostly to the drop in $PaCO_2$ secondary to hyperventilation, which right-shifts the O_2 dissociation curve. This is beneficial to O_2 delivery, but inhibits somewhat the O_2 uptake at the lungs. However, the left-shift due to blood alkalinization and drop in $PaCO_2$ outweighs the right shift due to increased 2,3-DPG; the resulting limited left-shift is beneficial, as it increases the O_2 uptake at the lungs.

In working muscles the capillary bed appears to increase, and both the concentration of oxidative enzymes and the myoglobin content rise. The combined effect of the increase in vascularity, myoglobin content and blood 2,3-DPG enables muscles to work efficiently in spite of severe hypoxemia. As previously mentioned, O_2 delivery to working muscles is also enhanced by the right-shifting effect of increased muscle temperature and PCO_2, and drop in pH (evidenced by increased $P\bar{v}CO_2$ and decreased $pH\bar{v}$).

Acute Mountain Sickness

People acutely exposed to high altitude may suffer from Acute Mountain Sickness (AMS). Symptoms of AMS include: dizziness, fatigue, palpitation, nausea, anorexia, insomnia and headache. The mechanisms involved are poorly understood, but these symptoms are likely to result from a cascade of events initiated by hypoxemia and alkalosis, which in extreme cases may result in cerebral edema. The hypoxemia-induced increase in cerebral blood flow, in spite of cerebral vasoconstriction secondary to hypocapnia, causes fluid to exit brain capillaries leading to edema.

Acute high altitude pulmonary edema (HAPE) is also a serious complication of high altitude exposure. It may occur at altitudes greater than 8,000-9,000 ft. (2400-2700 m). The symptoms include dyspnea, cough, weakness, and chest tightness. Chest auscultation will reveal crackles, and X-ray images will show bilateral areas of infiltration.

Administration of acetazolamide, a carbonic anhydrase inhibitor used for treating both metabolic and respiratory alkalosis, reduces the symptoms of AMS. By inhibiting HCO_3^- reabsorption in the kidneys, acetazolamide causes diuresis and urine alkalinization, and consequential blood acidification. Since its effect develops slowly, acetazolamide is more beneficial if it is administrated a day or two prior to high altitude exposure.

Chronic Mountain Sickness

Some people living for extensive periods of time at high altitude may experience symptoms of Chronic Mountain Sickness (CMS), also known as Monge's disease, in recognition of the work of the Peruvian physician Carlos Monge Medrano (1884-1970) who first described it in 1925. Its symptoms include: more severe hypoxemia, abnormally high levels of polycythemia, fatigue, inability to perform physical work, anorexia, mental confusion, sleep disorders, cyanosis and vein dilatation. The mechanisms involved are not fully understood, but increased blood viscosity caused by excessive polycythemia appears to be a major factor. CMS seems to occur when the number of erythrocytes increases above ~7 million/µl, hemoglobin concentration is above ~20 g/100ml blood, and hematocrit rises above ~60% [4, 5].

Adaptation to High Altitude

Populations living at high altitudes have increased pulmonary diffusing capacity, which appears to result from increased alveolar surface area and greater blood flow; both factors significantly increase O_2 transport. At the tissue level, O_2 delivery to cells is enhanced by greater capillary density, which reduces the distance between capillaries and cells for O_2 diffusion. Additionally, it has been found that the number of mitochondria is greater than in low-land people. This significantly enhances the efficiency of O_2 utilization for ATP synthesis.

Different populations living for thousands of years at high altitude have successfully adapted to the hypoxic environment by means of different mechanisms. While high altitude dwellers of the Andes appear to have been naturally selected to develop increased total lung capacity and hemoglobin concentration, Himalayans ventilate at higher frequency and have larger arteries and capillaries, but hemoglobin concentrations not much greater than low-land populations. In addition to increased ventilation at rest, Tibetans are known to have several other distinct physiological characteristics such as decreased arterial O_2-content, absence of pulmonary hypoxic vasoconstriction, and lower hemoglobin concentration.

These characteristics are based on evolutionary genetic adaptation, as high altitude Tibetans have been found to express at least ten oxygen-processing genes which are uncommon in low-land people. Recent studies [6] have reported that most Tibetans belong to three haplotypes selected for adaptation to life in hypoxic environments. Two of these haplotypes, EGLN1 and PPARA, are associated with decreased hemoglobin content and one, EPAS1, which is preferentially expressed in organs involved in O_2 diffusion such as lungs and placenta, is associated with the expression of genes like erythropoietin, vascular endothelial growth factor, and endothelial nitric oxide synthase (eNOS).

REFERENCES

[1] Sutton JR. *et al.* Operation Everest II: oxygen transport during exercise at extreme simulated altitude. J Appl Physiol 1988;64:1309-1321.

[2] Beyaert CA, Hill JM, Lewis BK, Kaufman MP. Effect on airway caliber of stimulation of the hypothalamic locomotor region. J App Physiol 1994;84:1388-1394.

[3] Bärtsch P, Gibbs JSR. Effect of altitude on the heart and the lungs. Circulation 2007;116:2191-2202.

[4] Reeves JT, Leon-Velarde F. Chronic mountain sickness: recent studies of the relationship between hemoglobin concentration and oxygen transport. High Alt. Med. Biol. 2004;5:147-155.

[5] Zubieta-Castillo G Sr, Zubieta-Castillo, GR Jr, Zubieta-Calleja L. Chronic mountain sickness: the reaction of physical disorders to chronic hypoxia. J Physiol Pharmacol 2006;57(Supp. 4): 431-442.

[6] Simpson TS *et al.* Genetic evidence for high-altitude adaptation in Tibet. Science 2010;329:72-75.

CHAPTER 10

Functional Consequences of Respiratory Diseases

Camillo Peracchia

Abstract: This chapter briefly details the major functional consequences of pulmonary diseases. In particular, respiratory disorders are reviewed in terms of their etiopathology and effects on alveolar dead space, conductive shunt, maldistribution shunt-like effect, diffusion impairment, partial pressure of arterial blood gases, acid-base balance, tissue oxygenation, pulmonary circulation, mechanics (static and dynamic) and control of breathing.

Keywords: Asthma, Bronchiectasis, Bronchiolitis, Chronic bronchitis, Chronic-Obstructive-Pulmonary-Disease (COPD), Control-of-Breathing Disorders, Cystic Fibrosis, Emphysema, Extra-thoracic Obstruction, Interstitial Pulmonary-Fibrosis, Mediastinal Diseases, Muco-Ciliary Clearance, Phagocytic-Inflammatory Cells, Pneumonia, Pneumothorax, Pulmonary Edema, Pulmonary Embolism, Pulmonary Hypertension, Respiratory Failure (ARDS, IRDS), Respiratory-Mechanics Disorders.

SYMBOLS, ACRONYMS AND NORMAL VALUES: See Appendix 3.

Obstructive Diseases

Chronic Obstructive Pulmonary Disease (COPD)

Pure Emphysema (COPD type A)

Etiopathology

Cigarette smoking is the most common cause of COPD type A. Most patients have been smokers for several decades, but the mechanism by which smoking causes alveolar destruction is not fully understood. Non-smokers who develop emphysema have a congenital enzymatic unbalance, involving elastase and anti-elastase; alveolar destruction is caused by the activity of the enzyme elastase, which degrades elastic fibers - a process inhibited by anti-elastase. Cigarette smoke is likely to inactivate the anti-elastase, which may be the reason for emphysema in smokers. In <1% of the cases emphysema develops in non-smokers if there is a congenital deficiency in α1-Antitrypsin (AAT), an anti-elastase.

In addition to AAT, other rare hereditary diseases that may cause emphysema include: cutis laxa (X-linked disease with defective synthesis of elastin or tropoelastin), Ehlers-Danos type IX syndrome (a form of cutis laxa with deficient synthesis of lysyl oxidase, an enzyme needed for collagen cross-linking), and Marfan syndrome (defective type I collagen). In rare cases emphysema develops in intravenous drug users, due to vascular damage from insoluble fillers, in patients with autoimmune deficiency syndrome, and in patients with Hypocomplementemic Urticarial Vasculitis Syndrome (HUVS; more prevalent in Caucasian women). Malnutrition and drastic weight loss have also been reported to cause emphysema, possibly *via* insufficient anti-elastase activity.

Emphysema can be classified as "centrilobular" or "panlobular". In the centrilobular form the damage is restricted to respiratory bronchioles, which become greatly enlarged, leaving alveolar ducts and sacs relatively undamaged; this form causes symptoms more consistent with COPD type B. In the panlobular form the destruction and distension affects the alveolar sacs; this generates areas of greatly enlarged air spaces, due to disruption of alveolar walls.

Pathophysiology

Alveolar Dead Space: Large increase in $\dot{V}Ad/\dot{V}\bar{A}$ in panlobular emphysema due to high $\dot{V}/\dot{Q}$ in diseased areas - enlarged air spaces have much reduced blood perfusion. $P\bar{A}CO_2 < PaCO_2$ because of increased $\dot{V}Ad/\dot{V}\bar{A}$.

Conductive Shunt: Minimal, because of absence or limited amount of unventilated alveoli.

Maldistribution Shunt-Like Effect: Small amount, due to partial shifting of blood flow from capillary deprived (emphysematous) air spaces to normal alveoli and consequential small drop in $\dot{V}/\dot{Q}$ in the latter.

Diffusion Impairment: Moderate, in spite of significantly decreased CO transfer factor, due to reduced surface area available for gas exchange.

Hypoxemia: Mild (PaO_2 = ~80 mmHg) due to low $\dot{V}/\dot{Q}$ regions (see above). $(Ai\text{-}a)PO_2$ = 10-15 mmHg (air breathing). More severe with exercise due to drop in $P\bar{v}O_2$ which increases the effect of shunt on hypoxemia (see Chapter 7).

Hypercapnia: None ($PaCO_2$ = 30-40 mmHg), as long as $\dot{V}E$ increases to properly compensate for $\dot{V}Ad$.

Acid/Base Problems: None, as long as $PaCO_2$ is near normal values.

Tissue Oxygenation: Normal, as long as the effect of mild hypoxemia on tissue O_2-delivery is compensated by an increase in $\dot{Q}$.

Mechanics: Due to decreased lung recoil (increased compliance) emphysema affects both static and dynamic lung mechanics.

Static: Left and upward shift in lung compliance curve. Increase in RV, TLC, FRC. The fraction RV/TLC may increase by 40%.

Dynamic: Drop in FEV_1, FVC, FEV_1/FVC and $FEF_{25\text{-}75\%}$.

Pulmonary Circulation: Increased pulmonary artery pressure due to decreased capillary bed and consequential increase in flow resistance.

Control of Breathing: Increased central drive resulting in increased VT. In later stages VT drops and respiratory frequency increases.

Pure Chronic Bronchitis (COPD Type B)

Etiopathology

Most common in cigarette smokers. Abundant mucous secretion in bronchial tree and narrowing of small airways due to inflammation and wall edema. Bronchial mucous glands become hypertrophic and goblet cells are more numerous (hyperplasia) and hypertrophic.

Some forms of COPD type B result from cenrilobular emphysema (bronchiolar distension), with symptoms of chronic bronchitis (airflow obstruction). In moderate forms of cenrilobular emphysema symptoms may be limited, while more severe cases are associated with bronchiolar obstruction and consequential hypoxemia due to $\dot{V}/\dot{Q}$ maldistribution (shunt-like effect).

Pathophysiology

Alveolar Dead Space: Small to moderate increase in $\dot{V}Ad$ due to small areas with high $\dot{V}/\dot{Q}$ ratio.

Conductive Shunt: Minimal. Absence, or minimal presence, of unventilated alveoli ($\dot{V}/\dot{Q}$ =0).

Maldistribution Shunt-Like Effect: Significant amount, due to excessive blood flow to poorly ventilated alveoli resulting in large drop in $\dot{V}/\dot{Q}$ ratio. Some compensation is provided by hypoxic vasoconstriction.

Diffusion Impairment: Minimal or absent.

Hypoxemia: Significant to severe (PaO_2 = 40-70 mmHg) due to low $\dot{V}/\dot{Q}$ regions. $(Ai\text{-}a)PO_2$ = 20-50 mmHg (air breathing). More severe with exercise due to drop in $P\bar{v}O_2$, which increases the effect of shunt on hypoxemia. Chronic hypoxemia results in polycythemia.

Hypercapnia: Moderate ($PaCO_2$ = ~50 mmHg). Increased airway resistance due to bronchial obstruction and narrowing of small airways result in chronic hypoventilation.

Acid/base Problems: Minimal to moderate acidosis, in spite of increased $PaCO_2$, due to compensatory retention of bicarbonate by the kidneys.

Tissue Oxygenation: Normal as long as hypoxemia is compensated by increased $\dot{Q}$.

Mechanics:

Static: Moderate increase in RV, FRC and RV/TLC.

Dynamic: Due to mucous buildup, increased size of mucous glands, inflammation of small airways (bronchiolitis) and increased smooth muscle mass, there is intra-luminal obstruction resulting in increased airway resistance. Drop in FEV1 and FEV1/FVC. Both may drop to less than 70% of normal.

Pulmonary Circulation: Moderate increase in pulmonary artery pressure due to hypoxic vasoconstriction, potentiated by hypercapnia. Right ventricular and atrial pressures are increased. If venous pressure also increases, peripheral edema may develop.

Oxygen therapy, commonly used in COPD patients, corrects the hypoxemia by eliminating the shunt-like effect of $\dot{V}/\dot{Q}$ maldistribution, it eliminates the hypoxic vasoconstriction, which reduces pulmonary hypertension and chance of developing right heart failure (cor pulmonale), and corrects the polycythemia. A drawback is the possible development of hypercapnia (respiratory acidosis), due to redistribution of blood flow to low $\dot{V}/\dot{Q}$ regions that follows the elimination of both hypoxic vasoconstriction, and loss of the hypoxic stimulus to the carotid bodies.

Control of Breathing: Normal, but increased work of breathing induces patients to hypoventilate. $PaCO_2$ increases, but the compensatory increase in bicarbonate maintains pHa to near normal values. When PaO_2 drops below ~70 mmHg, breathing is maintained by carotid body stimulation.

Mixed Emphysema and Chronic Bronchitis

Variable combinations of the functional consequences mentioned above. This is the most common occurrence in clinical practice, as pure COPD Types A and B are relatively rare.

Bronchiectasis

Etiopathology

Localized infection-related inflammatory processes affecting the airway wall may lead to irreversible dilatation (bronchiectasis) of the airway. The infection agents may be viruses or bacteria. Complications of measles and pertussis, as well as fungal infections (ex. bronchopulmonary aspergillosis), may also lead to bronchiectasis. A syndrome associated with bronchiectasis is known as the "Kartagener's syndrome", which involves sinusitis, bronchiectasis and situs inversus (dextrocardia). Damage to airway walls affects cilia function. The lack of cilia's propulsive movement impairs the normal removal of mucous and bacteria, allowing localized infections to develop.

Pathophysiology

Minimal functional abnormality in cases of small localized bronchiectasis, but greater tendency to develop airway infections leading to bronchitis and/or bronchopneumonia. Extensive bronchiectasis causes symptoms similar to COPD type B (see above).

Bronchiolitis

Etiopathology

The term bronchiolitis comprehends a variety of inflammatory diseases of bronchioles.

Bronchiolitis Obliterans Organizing Pneumonia (BOOP) and Obliterative

Bronchiolitis (OB): Both BOOP and OB occur mostly in patients with autoimmune diseases (lupus, rheumatoid arthritis, *etc.*), but while BOOP is an acute pneumonia leading to intraluminal fibroblastic plugs that extend from respiratory bronchioles all the way down to alveolar ducts and alveoli, OB is a chronic condition in which fibrous tissue only develops in terminal bronchioles. OB can also be idiopathic (unknown origin) or the consequence of inhaled toxins, radiation therapy, *etc.*

Respiratory Syncytial Virus (RSV) Infection: Most common in very young children (usually younger than 6 month old), this is the leading cause of infant mortality by viral infections. The disease causes swelling and inflammation of small airway walls (bronchioles) and consequential airway obstruction.

Follicular Bronchiolitis: Caused by lymphoid follicular formations that develop around bronchioles. This disorder is usually associated with diffuse lung disease, as a complication of rheumatoid arthritis or Sjögren's disease.

Complication of Hematopoietic Stem Cell Transplantation (HSCT), formerly known as "bone marrow transplantation"): Obliterative bronchiolitis may develop as consequence of immune-mediated injury to bronchiolar epithelium *via* expression of Ia antigens leading to activation of cytotoxic T-lymphocytes (treatment with methotrexate may be a co-factor).

Pathophysiology

The following functional consequences are particularly severe in infant bronchiolitis (RSV infection) and less so, to different degrees, in other forms of bronchiolitis.

Conductive Shunt: Significant. In areas where bronchioles become completely occluded $\dot{V}/\dot{Q} = 0$ (shunt).

Maldistribution Shunt-Like Effect: Significant, due to alveolar regions with low $\dot{V}/\dot{Q}$.

Hypoxemia: Significant, due to conductive shunt, maldistribution shunt-like effect and hypoventilation. Severe cyanosis in RSV infection.

Hypercapnia: Significant, due to hypoventilation. In infants with RSV infection, muscular fatigue may lead to respiratory failure (see below) with cyanosis and episodes of sudden apnea.

Acid/Base Problems: Respiratory acidosis, particularly severe in infants. If tissue hypoxia develops, there will be a metabolic component as well (lactic acid). Some renal compensation occurs in chronic bronchiolitis.

Tissue Oxygenation: Tissue hypoxia due to hypoxemia, unless significant compensatory increase in $\dot{Q}$ occurs.

Mechanics

Dynamic: Significant increase in airway resistance resulting in impaired expiration and, to a lesser extent, inspiration.

Pulmonary Circulation: Pulmonary hypertension develops due to generalized hypoxic vasoconstriction, potentiated by hypercapnia and acidosis.

Cystic Fibrosis

Etiopathology

Cystic fibrosis is based on a genetic defect in chromosome #7 in the site that codes for the Cystic Fibrosis Transport Regulator (CFTR), which plays a major role in epithelial chloride transport. The lack of three nucleotides coding for a phenyalanine residue results in altered chloride transport. The disease causes very thick, viscous, secretion with severe blockage of airways as well as ducts of various organs, especially pancreas.

The lungs display diffuse bronchiectasis, where dilated airways with thick, fibrous, walls are occupied by purulent mucous, and enlarged alveolar sacs with destroyed septa and extensive interstitial fibrosis. Frequent occurrence of pulmonary infections by *Staphylococcus aureus* and *Pseudomonas aeruginosa*, and consequential inactivation of β-defensins, results in severe damage to lung parenchyma and formation of bronchiectasis. This is due to chemicals released by the bacteria, which activate macrophages inducing them to secrete cytokines that attract polymorphonuclear leukocytes (neutrophils). As the neutrophils die, their DNA and proteases accumulate in the airways, increasing mucous viscosity and stimulating mucous gland secretion, which further impairs airway clearing.

Pathophysiology

Pathologically and functionally, cystic fibrosis is a combination of COPD type B, bronchiectasis, asthma and interstitial fibrosis.

Conductive Shunt: Frequent bronchial infections result in airway obstruction causing shunt.

Maldistribution Shunt-Like Effect: Significant in late stages, due to $\dot{V}/\dot{Q}$ maldistribution.

Diffusion Impairment:Minimal or absent. The diffusing capacity (DLCO) is near normal up to the latest stages in which large loss of alveolar septa has occurred.

Hypoxemia: Of late occurrence in the disease process and carries poor prognosis.

Hypercapnia: Often hypoxemia is accompanied by CO_2 retention.

Tissue Oxygenation: Tissue hypoxia is likely in late stages due to hypoxemia, unless significant compensatory increase in $\dot{Q}$ occurs.

Mechanics:

Static: Drop in lung compliance and VC. Increased FRC and RV.

Dynamic: Airway hyperactivity is of common occurrence, as in asthma; this results in increased airway resistance - decreased FEV1.

Pulmonary circulation: Hypoxia induced vasoconstriction results in pulmonary hypertension. Extreme cases result in right heart failure (cor pulmonale).

Asthma

Etiopathology

Increased airway sensitivity to a variety of stimuli, and greater hyper-response to histamine and methacholine are most commonly observed. One of the greatest risk factors for developing asthma is "atopy", a hereditary condition resulting in increased IgE; this can be confirmed by testing for IgE specific against the most obvious environmental allergens. Home dust mites and cat's hair are the most common asthma's risk factors.

Asthma symptoms results from contraction of hypertrophic airway smooth muscles (bronchoconstriction), increased wall thickness due to edema and eosinophil infiltration, and luminal obstruction due to mucous secretion. Aside from exposure to allergens, asthma attacks can be triggered by viral respiratory infections, indoor and outdoor pollutants, exercise, drugs such as β-blockers and aspirin, and pre-menstrual and menstrual periods.

Pathophysiology

Conductive Shunt: Minimal. In spite of airway obstruction the amount of unventilated alveoli is minimal because of collateral ventilation from neighboring air spaces.

Maldistribution Shunt-Like Effect: Significant, due to severely reduced ventilation (airway obstruction) of alveoli with normal blood flow. This results in severe drop of $\dot{V}/\dot{Q}$ ratio. Some compensation is provided by hypoxic vasoconstriction. Administration of beta-2 agonists drastically reduces the shunt-like effect by improving ventilation in hypoxic regions. This results from relaxation of airway smooth muscles and consequential reopening of narrowed airways.

Hypoxemia: Significant ($PaO_2 = \sim 70$ mmHg) due to low $\dot{V}/\dot{Q}$ regions. $(Ai\text{-}a)PO_2 =$ 20-25 mmHg (air breathing). Hypoxemia is often reduced by increased $P\bar{v}O_2$. This results from anxiety-induced increase in $\dot{Q}$ and secondary drop in O_2 extraction.

Hypercapnia: Absent. In contrast, there might be mild hypocapnia ($PaCO_2$ = 30-35 mmHg) compensatory to hypoxemia, as long as the patient is able to overcome the increased airway resistance. After several days of severe asthma (status asthmaticus) the patient may approach respiratory failure. In this case a progressive drop in ventilation causes hypercapnia and very severe hypoxemia that require urgent intervention.

Acid/Base Problems: Mild alkalosis, as long as the hypocapnia is not compensated by a drop in bicarbonate.

Tissue Oxygenation: Normal as long as hypoxemia is compensated by increased $\dot{Q}$.

Mechanics: Due to airway narrowing (see above), and consequential increase in air airway resistance, asthma affects mostly airway dynamics.

> *Static*: Increased RV due to narrowed airways. Increase in VC and TLC due to some loss of lung recoil (slight left and upward shift in the lung compliance curve).
>
> *Dynamic*: Reduced flow rate, FEV1, FEV1/FVC, $FEF_{25\text{-}75\%}$, $\dot{V}max_{50\%}$ and $\dot{V}max_{75\%}$

Pulmonary Circulation: Normal or mild decrease in pulmonary artery pressure. Regional drop in gas flow leads to regional alveolar hypoxia and consequential regional hypoxic vasoconstriction; this results in local increase in vascular resistance. However, this does not cause an increase in pulmonary artery pressure because blood flow is shifted from hypoxic to normoxic lung regions.

Control of Breathing: Hypoxemia stimulates peripheral chemoreceptors, resulting in hyperventilation which partially compensates for hypoxemia and causes hypocapnia. Hyperventilation is also caused to a lesser extent by stimulation of stretch receptors in smooth muscles of airways, which respond to changes in lung volume.

Impairment of Muco-Ciliary Clearance

Etiopathology:

Defects in ciliary structure such as absence of dynein arms in ciliary microtubules are the basis of the so called “Kartagener’s syndrome”, which is an autosomal recessive disease that involves sinusitis, situs inversus (dextrocardia), obstructive azoospermia and bronchiectasis. This syndrome is present in about 50% of the cases of primary ciliary dyskinesia.

Viral or bacterial infections cause transient structural changes in airway mucosa, impairing cilia function; if the infection kills the epithelial cells, cilia clearance is permanently lost. Other conditions that impair cilia activity include: cigarette smoke, pollutants such as sulfur dioxide (SO_2), nitrogen dioxide (NO_2) and ozone (O_3), and high FIO_2 (90-100%) breathing.

Pathophysiology

Pulmonary symptoms similar to chronic bronchitis (COPD type B) and/or bronchiectasis (see above).

Impairment of Phagocytic and Inflammatory Cells

Etiopathology

Impaired function (paralysis) of macrophages caused by certain viral infections and cigarette smoke. Impaired function of polymorphonuclear leukocytes, resulting from bone marrow diseases (leukemia) or chemotherapy.

Pathophysiology

The malfunction of macrophages or polymorphonuclear leukocytes may result in primary or secondary bacterial bronco-pulmonary infections (broncho-pneumonia).

Restrictive Diseases

Interstitial Pulmonary Fibrosis

Etiopathology

Thickening of alveolar wall due to interstitial infiltration with lymphocytes and plasma cells, and collagen formation. Aside from the well-known Idiopathic Pulmonary Fibrosis (IPF), fibrotic lung diseases comprehend a large variety of additional conditions bracketed under the general term: "Diffuse Lung Diseases". They include: inhalant-related diseases (asbestosis, silicosis, coal-pneumoconiosis, *etc.*), collagen diseases (lupus, rheumatoid arthritis, scleroderma, *etc.*), drug-related diseases, lung damage by physical agents (radiation, high FIO_2 breathing, *etc.*), sarcoidosis, neoplastic diseases, vasculitis, chronic infections, and so on.

Pathophysiology

Alveolar Dead Space: None or minimal.

Conductive Shunt: Minimal. Absence or minimal presence of unventilated alveoli.

Maldistribution Shunt-Like Effect: Moderate amount, due to some reduction of ventilation in alveoli with relatively normal blood flow.

Diffusion Impairment: Minimal at rest, in spite of several fold increase in the alveolar gas-to-blood distance, due to the great diffusion reserve available (normally blood gases equilibrate with alveolar gases in the first third of the time spent in an alveolar capillary). It can be greater if the disease causes extensive destruction of the alveolar walls (reduced alveolar surface for gas exchange). Diffusion impairment is moderate to severe with exercise, due to increased velocity of blood circulation (reduced time spent in alveolar capillary).

Hypoxemia: Moderate at rest (PaO_2 = ~80 mmHg), due to low $\dot{V}/\dot{Q}$ regions, but significant with exercise due to additional factors such as diffusion impairment and drop in $P\bar{v}O_2$, which increases the effect of maldistribution shunt-like effect on hypoxemia. In most cases, diffusion impairment is not extensive enough to cause severe hypoxemia.

Hypercapnia: Absent, unless lung compliance is extremely reduced such that the very fatigued respiratory muscles can no longer provide sufficient ventilation. Usually, there is mild hypocapnia ($PaCO_2$ = 30-40 mmHg), probably due to receptor stimulation in the lungs. Juxta-capillary receptors (J-receptors) are stimulated by distended pulmonary capillaries, and stretch receptors are activated by increased pressure gradient between airway lumen and intra-pleural space, due to increased lung recoil (decrease compliance).

Acid/Base Problems: Mild alkalosis, as long as hypocapnia is not compensated by a drop in bicarbonate.

Tissue Oxygenation: Normal as long as hypoxemia is compensated by increased $\dot{Q}$.

Mechanics: Thickening of alveolar wall affects primarily the static lung mechanics.

Static: Right and downward shift in the lung compliance curve (increased lung recoil, stiff lung). Large reduction in VC, TLC, FRC and RV.

Dynamic: Due to increased lung elastance the airways are stretched open, resulting in increased flow rate, FEV1/FVC and $FEF_{25-75\%}$.

Pulmonary Circulation: Moderate pulmonary hypertension. Interstitial fibrosis and hypertrophy of smooth muscles result in narrowing of arterioles with consequential increase in vascular resistance.

Control of Breathing: Stimulation of mechanoreceptors in alveolar and bronchial walls, due to increased lung elastance, results in a fast and shallow breathing pattern causing mild hypocapnia.

Pneumothorax

Etiopathology

Gas accumulation in the intra-pleural space causing lung collapse. Gas may enter the intra-pleural space from ruptured lung or through holes in the chest wall. Causes include: rupture of alveolar bulla (emphysema) or cyst near the pleural surface, necrosis of lung tissue caused by pneumonia or cancer, and chest traumas such as stab wounds or gun shots. In patients with superficial alveolar bullas, mechanical ventilation by Positive End Expiratory Pressure (PEEP) can cause pneumothorax as a result of the increased alveolar pressure.

If the pathway of gas diffusion into the intra-pleural space seals in "check-valve" fashion during expiration, progressively greater amounts of gas diffuse into the intra-pleural space at each inspiration. This condition is known as "tension pneumothorax" (valve-type). This is an acute and extremely dangerous form of pneumothorax that requires immediate treatment, as the great pressure buildup in the intra-pleural space collapses the lung completely, shifts the mediastinum and blocks venous return to the right heart, causing dramatic drop in cardiac output and systemic blood pressure.

Once the hole is sealed, pneumothorax air is spontaneously resorbed at a rate of approximately 1.5%/day. This slow-rate can be increased by supplying high FIO_2 - the consequential removal of N_2 from the system increases the rate of air removal, which depends on the partial pressure gradients between intra-pleural and venous gases.

Pathophysiology

Alveolar Dead Space: None or minimal.

Conductive Shunt: Significant, depending on amount of alveolar collapse ($\dot{V}/\dot{Q} = 0$). Significantly, the conductive shunt fraction is usually less than predicted; for example, in case of total collapse of one lung, one would expect $\dot{Q}Cs/\dot{Q}$ to be ~50%; in fact $\dot{Q}Cs/\dot{Q}$ is more likely to be 25-30%. The reason is that in the collapsed lung the severe hypoxic vasoconstriction reduces significantly blood flow, and so the fraction of venous admixture.

Maldistribution Shunt-Like Effect: Significant, due to greatly reduced ventilation in partially collapsed alveoli and shift of blood flow to non-collapsed lung (reduced $\dot{V}/\dot{Q}$). However, hypoxic vasoconstriction significantly reduces the shunt-like effect of low $\dot{V}/\dot{Q}$ regions.

Hypoxemia: Moderate to significant (PaO_2 = 70-80 mmHg), due to shunt from regions with $\dot{V}/\dot{Q} = 0$ and maldistribution shunt-like effect due to low $\dot{V}/\dot{Q}$ regions (see above).

Hypercapnia: Absent. There might be mild hypocapnia ($PaCO_2$ = 30-40 mmHg) due to stimulation of chemoreceptors by hypoxemia if PaO_2 drops below ~70 mmHg.

Acid/base Problems: None or mild alkalosis, if possible hypocapnia is not compensated by a drop in bicarbonate.

Tissue Oxygenation: Normal as long as hypoxemia is compensated by increased $\dot{Q}$.

Mechanics: Due to collapsed lung, pneumothorax affects mostly the static lung mechanics.

Static: Large reduction of VC and FEV_1. Decreased lung compliance.

Dynamic: Increased airway resistance due to reduced negativity of intra-pleural pressure – greater tendency of small-airway collapse in expiration.

Pulmonary Circulation: Shift of blood flow from collapsed lung due to hypoxic vasoconstriction in unventilated alveolar regions. The less negative, or positive, intra-pleural pressure reduces venous return from venae cavae, which also causes an increase in right atrial and ventricular pressures. If the foramen ovale opens, conductive shunt develops. The decreased venous return results in lower blood pressure and cardiac output. This is more prominent in tension pneumothorax.

***Control of Breathing*: No significant change.**

Pleural Effusion

Etiopathology

Pleural effusion is caused by diffusion into the intra-pleural space of either transudate or exudate.

Transudate effusion results from abnormal hydrostatic or oncotic pressure gradients between pleural capillary blood and perivascular fluid. The transudate is serous, low in protein and cells, and caused most often by increased pulmonary venous pressure due to cardiac failure. It is usually associated with pulmonary edema. Less common causes are: diffusion of abdominal fluid through diaphragmatic defects in patients with cirrhotic ascites, pleural effusion in patients with severe hypoalbuminemia, or the result of sizable atelectasis – more negative intra-pleural pressure.

Exudate effusion most often results from bacterial or fungal infections (pleural inflammation). Other cases result from pleural malignancies, such as mesothelioma, carcinoma, lymphoma *etc.*, and immunological disorders, such as lupus or rheumatoid pleurisy. Exudate is a fluid composed of red blood cells, neutrophils (pus), bacteria, blood proteins and various other blood components.

Pathophysiology

Minimal functional consequences in cases of limited effusion volumes. Large effusions affect pulmonary function similarly to pneumothorax, resulting in partial lung collapse and consequential regional atelectasis (see above).

Vascular Diseases

Pulmonary edema

Etiopathology

Accumulation of fluid in alveolar air space and in alveolar wall, most often caused by left ventricular failure resulting in increased hydrostatic pressure in left atrium, pulmonary capillaries and pulmonary veins. Edemas limited to the interstitial space have minimal effects on pulmonary functions. Fluid diffusion from capillaries to interstitial space is governed by a modified Starling equation (Eq. 1):

$$\dot{Q}f = Kf[P_{iv} - P_{is}] + \sigma(\pi_{is} - \pi_{iv})] \; \ldots \tag{1}$$

where $\dot{Q}f$ is the rate of fluid diffusion through the capillary wall (in ml/min), Kf is the filtration coefficient of the capillary wall, π is the oncotic pressure of the proteins in the interstitial fluid (is) or the capillary plasma (iv), P is the hydrostatic pressure in the interstitial fluid (P_{is}) or the capillary plasma (P_{iv}), and σ is the reflection coefficient (a correction factor for the fact that the capillary wall is not totally impermeable to solutes).

With a large increase in P_{iv} edema occurs, as the capacity of the lymphatic vessels to clear the system from the flood is overwhelmed. The resulting increase in interstitial pressure limits somewhat the fluid diffusion, but when pressure becomes excessive, fluid spills into the alveolar lumen.

Pathophysiology

Alveolar Dead Space: None or minimal.

Conductive Shunt: Significant, due to unventilated alveoli because of intra-alveolar fluid.

Maldistribution Shunt-Like Effect: Moderate amount, due to partial airway obstruction by fluid and regional $\dot{V}/\dot{Q}$ drop.

Diffusion Impairment: Minimal at rest, in spite of interstitial fluid, due to the great diffusion reserve available (see above).

Hypoxemia: Moderate (PaO_2 = 70 - 80 mmHg) due to maldistribution shunt-like effect (low $\dot{V}/\dot{Q}$ regions) and conductive shunt (regions with $\dot{V}/\dot{Q} = 0$).

Hypercapnia: Absent or mild hypocapnia due to stimulation of lung receptors and hypoxemia, if PaO_2 drops below ~70 mmHg.

Acid/base Problems: None or mild alkalosis, as long as the hypocapnia is not compensated by a drop in bicarbonate.

Tissue Oxygenation: Normal as long as hypoxemia is compensated by increased $\dot{Q}$.

Mechanics: Alveolar and interstitial flooding affects both static and dynamic lung mechanics.

> *Static*: Decreased lung compliance – right shift in the lung compliance curve, due to alveolar flooding and increased surface tension (reduced surfactant). Interstitial edema also contributes to increased lung stiffness.
>
> *Dynamic*: Reduced flow rate due to increased flow resistance brought about by intra- and extra-bronchial fluid accumulation (alveolar and interstitial edema). Some reflex constriction of airways due to stimulation of bronchial receptors may add to increased airway resistance.

Pulmonary Circulation: Increased pulmonary artery resistance due to hypoxic vasoconstriction in unventilated or poorly ventilated alveoli, and capillary compression. Inversion of flow gradient between basal and apical lung regions, due to greater vascular compression at the base of the lung.

Control of Breathing: Hypoxemia and stimulation of mechanoreceptors stimulate breathing, resulting in increased respiratory frequency, but decreased tidal volume.

Pulmonary Embolism

Etiopathology

Acute occlusion of branches of the pulmonary artery, most often caused by thrombi that came loose from the walls of deep veins of lower extremities, pelvic regions, inferior vena cava or right heart. Embolism may also be caused by amniotic fluid, air, tumor cells and fat; the latter usually results from fractures of long bones (femur). Embolism can cause ARDS (see above).

Pathophysiology

Alveolar Dead Space: Significantly increased, depending on the size of the affected area, due to drastic reduction of regional alveolar perfusion (large regional increase in $\dot{V}/\dot{Q}$). Some compensation occurs due to bronchial constriction in unperfused or poorly perfused (hypocapnic) regions.

Conductive Shunt: Significant, due to blood flow through unventilated alveoli in infarcted regions (hemorrhagic atelectasis) and unventilated regions where loss of surfactant leads to alveolar collapse ($\dot{V}/\dot{Q} = 0$).

Maldistribution Shunt-Like Effect: Significant amount, due to redistribution of blood flow from obstructed arteries to normal lung regions. This results in excessive perfusion of normally or poorly ventilated alveoli with sizable drop in regional $\dot{V}/\dot{Q}$.

Diffusion Impairment: Minimal to moderate, due to increased regional blood flow velocity resulting in reduced transit time.

Hypoxemia: Moderate (PaO_2 = 70-80) due to maldistribution/diffusion shunt-like effects and conductive shunt (regions with $\dot{V}/\dot{Q}$ = 0). Hypoxemia is partially compensated by hypocapnia. Large emboli may cause additional venous admixture and more severe hypoxemia if an acute increase in pulmonary artery pressure develops, leading to increased right heart pressures and opening of the foramen ovale.

Hypercapnia: Absent. In contrast, there is moderate hypocapnia due to the effect of hypoxemia on chemoreceptors, especially if PaO_2 drops below ~70 mmHg.

Acid/base Problems: Moderate respiratory alkalosis. If tissue hypoxia occurs, alkalosis will be reduced by formation of lactic acid.

Tissue Oxygenation: Tissue hypoxia develops if the embolus is large enough to cause a sizable drop in $\dot{Q}$, which contributes to the effect of hypoxemia in lowering $P\bar{v}O_2$.

Mechanics: Small effect on static lung mechanics

Static: Hemorrhagic atelectasis and some loss of surfactant contribute to regional increase in lung stiffness (decreased compliance).

Dynamic: No significant change.

Pulmonary Circulation: Moderate increase in pulmonary artery pressure unless embolus is very large. Release of humoral factors from platelets also contribute to pulmonary hypertension by their vasoconstrictive action. If the embolism occludes 50% or more of the circulation, the consequential large increase in vascular resistance causes a dramatic increase in right ventricular pressure, leading to life-threatening cardiac failure.

Control of Breathing: Stimulation of peripheral chemo-receptors results in hyperventilation if PaO_2 drops below ~70 mmHg.

Pulmonary Hypertension

Etiopathology

Several potential causes: increase in left atrial pressure (mitral stenosis, left ventricular failure), increase in pulmonary blood flow (ex. left-to-right shunt due to inter-atrial or inter-ventricular communication, patent ductus arteriosus, *etc.*), primary pulmonary hypertension of unknown cause, and hypoxic vasoconstriction resulting in increased vascular resistance. Pulmonary hypertension may also develop as a complication of autoimmune diseases, especially in patients affected by Raynaud's disease (possible neurohumoral mechanism), pulmonary embolism, and in rare cases of pulmonary veno-occlusive disease (diffuse occlusion of pulmonary veins caused by increased elastic fibers).

In primary pulmonary hypertension, the arterial wall shows fibrotic proliferation of the intima and medial layer hypertrophy. Dilatation of the pulmonary artery and plexiform lesions, also known as glomangiomas (multiple complexes of small arterial vessels, each forming a glomus) are also common.

Pathophysiology

Conductive Shunt: Usually minimal. However, in some cases the right atrial pressure may increase to a level that opens the foramen ovale (secondary inter-atrial communication). This causes significant right-to-left shunt. In cases of primary inter-atrial or inter-ventricular communication and patent ductus arteriosus, shunt is usually left-to-right.

Maldistribution Shunt-Like Effect: Moderate, due to uneven distribution of blood flow.

Diffusion Impairment: Minor diffusion impairment may occur due to some regional loss of pulmonary vessels.

Hypoxemia: Moderate due to uneven regional perfusion – lung regions with low $\dot{V}/\dot{Q}$. However, it might be significant if right atrial pressure increases, due to right ventricular failure, causing secondary opening of the foramen ovale and consequential blood shunt (venous admixture).

Hypercapnia: Absent or mild hypocapnia, probably caused by activation of juxta-capillary stretch receptors (J-receptors), and by hypoxemia if shunt develops through the foramen ovale and PaO_2 drops below ~70 mmHg.

Acid/Base Problems: None or mild alkalosis.

Tissue Oxygenation: Normal as long as the potential hypoxemia is compensated by increased $\dot{Q}$.

Mechanics: No significant change.

Pulmonary Circulation: In primary pulmonary hypertension, the increased flow resistance in pulmonary arteries, especially in arterioles, raises both systolic and diastolic pulmonary artery pressures, while capillary pressure is unchanged. In hypertension due to left cardiac failure or mitral stenosis pulmonary capillary pressure increases as well. Pressure also increases in the right ventricle. Pressures in the right atrium and venae cavae will also increase in case of right ventricular failure, and peripheral edema may develop.

Control of Breathing: Simulation of respiratory centers by activation of J-receptors, and peripheral chemo-receptors if PaO_2 drops below ~70 mmHg.

Infectious Diseases

Pneumonia

Etiopathology

There are two major types of pneumonia: bacterial and atypical.

Bacterial pneumonia is most often caused by Streptococcus pneumoniae (pneumococcus); less frequently, by Klebsiella pneumoniae or Staphylococcus aureus. Pneumonia by Streptococcus is usually a complication of a viral respiratory infection causing impaired mucous clearance (malfunction of ciliated cells) and phagocytosis (impaired function of macrophages and/or polymorphonuclear leukocytes). This type of pneumonia begins with interstitial inflammation and capillary damage, followed by alveolar flooding with exudate (fluid composed of erythrocytes, neutrophil "pus", bacteria, blood proteins and various other blood components), manifested by a rusty-purulent expectorate. Spread of the infection to contiguous alveolar sacs, *via* Kohn's pores, results in "lobar pneumonia", while spread *via* airways results in "bronchopneumonia".

Atypical pneumonia can be caused by Mycoplasma pneumoniae as well as by various fungal and viral agents including: Chlamydia psittaci (from birds), Chlamydia pneumonia, Coxiella burnetii (Q-fever), Aspergillus fumigatus, Histoplasma capsulatum, Legionella pneumonia, and viruses such as: adenovirus, influenza viruses (types A and B), Respiratory Syncytial Virus (RSV; which most often causes bronchiolitis) and, less frequently, measles, chickenpox and hantavirus infection. These agents cause inflammation and damage to airway's epithelial cells at various levels of the bronchial tree. Mycoplasma pneumoniae organisms bind to the surface of epithelial cells and multiply, releasing toxic products. Since these organisms are unaffected by macrophages and leukocytes, the disease continues until the immunitary system generates sufficient amounts of specific antibodies.

Pathophysiology

Alveolar Dead Space: None or minimal.

Conductive Shunt: Significant, due to unventilated alveoli because of intra-alveolar exudate.

Maldistribution Shunt-Like Effect: Moderate amount, due to partial airway obstruction by fluid and regional $\dot{V}/\dot{Q}$ drop.

Diffusion Impairment: None.

Hypoxemia: Moderate to severe (PaO_2 = 50-70 mmHg), depending on size of affected area, due primarily to conductive shunt (regions with $\dot{V}/\dot{Q} = 0$) and to a lesser extent to maldistribution shunt-like effect (low $\dot{V}/\dot{Q}$ regions). Some compensation resulting from hypoxic vasoconstriction.

Hypercapnia: Mild hypocapnia due to stimulation of chemoreceptors by hypoxemia.

Acid/base Problems: None or mild alkalosis, if hypocapnia is not compensated by a drop in bicarbonate.

Tissue Oxygenation: Normal as long as hypoxemia is compensated by increased $\dot{Q}$.

Mechanics:

Static: Drop in TLC and FRC. Decreased compliance due filling of alveoli with liquid exudate.

Control of Breathing: Simulation of peripheral chemo-receptors by hypoxemia results in hyperventilation.

Pulmonary Tuberculosis

Etiopathology

Infection caused by Mycobacterium tuberculosis (rod-shaped aerobic bacterium), transmitted by aerosol droplets. Most often the infection occurs in the upper lobe, near the posterior side of the apex; in this high $\dot{V}/\dot{Q}$ area the greater PAO_2 favors the growth of this aerobic bacterium. The infection generates granulomas - aggregates of phagocytic cells (epithelioid histiocytes), cheese-like necrosis – which destroy the alveolar tissue leaving cavities, areas of fibrosis and calcium deposits. Pleural exudate effusion may occur.

Pathophysiology

In spite of the alveolar destruction, cavity formation and scarring, the functional consequences are relatively mild, because the infection is usually restricted to the upper-posterior lung regions, leaving most of the lung tissue fully functional. The $\dot{V}/\dot{Q}$ ratio is minimally affected because the regional drop in ventilation is matched by a drop in blood perfusion. Consequently, hypoxemia is minimal or absent. Cases of extensive scarring and/or pleural effusion result in functional consequences similar to restrictive diseases – drop in lung compliance, reduction in VC, TLC, FRC and RV, and increase in flow rate, FEV1/FVC and $FEF_{25\text{-}75\%}$.

Respiratory Failure

Respiratory failure occurs when respiration becomes inadequate in its function of supplying enough O_2 to arterial blood and removing sufficient CO_2 from mixed venous blood. Several conditions may lead to respiratory failure. Aside from Adult and Infant Respiratory Distress Syndromes (ARDS and IRDS), which will be discussed below, respiratory failure can be the consequence of pneumonias, pulmonary embolism, exposure to toxic air pollutants, neurological diseases that depress the centers of the control of breathing, such as drugs (heroin, barbiturates, *etc.*), encephalitis, poliomyelitis, Guillain-Barré syndrome, and muscular dystrophy. Severe cases of bronchitis, emphysema, prolonged asthma attacks, and late stages of cystic fibrosis can also lead to respiratory failure.

Adult Respiratory Distress Syndrome (ARDS)

Etiopathology

Diffuse lung injury resulting in capillary damage, engorgement and inflammation, and leakage of fluid into interstitial space and alveoli. The so called "hyaline membrane" develops as a result of alveolar filling with blood, cell debris and protein-rich fluid (fibrin and other blood components), surfactant inactivation, and alveolar collapse (atelectasis). In response to lung injury, Epithelial Cells Type 2 (surfactant producers) proliferate, and some differentiate into Epithelial Cells Type 1, which initiate the capillary membrane repair; a drawback of this process is the formation of fibrosis. ARDS has multiple causes: lung trauma, large body trauma, septicemia, aspiration, shock, fat pulmonary embolism (release of free fatty acids), *etc.*

Pathophysiology

Alveolar Dead Space: Minimal, but can be significant if patients are ventilated with Positive End Expiratory Pressure (PEEP), due to alveolar capillary compression by PEEP and consequential reduction of capillary blood flow in well ventilated alveoli (increase in $\dot{V}/\dot{Q}$).

Conductive Shunt: Significant, due to unventilated alveoli (alveolar atelectasis due to loss of surfactant - hyaline membrane formation), intra-alveolar fluid and blood.

Maldistribution Shunt-Like Effect: Significant, due to partial airway obstruction by fluid, causing regional $\dot{V}/\dot{Q}$ drop.

Diffusion Impairment: Not significant.

Hypoxemia: Severe (PaO_2 < 60 mmHg), due to conductive shunt and maldistribution shunt-like effect.

Hypercapnia: Absent. Usually, significant hypocapnia ($PaCO_2$ = 20-30 mmHg) due to stimulation of mechano-receptors in the lungs (caused by interstitial edema) and hypoxemia-induced stimulation of chemo-receptors.

Acid/base Problems: Various possibilities. Acidosis, if severe hypoxemia causes tissue hypoxia (lactic acid). Alkalosis, if hypocapnia is not compensated by decreased bicarbonate.

Tissue Oxygenation: Normal or low $P\bar{v}O_2$ depending on compensation of hypoxemia by increased $\dot{Q}$.

Mechanics: Major effect on static pulmonary mechanics, as lung stiffness increases due to interstitial and alveolar edema. The latter causes drop in compliance due to reduced effect of surfactant on surface tension.

Static: Large drop in FRC, and both downward and right shift in the lung compliance curve.

Dynamic: No significant change.

Pulmonary Circulation: Increased vascular resistance due to hypoxic vasoconstriction and fluid buildup in the interstitial space, which decreases the size of small vessels. The redistribution of blood flow to regions of lower flow resistance adds to the maldistribution shunt-like effect and consequential hypoxemia.

Control of Breathing: Stimulation of mechano-receptors, and peripheral chemo-receptors by hypoxemia, results in hyperventilation.

Infant Respiratory Distress Syndrome (IRDS)

Etiopathology

Interstitial and alveolar edema as well as alveolar filling with blood, cell debris and protein-rich fluid. Regional atelectasis. Hyaline membrane, resulting from proteinaceous liquid and cell debris accumulated in alveoli. Major cause: luck of pulmonary surfactant. While in ARDS the surfactant abnormality is the consequence of lung damage, in IRDS it is the primary cause of lung malfunction.

Pathophysiology: *see ARDS.*

Disorders of Respiratory Mechanics

These disorders can be classified in three groups: neuromuscular, chest-wall and obesity-related. The first most commonly include: Guillain-Barré syndrome, myasthenia gravis, poliomyelitis, amyotrophic lateral sclerosis, quadriplegia, polymyositis, and muscular dystrophy. Most frequent among the chest-wall related group are: kyphoscoliosis, ankylosis spondylitis and flail chest.

Neuromuscular Diseases (Weakness in Respiratory Muscles)

Etiopathology

Guillain-Barré syndrome is an acute polyneuropathy, usually triggered by an infection, which affects the peripheral nervous system. Life-threatening cases severely weaken the respiratory muscles.

Myasthenia gravis is an autoimmune disease which generates antibodies to acetylcholine receptors of neuromuscular junctions; the receptor blockage causes severe muscle weakness.

Poliomyelitis is an acute infection by an Enterovirus known as poliovirus; three serotypes of poliovirus have been identified: PV1, PV2 and PV3. The virus spreads along nerve fibers and once it reaches the spinal cord it destroys motor neurons, leading to paralytic poliomyelitis.

Amyotrophic Lateral Sclerosis (ALS, Lou Gehrig's disease) is a motor neuron disease characterized by progressive muscle weakness, atrophy and spasticity. When it compromises respiratory muscles it causes dyspnea. A few cases are hereditary, but in the majority of cases there is no known cause.

Quadriplegia (tetraplegia) results from spinal cord damage at the vertebral levels C1–C7. The injury causes total or partial loss of function in all of the limbs. Patients with an injury at C1 most often lose respiratory function as well and need to be mechanically ventilated.

Polymyositis is an autoimmune disease (related to dermatomyositis) that causes chronic muscular inflammation. Respiratory muscle weakness impairs breathing as vital capacity, total lung capacity, and maximum voluntary ventilation are reduced.

Muscular dystrophy (Duchenne's disease, DMD) is a recessive X-linked hereditary disease resulting in progressive skeletal muscle weakness, muscle defects, and myocyte death. The malfunction of muscle's dystrophin and the dystrophin-associated protein complex affects a variety of systems. As the disease progresses, loss of respiratory muscle strength occurs and death may result from respiratory insufficiency. The majority of patients also develop cardiomyopathy.

Pathophysiology

Conductive Shunt: Significant if atelectasis develops.

Maldistribution Shunt-Like Effect: Significant if respiratory infection develops, due to insufficient mucous clearing.

Hypoxemia: Due to hypoventilation. More severe if conductive shunt (atelectasis) and low $\dot{V}/\dot{Q}$ regions, due to mucous obstruction of airways, are present.

Hypercapnia: Due to hypoventilation - shallow breathing.

Acid/base Problems: In spite of increased $PaCO_2$, acidosis is moderate due to compensatory retention of bicarbonate by the kidneys.

Tissue Oxygenation: Normal as long as hypoxemia is compensated by increased $\dot{Q}$.

Mechanics:

> *Static*: Reduction in VT, TLC and VC due to inspiratory muscle weakness, and increase in RV due to expiratory muscle weakness. Increase VCd/VT due to shallow breathing. Reduced lung compliance if atelectasis develops. Reduced chest compliance in chronic neuromuscular diseases due to stiffness of joints, ligaments and tendons. Significant drop in peak inspiratory and expiratory pressures.
>
> *Dynamic*: Shallow breathing. Reduced FEV1/FVC and peak expiratory flow rate in forced expiration.

Chest Wall Diseases

Etiopathology

Kyphoscoliosis is a musculoskeletal disorder causing pathological curvature of the spine in sagittal and coronal planes (combination of scoliosis and kyphosis). It results from asymmetric weakening of back muscles that can be caused by diseases such as syringomyelia (cystic formation within the spinal cord), ataxia and muscular dystrophy. The degree of lateral curvature of the spine is usually determined by calculating the "Cobb angle" from X-ray images.

Ankylosing spondylitis is an inflammation of spinal joints resulting in fusion of vertebral bodies and costovertebral joints.

Pathophysiology

Conductive Shunt: Moderate, due to some atelectasis in compressed regions.

Maldistribution Shunt-like effect: Moderate, due to regional drop in $\dot{V}/\dot{Q}$.

Hypoxemia: Moderate. Due to hypoventilation, maldistribution shunt-like effect, and conductive shunt caused by regional micro- and macro-atelectasis.

Hypercapnia: Significant, because of hypoventilation.

Diffusion Impairment: Reduced diffusion capacity for carbon monoxide (DLCO). However, the transfer coefficient (KCO) increases because the alveolar compression reduces regional ventilation more than blood perfusion.

Acid/base Problems: Moderate acidosis, in spite of significant increase in $PaCO_2$, due to compensatory retention of bicarbonate by the kidneys.

Tissue Oxygenation: Normal as long as hypoxemia is compensated by increased $\dot{Q}$.

Mechanics: Functional consequences somewhat similar to those of restrictive diseases.

Static: Reduced VC, TLC, FRC and ERV.

Flail Chest

Etiopathology

Multiple rib fractures cause the so called "flail chest", a condition that compromises normal chest expansion during inspiration. In flail chest, three or more adjacent ribs have fractured in two or more places, causing the loss of chest-wall functional integration during the breathing cycle. If the fractured ribs puncture the lung, pneumothorax may develop. Pulmonary contusion my cause lung edema and/or lobar collapse. In many cases, spleen or liver injuries may also occur.

Pathophysiology

Conductive Shunt: Moderate, due to some atelectasis, edema or lobar collapse in injured lung.

Maldistribution Shunt-Like Effect: Moderate. The much reduced lung expansion of the affected side will create areas of very low $\dot{V}/\dot{Q}$. Partial compensation will occur as a result of hypoxic vasoconstriction, which will shift some blood flow to the contralateral lung.

Hypoxemia: Moderate, due to maldistribution shunt-like effect, hypoventilation, and some conductive shunt if atelectasis, edema or lobar collapse occurs.

Hypercapnia: Due to hypoventilation

Acid/base Problems: Acute respiratory acidosis due to acute hypoventilation.

Tissue Oxygenation: Tissue hypoxia is unlikely in spite of hypoxemia, because the hypercapnia-induced acidemia will favor O_2 unloading at the tissue. Increase in cardiac output may also compensate for hypoxemia.

Mechanics:

Static: In the case of flail chest, the chest wall moves paradoxically during the breathing cycle, being sucked in during inspiration due to more negative intra-pleural pressure as the diaphragm contracts. PEEP ventilation is required up to healing of the fractured ribs.

Obesity-Related

Etiopathology

Obesity results either from abnormal eating habits that alter the balance between ingested and expended calories or from genetic defects in the mechanism that regulates caloric intake and/or energy expenditure. The major signaling molecules [1] that increase either energy expenditure (catabolic mechanism) or food intake (anabolic mechanism) are the corticotropin-releasing hormone and the neuropeptide-Y, respectively; they act by stimulating or inhibiting, respectively, the central nervous system's activity. Other catabolic stimulants include: thyrotropin-releasing hormone (TSH), bombesin, somatostatin, cholecystokinin, calcitonin-gene-related-peptide, neurotensin, serotonin, and glucagon-like peptide-1. Other anabolic stimulants include: galanin, β-endorphin, dynorphin, growth-hormone-releasing hormone, and norepinephrine.

Pathophysiology

Obesity increases $\dot{V}O_2$ and $\dot{V}CO_2$ both at rest and during work, requiring increased ventilation and cardiac output, and has a major effect on respiratory mechanics.

Conductive Shunt: Moderate. Small airway closure may result in areas of atelectasis.

Maldistribution Shunt-Like Effect: Moderate, due to altered ventilation-perfusion ratio brought about by breathing at low lung volumes. In compressed alveolar regions there is reduced ventilation but normal perfusion (decreased $\dot{V}/\dot{Q}$).

Hypoxemia: Moderate, due to combination of hypoventilation, maldistribution shunt-like effect and conductive shunt.

Hypercapnia: Due to hypoventilation.

Acid/base Problems: Mild chronic respiratory acidosis, partially compensated by increased bicarbonate retention.

Tissue Oxygenation: Normal as long as the effect of hypoxemia is corrected by increased cardiac output.

Mechanics:

Static: Reduced FRC, ERV and VT due to chest wall restriction (increased weight of abdominal and thoracic walls) causing increased inspiratory muscle work. Drop in VT is partially compensated by increased respiratory frequency.

Dynamic: Lung compression results in reduced airway diameter and consequential increased airway flow resistance, more severe in expiration (airway collapse). Upper airway obstruction is likely, causing sleep apnea-hypopnea syndrome (SAHS).

Pulmonary Circulation: Lung compression and breathing at low volumes cause increased vascular resistance and consequential mild pulmonary hypertension.

Control of Breathing: Hypoventilation is not due to decreased ventilatory response to PaO_2, $PaCO_2$ or pHa, but rather to increased work of breathing for which heavily obese subjects, as patients with COPD type B, adapt to tolerate mild hypercapnia and hypoxemia. Hypoventilation is also due to kidney compensation of respiratory acidosis which increases pHa by retaining bicarbonate.

Mediastinal Diseases

Pneumomediastinum

Etiopathology

Pneumomediastinum results from conditions that allow gas to gain access into the mediastinum. The source of gas influx includes: stub wounds through skin and chest wall, and tears in esophagus or airways (trachea, bronchi or alveoli). Gas easily diffuses from the environment through chest wounds or from the airway-alveolar cavities, because the mediastinum is subjected to negative pressure caused by lung recoil.

Pathophysiology

Impaired venous return from venae cavae. Major symptoms are dyspnea, and hypotension.

Mediastinal Masses

Etiopathology

Anterior masses may result from thymomas, lymphomas (Hodgkin and non-Hodgkin types), thyroid enlargements and teratomas (tumors with cells of ectodermal, endodermal and mesodermal origin).

Middle masses include: lymphomas, enlarged lymph nodes from diseases such as sarcoidosis and tuberculosis, and both pericardial and bronchial cysts.

Posterior masses are usually of neurogenic origin, including: Schwannomas, ganglioneuromas and neuroblastomas, but may also result from diaphragmatic hernias.

Pathophysiology

Mediastinal masses may cause esophageal compression, resulting in swallowing difficulties (dysphagia), and compression of the superior vena cava, with consequential facial and upper extremity edema caused by impaired venous return.

Lung Cancer

Etiopathology

There are two major groups of lung cancers: Small-Cell Lung Cancer (SCLC) and Non-Small-Cell Lung Cancer (NSCLC). The latter is subdivided into three subtypes: squamous cell carcinoma, adenocarcinoma and large cell carcinoma. Subgroups of small cell carcinoma and adenocarcinoma are the oat-cell carcinoma (from transformed Feyrter's cells) and the bronchioalveolar carcinoma, respectively. Both squamous and small cell carcinomas are strongly associated with history of smoking. Adenocarcinoma and large cell carcinoma are more frequent in smokers, but may also develop in non-smokers.

Pathophysiology

Most types of lung cancer have little effect on respiratory function in early stages. Cancers of bronchial origin, such as squamous cell and small cell carcinomas, may cause airway obstruction and consequential respiratory infection (pneumonia). Early symptoms of bronchitis may include: cough, hemoptysis, chest pain and dyspnea. Atelectasis, pleural effusion and pneumothorax may also occur. Bronchogenic carcinoma may occlude the superior vena cava, causing swollen neck veins, and facial edema.

Cancers that invade the pleura can cause pleural effusion and partial lung collapse. If pleural invasion occurs toward the mediastinum, cardiac compression and consequential arrhythmias may result from pericardial effusion; compression of the esophagus may cause dysphagia.

Cancers localized at the lungs' apex, such as "Superior Sulcus Tumors ", are also known as Pancoast tumors (first described by the American radiologist Henry Khunarath Pancoast, 1875-1939). These tumors, which most often belong to the NSCLC category, may compress nerve branches of the brachial plexus or cervical sympathetic nerves, causing arm weakness and pain. Compression of the sympathetic branches produces the so called Horner's syndrome (first described by the Swiss ophthalmologist Johann Friedrich Horner, 1831-1886) characterized by eyelid ptosis, miosis and hemi-facial loss of sweat.

Extra-Thoracic Obstruction

Etiopathology

Pharingo-laryngeal inflammation, paralysis of vocal cords, swollen lymph nodes and tumors are the most common causes of extra-thoracic airway obstruction. In addition, conditions that cause sleep apnea may also play a role (see below); they include: excessive soft tissue in the upper airways, extreme obesity, large tongue or tonsils, and defects in the genioglossus, a muscle which keeps the tongue from falling back onto the pharynx.

Pathophysiology

The partially obstructed airways become further constricted during inspiration because of the negative intra-airway pressure that develops below the obstruction, as inspiratory muscles contract to create a pressure gradient between alveoli and environment (see Chapter 3). The increased gas velocity at the constricted site causes stridor, an abnormal high-pitch grating sound caused by turbulent gas flow. In contrast, in expiration the increased intra-airway pressure below the obstruction tends to enlarge the constricted airway. Thus, expiration is easier than inspiration.

Disorders of Control of Breathing

Primary Neurological Diseases

Neurogenic Hyperventilation

Etiopathology

Causes include: CNS infections such as meningitis or encephalitis, stroke and CNS traumas.

Pathophysiology

The drop in $PaCO_2$, secondary to hyperventilation, results in alkalosis. Prolonged hyperventilation is compensated by reduced HCO_3 retention (renal compensation) resulting in pHa normalization.

Neurogenic Hypoventilation

Etiopathology

Causes include: idiopathic hypoventilation (primary alveolar hypoventilation) from previous CNS infections (encephalitis, meningitis, bulbar poliomyelitis, *etc.*), chemical damage to control centers sensitive to pH and/or hypoxia, Ondine's curse (idiopathic hypoventilation) - impaired automatic control, but normal voluntary breathing, Arnold-Chiari malformation, and displacement of the cerebellar tonsils through the foramen magnum.

Pathophysiology

The resulting hypercapnia causes acidosis. In chronic conditions, renal compensation (HCO_3-retention) brings pHa to near normal values.

Abnormal Breathing Patterns

<u>Ataxic Breathing</u>

Etiopathology

Caused by various types of medullary lesions.

Pathophysiology

Very irregular breathing patterns.

<u>Apneustic Breathing</u>

Etiopathology

Caused by lesions of the pons.

Pathophysiology

Extended inspiratory pauses.

<u>Cheyne-Stokes Breathing</u>

Etiopathology

Causes include: congestive heart failure and CNS diseases resulting in problems with the feedback system.

Pathophysiology

Periods of gradual increase in ventilation alternating with periods of gradual decrease, due to instability of control of breathing with cycles of ventilatory over- and under-shooting. The mechanism may involve delayed responses to PCO_2 and PO_2 and/or excessive response to stimuli. In the case of congestive heart failure, the prolonged circulatory time causes a delay between pulmonary changes and chemoreceptors' response to PCO_2 (pH). The consequence of Cheyne-Stokes breathing is sizable oscillations in PaO_2 and $PaCO_2$ values.

Kussmaul's Respiration

Etiopathology

Caused by late stages of severe metabolic acidosis, especially in cases of acute diabetic ketoacidosis (see Chapter 3).

Pathophysiology

Breathing pattern characterized by labored hyperventilation - large tidal volumes and increased frequency.

Cluster Breathing (Biot's Respiration)

Etiopathology

Caused by damage to the medulla oblongata resulting from stroke, trauma or compression due to herniation of uncus or tenorium cerebelli; it can also occur after prolonged addiction to opioid drugs.

Pathophysiology

Periods (clusters) of fairly rapid breathing alternating with periods of apnea that can last up to a couple of minutes. This breathing pattern is similar to Cheyen-Stokes except that the tidal volume does not change during the breathing period.

Secondary to Lung Diseases

Etiopathology

In type B COPD the control mechanism is reset to operate at higher $PaCO_2$ values

Pathophysiology

Chronic hypoventilation with near normal pHa due to renal compensation, which complements the effect of control center resetting.

Sleep Apnea-Hypopnea Syndrome (SAHS)

Etiopathology

Several conditions can result in sleep apnea. They include: excessive soft tissue in the upper airways, which reduces the size of pharyngeal air passages, obesity, small jaw, large tongue and/or tonsils, or defects in the upper airway musculature, particularly the genioglossus muscle, which prevents the tongue from falling onto the posterior wall of the pharynx, occluding it.

Pathophysiology

Hypoxemia. Approximately 5% of the patients are also hypercapnic, with consequential acute respiratory acidosis. Alveolar hypoxia causes pulmonary hypertension due to diffuse pulmonary vasoconstriction; this may lead to cardiac arrhythmias, especially when $\%SaO_2$ drops below 60%.

REFERENCE

[1] Kaiyala KJ, Woods SC, Schwartz MW. New model for the regulation of energy balance and adiposity by the central nervous system. Am J Clin Nutr 1995;62(Suppl):S1123-1134.

Lung Function In Health And Disease, 2014, 270-353

Clinical Cases

Camillo Peracchia

For Methods Used in Calculations (See Appendix 4)

For Symbols, Acronyms and Normal Values (See Appendix 3)

In this section we present ten case-studies. Each case is analyzed in detail for the purpose of training students on the methods used to evaluate qualitatively and quantitatively the functional consequences of pulmonary diseases. While the quantitative analysis of the cases is important, we feel that even greater emphasis should be given to a careful qualitative analysis of patient's medical history and lab reports. For this purpose, the quantitative analysis of each of the present cases is preceded by the following question: *"Based on the history and the given values, what can one say"?*

The student should train himself/herself to become a meticulous medical detective - which indeed is what a good physician should be. Before performing any calculations, the student should proceed as follows:

- Read carefully the patient's history making sure that even minor details are not overlooked
- Analyze carefully lab and other test reports.
- Recognize normal *versus* abnormal values.
- Relate each value to other relevant values.
- Determine whether the abnormal values are primary abnormalities or compensatory changes.
- Before performing calculations, make an educated guess on the major problems in terms of ventilation, perfusion, venous admixture, alveolar dead space, tissue oxygenation, acid-base balance, respiratory mechanics, control of breathing, and so on.

For example, let's assume that a patient has the following values while breathing ambient air at sea level: PaO_2 = 70 mmHg, $PaCO_2$ = 30 mmHg, $P\bar{A}CO_2$ = 25 mmHg, pHa = 7.3, $\dot{V}O_2$ = 0.25 l/min and $\dot{Q}$ = 3.5 l/min. From these data one can say that there is hypoxemia, hypocapnia, metabolic acidosis, normal oxygen consumption and reduced cardiac output. The hypoxemia is caused by a large right-to-left shunt (as both PaO_2 and $PaCO_2$ have dropped relative to normal values), and is partially compensated by hyperventilation. The case is complicated by circulatory problems, which cause an abnormally high O_2-extraction (normal $\dot{V}O_2$, but low $\dot{Q}$); this, combined with hypoxemia, suggests the likelihood of tissue hypoxia. This is consistent with metabolic acidosis (the anaerobic metabolism due to tissue hypoxia generated lactic acid), which is partially compensated by hyperventilation. There is also sizable alveolar dead space ventilation because $PaCO_2 \neq P\bar{A}CO_2$.

CASE #1 - PULMONARY FIBROSIS COMPLICATED BY PNEUMONIA

A seventy year old man (123 lb.) with a long history of chronic respiratory problems developed upper respiratory symptoms and noticed that his shortness of breath had worsened. A day before admission he suffered an episode of extreme shortness of breath. At the time of admission (March 21) samples of arterial and mixed venous blood were obtained (Table **1**). Based on the data, he was given oxygen and was treated with antibiotics. On March 23, other blood samples were taken (Table **1**).

Table 1: Laboratory blood and gas data.

	March 21	March 23
pHa	7.3	7.43
pH$\bar{v}$	7.25	7.38
$PaCO_2$ (mmHg)	36	31
PaO_2 (mmHg)	36	83
Hb (g/ml blood)	14	14
VT (liters, BTPS)	0.37	0.37
F (breaths/min)	26	23
VCd (liters, BTPS)	0.123	0.123
PB (mmHg)	747	747
R	0.8	0.8
FIO_2 (%)	21	50
$\dot{V}O_2$ (liters/min, STPD)	0.32	0.25
O_2 extraction (vol%)	4	5
Heart Rate	130	80
Body Temperature (°C)	39	37
At Body Temperature = 39°C, the constant "863" becomes "868.6", and PH_2O is 51.6 mmHg at 100% saturation		

A year before the acute episode, a lung function test gave the following results (Table **2**):

Table 2: Pulmonary function test data

	Observed	Predicted
Vital capacity (liters, BTPS)	2.56	3.51
FEV1/VC (%)	87	69
Compliance (ml/cm H_2O)	50	100

Based on the History and the Given Values, What Can One Say?

<u>March 21</u>

- Mild acidosis, hypocapnia (hyperventilation), severe hypoxemia, small tidal volume, high respiratory frequency, increased oxygen consumption, and tachycardia (consistent with fever and severe hypoxemia).

- A pHa of 7.3, in conjunction with a $PaCO_2$ of 36, indicates the presence of a base deficit (metabolic acidosis), partly compensated by hyperventilation - full compensation (pHa = 7.4) would have resulted in the reduction of $PaCO_2$ to ~27 mmHg.

- Since there is severe hypoxemia, hyperventilation is compensatory to both acidosis and hypoxemia. However, note that such a severe hypoxemia would be expected to stimulate ventilation to a much greater extent - a $PaCO_2$ of 36 mmHg is still pretty much within the normal range. This indicates that the patient is approaching respiratory failure, as breathing is becoming increasingly harder - note the high respiratory frequency. The reason why breathing is so hard for this patient may seem puzzling at first, but it becomes clear if one looks at the mechanics data and considers evidence of respiratory infection.

- The small vital capacity, low compliance and increased FEV1/VC indicate that the patient may be suffering from an interstitial lung disease (fibrosis); fibrosis causes an increase in lung recoil (the lungs are stiff) and a drop in airway resistance (opposite to emphysema). In this case, the elastic work is greatly increased, while the resistive work is slightly decreased.

- The great increase in respiratory demand is due to the severe hypoxemia that, in association with hypocapnia, clearly indicates the presence of a large right-to-left blood shunt (venous admixture), as well as to the fever – increased metabolic rate due to respiratory infection.

March 23

- Virtually normal pHa, increased hypocapnia (greater hyperventilation), mild hypoxemia, small tidal volume, lower but still high respiratory frequency, and normal oxygen consumption, heart rate and extraction.
- Most of the data appear normal or close to normal, but one has to keep in mind that the patient is breathing a 50% oxygen mixture - in a normal subject this would result in a PaO_2 of 280-300 mmHg - thus, a PaO_2 of 83 mmHg clearly indicates the persistence of a large right-to-left blood shunt.
- One may wonder why with a pHa of 7.43 the patient is hyperventilating ($PaCO_2$ = 31); the reason for this is the persistent hypoxemia, now reasonably well compensated by hyperventilation and 50% O_2 breathing. In fact, in the absence of hyperventilation PaO_2 would be ~70 mmHg and would drop to ~60 mmHg, if the patient were breathing room air.

Shunt Fraction, (Ai-a)PO_2 Gradient, Cardiac Output and Stroke Volume

March 21:

$CaO_2 = 10.43$ vol% $C\bar{v}O_2 = 6.43$ vol%

$\frac{\dot{Q}Ps}{\dot{Q}} = \mathbf{66.4\%}$ (Ai-a)PO_2 = 66.5 mmHg $\dot{Q} = \mathbf{8\ l/min}$ SV = 61.5 ml

Very large physiological shunt fraction, large (Ai-a)PO_2,

increased cardiac output, and relatively normal stroke volume

March 23:

Even though the patient is not breathing 100% O_2, we can assume that 50% O_2 breathing eliminates virtually all of the maldistribution/diffusion shunt-like effect. Therefore, we can reasonably estimate the conductive shunt fraction:

$CaO_2 = 18.27$ vol% $C\bar{v}O_2 = 13.27$ vol%

$\frac{\dot{Q}Cs}{\dot{Q}} = \mathbf{22.7\%}$ $(Ai\text{-}a)PO_2 = 23$ $\dot{Q} = 5$ l/min SV = 62.5 ml

Reduced $(Ai\text{-}a)PO_2$, sizable residual conductive shunt fraction,

normal cardiac output and stroke volume.

Alveolar Dead Space Ventilation

March 21:

Since $P\bar{A}CO_2$ is not given, the alveolar dead space fraction can be calculated by determining $\dot{V}\bar{A}$ and $\dot{V}Ai$.

$\dot{V}E = 9.62$ l/min (BTPS) $\dot{V}Cd = 3.2$ l/min (BTPS) $\dot{V}\bar{A} = 6.42$ l/min (BTPS)

$\dot{V}CO_2 = 0.256$ l/min (STPD) $\dot{V}Ai = 6.18$ l/min (BTPS) $\dot{V}Ad = 0.245$ l/min (BTPS)

$$\frac{\dot{V}Ad}{\dot{V}\bar{A}} = \mathbf{3.8\%}$$

Small fraction of alveolar dead space ventilation

March 23:

$\dot{V}E = 8.51$ l/min (BTPS) $\dot{V}Cd = 2.83$ l/min (BTPS) $\dot{V}\bar{A} = 5.68$ l/min (BTPS)

$\dot{V}CO_2 = 0.2$ l/min (STPD) $\dot{V}Ai = 5.57$ l/min (BTPS) $\dot{V}Ad = 0.11$ l/min (BTPS)

$$\frac{\dot{V}Ad}{\dot{V}\bar{A}} = \mathbf{1.94\%}$$

Minimal (normal) alveolar dead space ventilation

Base Excess (BE)

March 21:

Since we know the values of $PaCO_2$ and pHa, we can calculate the $[HCO_3^-]_{actual}$ by means of the Henderson-Hasselbalch equation:

$$BE = -7.8 \text{ mEq/l}$$

Metabolic acidosis (pHa = 7.3) without significant respiratory compensation ($PaCO_2$ = 36 mmHg)

March 23:

$$BE = -3.75 \text{ mEq/l}$$

Residual base deficit slightly overcompensated by ventilation (pHa = 7.43, $PaCO_2$ = 31 mmHg)

Average Tissue Oxygenation ($P\bar{v}O_2$)

On March 21:

$$P\bar{v}O_2 = \sim 27 \text{ mmHg}$$

Low $P\bar{v}O_2$ (tissue hypoxia) due to severe hypoxemia (PaO_2 = 36 mmHg) and increased $\dot{V}O_2$ (fever). The $P\bar{v}O_2$ would have been much lower had the $\dot{Q}$ not increased to 8 l/min, decreasing the O_2 extraction to 4 vol%. Note that the low $P\bar{v}O_2$ increases the effect of shunt on hypoxemia, as the O_2-content of shunted (mixed venous) blood is lower than normal.

March 23:

$P\bar{v}O_2$ = ~38 mmHg Virtually normal tissue oxygenation

It might seem strange that $P\bar{v}O_2$ differs by only 11 mmHg between March 21st and 23rd despite a marked rise in PaO_2 (36 and 83 mmHg) and in O_2 content in both arterial (10.43 and 18.27 vol%) and mixed venous (6.43 and 13.27 vol%) blood. The explanation lies in the difference in behavior of the oxyhemoglobin dissociation curve in response to the differences in pH$\bar{v}$'s and body temperature between the two situations (Table **1**, March 21st and 23rd). The curve is greatly shifted to the right on March 21st, favoring O_2 dissociation from oxyhemoglobin. Therefore, dissolved O_2 and $P\bar{v}O_2$ are disproportionally low on March 23, in spite of the much greater $C\bar{v}O_2$.

What the Data on Lung Mechanics Tell You in Regard to:

The Type of Chronic Lung Disease of This Patient

All the data point to a disease that increases lung stiffness. Most compelling among them is the low compliance (50 ml/cm H_2O, half normal). A type of interstitial lung disease seems likely. Since there is no evidence from the history of a work related interstitial lung disease such as silicosis, coal-worker's pneumoconiosis, asbestosis, *etc.*, it is likely that the patient suffers from an interstitial lung disease of unknown origin, such as idiopathic pulmonary fibrosis.

The Elastic Properties of his Lungs

The low compliance indicates that the lungs are stiffer than normal, *i.e.* they have greater elastance, consistent with pulmonary fibrosis.

The Expiratory Resistance of his Airways

The greater than normal FEV1/FVC indicates that the airway resistance during expiration is reduced below normal. This is consistent with decreased compliance. The stiff lungs have greater recoil – they generate a more negative intra-pleural pressure than normal lungs at comparable volumes. Consequently, the intra-thoracic airways are stretched open more than normal at any phase of the breathing cycle, such that trans-airway pressure (pressure inside the airway minus intra-pleural pressure) is more positive than normal at any level of the intra-thoracic bronchial tree.

The Work of Breathing (Elastic *versus* Resistive)

Low compliance causes an increase in elastic work - it is harder to expand stiffer lungs. In contrast, the decreased airway resistance reduces the resistive work. To minimize elastic work, tidal volume is reduced (VT = 0.37 l) and to compensate for the smaller than normal tidal volume, breathing frequency is increased. An increase in frequency results in increased gas velocity, that in normal people (and even more so in emphysematous patients) would favor airway collapse (Bernoulli's principle). However, the effect of increased gas velocity on airway resistance is offset by a significantly more negative intra-pleural pressure (stiff lungs).

Why is $PaCO_2$ lower on March 23 than on March 21, in spite of the same tidal volume and greater respiratory frequency on March 21?

The reason is that the body temperature has returned to normal (37^0C from 39^0C) - metabolic rate is now normal, as indicated by the drop in $\dot{V}O_2$ (Table **1**) and consequently in $\dot{V}CO_2$. Therefore, less $\dot{V}Ai$ is needed to maintain the same $PaCO_2$. While $\dot{V}CO_2$ declined by 22% (from March 21st to the 23rd) $\dot{V}Ai$ decreased by only 10%. The ratio of $\dot{V}Ai$ to $\dot{V}CO_2$ rose from 24 on March 21st to 28 on March 23rd, resulting in greater CO_2 elimination rate and consequently a lower $PaCO_2$.

Why is the heart rate (HR) greater on March 21 than on March 23?

The higher HR on March 21st is probably related primarily to the patient's fever and the resulting rise in $\dot{V}O_2$. There is a linear relationship between $\dot{V}O_2$ and $\dot{Q}$ (especially HR); the greater the $\dot{V}O_2$ the greater is the HR. In addition, hypoxemia complements the effect of fever in increasing HR.

Challenging Questions

On March 23, just after the data were collected, the patient suffered a pulmonary embolism that caused a large alveolar dead space ventilation ($\dot{V}Ad/\dot{V}\overline{A}$ = 50%). Assuming: pHa = 7.24, pH$\bar{v}$ = 7.20, and no change in the other given values (March 23), what would $PaCO_2$ and $P\bar{v}CO_2$ be?

$\dot{V}Ad/\dot{V}\overline{A} = 1/2$. Therefore, $\dot{V}Ai$ and $\dot{V}Ad$ are each ½ of $\dot{V}\overline{A}$. Thus:

$$\dot{V}\overline{A} = \dot{V}Ai + \dot{V}A \qquad \dot{V}Ai = \dot{V}Ad \qquad \dot{V}Ad = \dot{V}\overline{A}/2 \qquad \dot{V}Ad = 5.68/2 = 2.84 \text{ l/min}$$

Since the values of $\dot{V}Ai$ and $\dot{V}CO_2$ are available, $PaCO_2$ can be calculated:

$$\mathbf{PaCO_2 = \frac{863 \times 0.2}{2.84} = 61\ torr}$$

With a $PaCO_2$ of 61 mmHg and a pH_a of 7.24, the arterial $[HCO_3^-]$ = 25.34 mEq/l.

Due to the "acute" change in pH and PCO_2 that the arterial blood experiences as it perfuses tissue capillaries, the mixed venous $[HCO_3^-]\bar{v}$ will be:

$$-10 = \frac{25.34 - [HCO_3^-]\bar{v}}{7.24 - 7.2} \quad [HCO_3^-]\bar{v} = 25.74 \text{ mEq/l}$$

With $[HCO_3^-]\bar{v}$ = 25.74 mEq/l and $pH\bar{v}$ = 7.2

$$P\bar{v}CO_2 = 67.9 \text{ mmHg}$$

Assuming no change in respiratory frequency, what VT would be needed to maintain the original $PaCO_2$ (31 mmHg) and $P\bar{v}CO_2$?

To maintain the original $PaCO_2$ with the same metabolic rate, $\dot{V}Ai$ needs to remain unchanged. Since the original $\dot{V}Ai$ was 5.57 l/min and $\dot{V}Ad = \dot{V}\overline{A}/2$, $\dot{V}\overline{A}$ will need to double:

$$\dot{V}Ai + \dot{V}Ad = 5.57 + 5.57 = 11.14 \text{ l/min. Thus:}$$

$$\mathbf{VT} = \frac{\dot{V}\overline{A} + \dot{V}Cd}{f} = \frac{11.14 + 2.83}{23} = \mathbf{0.607\ liters}$$

SEQUENCE OF EVENTS AND CONCLUSIONS

The patient's history of chronic respiratory problems, causing shortness of breath, coupled with data on lung mechanics, points to an interstitial lung disease (fibrosis). Fibrosis causes diffusion impairment at the alveolar-capillary barrier and ventilation-perfusion maldistribution, resulting in shunt and hypoxemia. The hypoxemia stimulates the peripheral chemoreceptors causing the patient to hyperventilate on chronic basis. This leads to mild hypocapnia and respiratory alkalosis with some degree of renal compensation (urinary loss of bicarbonate, negative BE). At this point, the patient's hypoxemia is not severe enough to cause significant tissue hypoxia and trigger anaerobic metabolism.

A week before the admission the patient developed upper respiratory symptoms, which worsened to extreme shortness of breath and chill on the night prior to admission. On March 21 there is a very large shunt (66.7%) and a metabolic acidosis with minimal respiratory compensation. Since at the time of blood sampling the patient was breathing room air, the shunt is likely to result from $\dot{V}/\dot{Q}$ maldistribution and diffusion impairment, as well as additional (conductive) shunt due to lung regions with a $\dot{V}/\dot{Q} = 0$ - the acute respiratory symptoms, the fever, and the large shunt point to a lung infection (pneumonia) that might have caused blockage of airways and alveolar exudates, resulting in perfused but unventilated alveoli (conductive shunt).

The large base deficit is probably the sum of a preexisting deficit (compensatory to chronic, hypoxemia-induced, hyperventilation) and acute metabolic acidosis caused by tissue hypoxia ($P\bar{v}O_2 = 27$ mmHg). This value of $P\bar{v}O_2$, however, is not as low as one would expect in view of the severe hypoxemia, due to right shift of the O_2 dissociation curve, induced by low $pH\bar{v}$ and increased temperature, and to increased cardiac output (decreased extraction). The patient is severely hypoxemic ($PaO_2 = 36$ mmHg) but little compensation is provided by ventilation ($PaCO_2 = 36$ mmHg). The reason for it is that the patient is approaching respiratory failure - due to increased elastic work of breathing and the effects of respiratory infection, it has become so hard to breathe that the patient is unable to adequately compensate for hypoxemia and metabolic acidosis.

The administration of antibiotics and 50% O_2 breathing must have partially cleared the affected alveoli, and has virtually eliminated the maldistribution-diffusion shunt-like effect. Thus, the residual 22.7% shunt fraction is probably only conductive, due to still unventilated alveoli and/or extra-alveolar shunts. The acid-base status has improved as well. Now, there is a smaller base deficit (-3.75 mEq/l) and normal pHa. The drop in base deficit could have occurred spontaneously over two and a half days (~2 mEq/l per day). There is now significant hyperventilation ($PaCO_2 = 31$ mmHg). Since pHa is now 7.43, hyperventilation is now caused entirely by hypoxemia. Hypoxemia is still present in spite of hyperventilation and 50% O_2 breathing, because of the still sizable shunt.

CASE #2 – CARDIAC FAILURE FOLLOWING ACUTE CHOLECYSTECTOMY IN A COPD PATIENT WITH MITRAL VALVE REGURGITATION

On February 28, a 76 year old man (160lb) with a history of chronic pulmonary disease and mitral valve regurgitation was brought to an Emergency Department for acute cholecystitis. He was immediately transferred to the operating room. During the operation the following values were recorded (Table **3**, February 28). Following the operation the patient was kept in the intensive care unit with naso-gastric suction and oxygen by mask. Another set of values was recorded three days later (Table **3**, March 3).

Table 3: Laboratory blood and gas data.

	February 28	March 3
pHa	7.3	7.45
$pH\bar{v}$	7.25	7.4
$PaCO_2$ (mmHg)	38	46
$P\bar{A}CO_2$ (mmHg)	28	---
PaO_2 (mmHg)	288	97
Hb (g/ml blood)	10	12
VT (liters, BTPS)	---	0.53
VCd (liters, BTPS)	0.160	0.160
F (breaths/min)	26	14
PB (mmHg)	749	747
R	0.8	0.8
FIO_2 (%)	100	30
$\dot{V}O_2$ (liters/min, STPD)	0.32	0.28
O_2 extraction (vol%)	6.7	5.4
Heart Rate	120	104
Body Temperature (°C)	38	37
At Body Temperature = 38°C, the constant "863" becomes "866", and PH_2O is 49 mmHg at 100% saturation		

Based on the History and the Given Values, What Can One Say?

<u>February 28</u>

- Lower than normal pHa and virtually normal $PaCO_2$, indicating the presence of base deficit not compensated by the setting of the respirator.

- $P\bar{A}CO_2$ is different from $PaCO_2$, indicating substantial alveolar dead space ventilation.

- PaO_2 is greater than normal, but still lower than what one would expect for a patient breathing 100% O_2. This, combined with a fairly normal $PaCO_2$, indicates the presence of a sizable conductive shunt.

- Low Hb concentration - anemia.

- High breathing frequency with relatively normal $PaCO_2$. In a normal subject this would suggest very shallow breathing (small VT); in this case, however, there is significant alveolar dead space ventilation (see above), so the ventilator is likely to be delivering a larger VT to compensate for the wasted ventilation.

- Oxygen consumption is elevated, but consistent with an increase in body temperature (metabolic rate increases ~13% per °C).

- High extraction, indicating that cardiac output is too low to properly compensate for the increased metabolic rate (fever). The combination of anemia and increased extraction would be expected to cause a drop in $C\bar{v}O_2$ and tissue hypoxia. However, low $pH\bar{v}$ and increase in body temperature shift the oxygen dissociation curve to the right, so that tissue oxygenation is likely to be adequate.

- Heart rate is high in spite of evidence for insufficient cardiac output, which points to small stroke volume, most likely due to mitral valve regurgitation.

March 3

- Both pHa and $PaCO_2$ are above normal - metabolic alkalosis partly compensated by hypoventilation.

- PaO_2 is slightly lower than expected for 30% O_2 breathing, due to hypoventilation and abnormal shunt.

- Tidal volume is normal, but frequency is slightly higher than normal. Since there is hypoventilation (hypercapnia, $PaCO_2$ = 46 mmHg) and normal metabolic rate, this indicates the presence of abnormal alveolar dead space ventilation.

- Since O_2 extraction and $\dot{V}O_2$ are fairly normal, cardiac output is also normal. However, the heart rate is high indicating that the stroke volume is lower than normal.

Shunt Fraction

February 28:

$CaO_2 = 14.3$ vol% $\quad C\bar{v}O_2 = 7.6$ vol% $\quad (Ai\text{-}a)PO_2 = 374$ mmHg

$$\frac{\dot{\mathbf{Q}}\mathbf{Cs}}{\dot{\mathbf{Q}}} = \mathbf{14}$$

March 3:

$CaO_2 = 16.1$ vol% $\quad C\bar{v}O_2 = 10.7$ vol% $\quad (Ai\text{-}a)PO_2 = 59$ mmHg

$$\frac{\dot{\mathbf{Q}}\mathbf{Ps}}{\dot{\mathbf{Q}}} = \mathbf{6\%}$$

Alveolar Dead Space Ventilation

February 28:

$$\frac{\dot{\mathbf{V}}\mathbf{Ad}}{\dot{\mathbf{V}}\bar{\mathbf{A}}} = \frac{PaCO_2 - P\bar{A}CO_2}{PaCO_2} = \frac{38 - 28}{38} = \mathbf{26\%}$$

March 3:

Since $P\bar{A}CO_2$ is not given, the alveolar dead space fraction is calculated by determining $\dot{V}\bar{A}$ and $\dot{V}Ai$.

$\dot{V}E = 7.42$ l/min $\quad \dot{V}Cd = 2.24$ l/ min $\quad \dot{V}\bar{A} = 5.18$l/min;

$$\dot{V}CO_2 = 0.224 l/min \qquad \dot{V}Ai = 4.2 \; l/min$$

$$\frac{\dot{V}Ad}{\dot{V}\bar{A}} = 18.9\%$$

Base Excess (B.E.)

February 28:

BE = - 6.7 mEq/l

Virtually uncompensated metabolic acidosis ($PaCO_2$ = 38 mmHg)

March 3:

BE = 7.45 mEq/l

Metabolic alkalosis almost fully compensated by hypoventilation ($PaCO_2$ = 46 mmHg)

Average Tissue Oxygenation ($P\bar{v}O_2$)

February 28:

$P\bar{v}O_2$ = ~37 mmHg

March 3:

$P\bar{v}O_2$ = ~37 mmHg

It might seem strange to find that the values of $P\bar{v}O_2$ are the same in spite of very different PaO_2 (288 and 97 mmHg), CaO_2 (14.3 and 16.1 vol%) and $C\bar{v}O_2$ (7.6 and 10.7 vol%). The explanation lies in the difference in the behavior of the oxyhemoglobin dissociation curve in response to the differences in $pH\bar{v}$ and body temperature between the two situations (Table **3**, Feb 28th *vs.* March 3rd). On February 28th, the O_2 dissociation curve is greatly shifted to the right, favoring the unloading of O_2 off oxyhemoglobin. On March 3rd, the curve is shifted leftward, which favors slightly the O_2 association with Hb at the level of the alveoli because at the high PO_2 the curve is virtually flat. However, at the same time the leftward shift hinders the unloading O_2 off oxyhemoglobin at the level of peripheral tissue. Hence the observation that dissolved O_2 and $P\bar{v}O_2$ are disproportionally low on March 3, relative to the much greater $C\bar{v}O_2$ on that day.

Stroke Volume (SV) (normal SV = 60-80 ml)

February 28:

$$\dot{Q} = \frac{\dot{V}O_2}{\text{extraction}} = \frac{0.32}{0.067} = 4.9\ \text{l/min}$$

SV = 4.9/120= ~40 ml

March 3:

$$\dot{Q} = \frac{0.28}{0.054} = 5\ \text{l/min}$$

SV = 5/104 = 50 ml

Low stroke volume on both days due to mitral valve regurgitation.

Tidal volume (VT) on February 28 (assume an added dead space of 80 ml, BTPS, due to the respirator)

$$\dot{V}Ai = 5.8\ \text{l/ min}$$

$$\frac{\dot{V}Ad}{\dot{V}\bar{A}} = 0.26$$

$$\frac{\dot{V}Ai}{\dot{V}\bar{A}} = 1 - 0.26 = 0.74$$

$$\dot{V}\bar{A} = \frac{5.8}{0.74} = 7.87\ \text{l/min}$$

$$\dot{V}E = \dot{V}\bar{A} + \dot{V}Cd_{(patient)} + \dot{V}Cd_{(respirator)}$$

$$\dot{V}E = 7.87 + (0.16 \text{ x } 26) + (0.08 \text{ x } 26) = 14.11\ \text{l/min}$$

$$\mathbf{VT} = \frac{14.11}{26} = \mathbf{543\ ml}$$

Normal tidal volume

On February 28 the static pressure at the respirator, after inflation of VT from FRC, was 3.6 cm H_2O (static pressure is the pressure measured in the absence of air flow)

What this tells you about:

Type of chronic lung disease

Lungs' elastic properties

Expiratory resistance of airways

Work of breathing (elastic *versus* resistive)

$$\textbf{Compliance} = \frac{\Delta V}{\Delta P} = \frac{540}{3.6} = \mathbf{150\ ml/cmH_2O}$$

Compliance is greater than the normal value of 100 ml/cm H_2O, pointing to a disease like emphysema. The greater compliance indicates that the lungs are not as stiff as normal, *i.e.* they have lower elastance. Although we do not have a value for FEV1/VC, the increased compliance suggests that airway resistance during expiration is greater than normal. With a less negative intra-pleural pressure the airways are not stretched open as much as in normal subjects at any phase of the breathing cycle, such that the trans-pulmonary pressure (TPP) across the airway wall (pressure inside the airway minus intra-pleural pressure) is less positive than normal at any level of the intra-thoracic bronchial tree. Increased compliance reduces the elastic work, as it is easier to expand the "floppy" lungs at inspiration, but increased airway resistance increases the expiratory work.

Challenging Question

Let's assume that on February 28 at 9:30 p.m., while the patient was still being operated on, a new arterial blood sample had given a $PaCO_2$ value of 70 mmHg, in spite of the absence of changes in respirator setting, body temperature, Hb and shunt fraction. What could have caused the increase in $PaCO_2$? What would PaO_2 be?

The reason for an increase in $PaCO_2$ is a drop in alveolar ideal ventilation ($\dot{V}Ai$). This could result from pulmonary embolism or significant drop in pulmonary artery pressure. Both would drastically increase the alveolar dead space ventilation.

$$\dot{V}Ai = \frac{866 \text{ x } 0.256}{70} = 3.17 \text{ 1/min} \qquad \frac{\dot{V}Ai}{\dot{V}\bar{A}} = \frac{3.17}{7.87} = 40.3\%$$

$$\frac{\dot{V}Ad}{\dot{V}\bar{A}} = 1 - 0.403 = 59.7\%$$

The fraction of alveolar ventilation wasted in alveolar dead space

has increased from 26.3% to 59.7%.

For calculating PaO_2 we need to calculate CaO_2.

$$PAiO_2 = 630 \text{ mmHg} \quad CAiO_2 = 15.35 \text{ vol\%}$$

$$\frac{\dot{Q}Cs}{\dot{Q}} = 0.148 = \frac{15.35 - CaO_2}{15.35 - (CaO_2 - 6.7)}$$

$$CaO_2 = 14.2 \text{ vol\%}$$

Since O_2 capacity is 13.4 vol%, the O_2 content is greater than capacity:

14.2-13.4 = 0.8 vol%

Hemoglobin is virtually 100% saturated at PO_2 >150. Therefore, we can approximate the lowest possible PaO_2 by assuming that the volume of O_2 above capacity is entirely dissolved O_2.

Thus:

$$\mathbf{PaO_2} = \frac{\text{dissolved } O_2}{0.0031} = \frac{0.8}{0.0031} = \mathbf{258 \text{ torr}}$$

Due to 100% O_2 breathing, PaO_2 remains significantly above normal in spite of drastically reduced $\dot{V}Ai$ ($PaCO_2$ = 70 mmHg)

SEQUENCE OF EVENTS AND CONCLUSION

Before the acute episode the patient had a history of chronic pulmonary disease which, based on compliance data, is likely to be emphysema. Emphysematous patients are known to chronically hypoventilate, and consequently they develop respiratory acidosis with some "metabolic" (renal) compensation (base excess). In contrast, this patient during the operation has a base deficit, indicative of metabolic acidosis. The most likely reason for this is that the patient is in cardiac failure, brought about by the acute cholecystitis with fever. The consequential increase in metabolic rate overloaded the circulatory system, already chronically stressed by mitral valve regurgitation and anemia. Oxygen delivery became insufficient, tissue hypoxia developed and the lactic acid produced turned a base excess into a base deficit.

During the operation, the respirator setting provided some compensation, albeit inadequate, for the metabolic acidosis, eliminated the hypoxemia that must have been present, and brought the tissue to a reasonably normal level of oxygenation. However, giving 100% O_2 was unnecessary (PaO_2 = 288 mmHg). In fact, it might have caused alveolar collapse in low $\dot{V}/\dot{Q}$ regions, resulting in conductive shunt. This usually happens in COPD patients given 100% O_2 while breathing on their own. It is rare, however, in patient on a respirator, unless VT is set too low.

On March 3 things look much better. Collapsed alveoli are now ventilated, resulting in decreased shunt fraction to a fairly normal value, and alveolar dead space has decreased, probably because of the reestablishment of compensatory vasoconstriction in low $\dot{V}/\dot{Q}$ regions, likely to be partly hypoxic - 30% oxygen is not that much greater than normal and oxygen masks are leaky. The acid/base situation has completely reversed. Now we have a metabolic alkalosis, brought about by the removal of hydrogen ions through nasal gastric suction, and compensatory hypoventilation. The return to normal body temperature (and thus normal metabolic rate), coupled to good oxygenation (30% oxygen) and increased hemoglobin concentration, has reduced the burden on the circulatory system, such that cardiac output and extraction have returned to normal. Heart rate is still above normal because of valve regurgitation, even though stroke volume has increased by 25%. In spite of all this, tissue oxygenation is about the same as during the operation because the pHa is greater than normal causing a left shift in the oxygen dissociation curve.

CASE #3 – RESPIRATORY FAILURE IN ASTHMATIC PATIENT WITH PATENT FORAMEN OVALE

(Modified and adapted from: Robert, R., Ferrandis, J., Malin, F., Herpin, D. and Pourrat, O. Enhancement of hypoxemia by right-to-left atrial shunting in severe asthma. Intensive Care Med. 20, 585-587, 1994. Permission granted by Springer)

Table 4: Laboratory blood and gas data.

	March 1	March 6
pHa	7.3	7.47
$pH\bar{v}$	7.25	7.42
$PaCO_2$ (mmHg)	45	22
PaO_2 (mmHg)	130	52
Hb (g/ml blood)	13	13
VT (liters, BTPS)	0.5	0.58
F (breaths/min)	10	15
VCd (liters, BTPS)	0.145	0.145
PB (mmHg)	747	747
R	0.8	0.8
FIO_2 (%)	40	100
$\dot{V}O_2$ (liters/min, STPD)	0.23	0.2
$\dot{Q}$ (liters/min)	4.6	4.0
Body Temperature (°C)	37	37

Note: Assume no added conductive dead space by the ventilator.

A 33 year old woman (weighing 145 lb) was admitted on March 1 for an acute asthma attack that required tracheal intubation and ventilation with a positive end expiratory pressure (PEEP) of 15 cm H_2O (**Note:** In the original case described by Robert, R. *et al.* in 1994, see above, the application of PEEP was not mentioned). Peak airway pressure (peak PAW) measured at the ventilator during lung inflation was 50 cm H_2O (normal: 18-22 cm H_2O) - the peak PAW is the pressure measured by the ventilator in the largest airways, and reflects the level of airway resistance. The patient was treated with aminophylline, terbutaline and corticosteroids, which resulted in rapid improvement. Blood gas analysis performed at that time gave the values shown in Table **4** (March 1). Four days after admission, however, PaO_2 had dropped to 57 mmHg in spite of continued ventilation at the same rate and VT with 40% O_2. On the 5th day PaO_2 had dropped to 47 mmHg and even an increase in FIO_2 to 100% did not increase PaO_2 (Table **4**, March 6). Pulmonary angiography was performed with the hypothesis of pulmonary embolism. During the procedure, the catheter (inserted into the right jugular vein) easily crossed to the left atrium. This was a clear indication that the foramen ovale was open and blood could freely flow across the inter-atrial septum. Despite persisting hypoxemia, the patient was weaned from the ventilator on the 7th day. Three days later PaO_2 returned to normal values.

Based on the History and the Given Values, What Can One Say?

<u>March 1</u>

From the history we know that this patient suffers from chronic asthma and was obviously in respiratory failure on admittance, as she required intubation and mechanical ventilation. Asthmatic patients usually hyperventilate, such that $PaCO_2$ is low and PaO_2 is normal or low due to shunts, as long as they can do it. Chronic hyperventilation causes alkalosis which is compensated by a negative base excess. When the respiratory work becomes exhausting these patients undergo respiratory failure - $PaCO_2$ rises and PaO_2 drops to dangerously low levels. Based on this, we notice the following abnormal values in the blood and gas analyses:

- Severe acidosis in spite of slightly higher $PaCO_2$, indicating a mixed metabolic and respiratory acidosis.

- PaO_2 is higher than normal, but it is not as high as one would expect for someone breathing 40% O_2, indicating the presence of sizable shunt. Asthmatic patients have usually a significant amount of maldistribution shunt like effect, and it is unlikely that all of the maldistribution/diffusion shunt-like effect has been eliminated by just doubling the FIO_2. Note, however, that conductive shunt often develops during acute asthma attacks due to the opening of the foramen ovale.

- Slight anemia.

- Fairly normal tidal volume and frequency, insufficient to compensate for acidosis.

- A high peak PAW could indicate decreased compliance and/or increased airway resistance. We do not have any data on compliance, but since the patient has asthma we know that she has increased airway resistance in both inspiration and expiration.

March 6

- Mild alkalosis in spite of a very low $PaCO_2$, indicative of a sizable negative base excess.

- PaO_2 had progressively dropped over five days from 130 to 57 and then to 47 in spite of constant ventilator settings, and even with 100% O_2 PaO_2 did not increase significantly (52 mmHg). If we did not know that $PaCO_2$ is also low (22 mmHg), we would think that the severe hypoxemia is due to hypoventilation and/or shunt, but in view of the low $PaCO_2$ there is no doubt that a large shunt has developed. The shunt is entirely conductive because with 100% O_2 breathing the maldistribution shunt-like effect and/or the diffusion impairment are eliminated. Evidence for patent foramen ovale indicates that the shunt across the inter-atrial septum has increased during mechanical ventilation with PEEP, as PEEP might have increase the pulmonary vascular resistance and the right atrial pressure.

- The very low $PaCO_2$ indicates that the attending physicians increased ventilation as much as possible to compensate for the hypoxemia, which in fact would be much worse if the ventilator settings had not been increased from 5 to 8.7 l/min.

- In view of severe hypoxemia, absence of change in O_2 extraction, alkaline arterial and mixed venous pH values and mild anemia, one would expect some tissue hypoxia. This would be expected to increase the base deficit.

Is there an abnormal physiological and/or conductive shunt fraction on March 1 and on March 6? Is there a difference between the two days?

March 1:

$CaO_2 = 17.47$ vol% $(CaO_2 - C\bar{v}O_2) = 5$ vol%

$$\frac{\dot{Q}Ps}{\dot{Q}} = 11\%$$

$C\bar{v}O_2 = CaO_2 - 5 = 12.47$ vol% $(Ai\text{-}a)PO_2 = 98$ mmHg

March 6:

$CaO_2 = 15.49$ vol% $(CaO_2 - C\bar{v}O_2) = 5$ vol%

$$\frac{\dot{Q}Cs}{\dot{Q}} = 44.6\%$$

$C\bar{v}O_2 = CaO_2 - 5 = 10.49$ vol% $(Ai\text{-}a)PO_2 = 626$ mmHg

Is there abnormal alveolar dead space ventilation on March 1 and on March 6? Is there a difference between the two days?

March 1:

$$\frac{\dot{V}Ad}{\dot{V}\bar{A}} = 0.5\%$$

March 6:

$$\frac{\dot{V}Ad}{\dot{V}\bar{A}} = 3.8\%$$

Is there a base excess (B.E.) on March 1 and on March 6? Is there a difference between the two days?

March 1:

$$BE = -3.8 \text{ mEq/l}$$

Respiratory and metabolic acidosis. The negative BE is likely to represent metabolic compensation for a pre-existing chronic respiratory alkalosis, but could also be the consequence of pre-existing tissue hypoxia due to respiratory failure. Mild respiratory acidosis is caused by slightly low ventilation-setting at respirator.

March 6:

$$BE = -7.81 \text{ mEq/l}$$

Mild alkalosis resulting from respiratory overcompensation for severe metabolic acidosis. In view of the severe hypoxemia without reduced oxygen extraction, the base deficit is likely to result from tissue hypoxia and formation of lactic acid.

What can you tell about the average tissue oxygenation ($P\bar{v}O_2$) on March 1 and on March 6? Are the values predictable based on CaO_2, $C\bar{v}O_2$, Hb and $\dot{Q}$?

March 1:

$$\%S\bar{v}O_2 = C\bar{v}O_2/\text{capacity} = 12.47/(13 \text{x} 1.34) = 71.6\%$$

$$\text{At pH}\bar{v} = 7.25, \mathbf{P\bar{v}O_2 = \sim 44 \text{ mmHg}}$$

March 6:

$$\%S\bar{v}O_2 = 10.5/(13 \text{x} 1.34) = 60.3\%$$

$$\text{At pH}\bar{v} = 7.42, \mathbf{P\bar{v}O_2 = \sim 31 \text{ mmHg}}$$

It might seem strange to find $P\bar{v}O_2$ on March 6 almost 30% lower than on March 6, in spite of decrease in $C\bar{v}O_2$ of only ~16%. The reason is the very different $pH\bar{v}$ (7.25 *versus* 7.42), that results in different Bohr shifts. The O_2 dissociation curve is greatly shifted to the right on Mach 1, favoring O_2 dissociation from Hb. The left shift of the O_2 dissociation curve on March 6 favors minimally O_2 association with Hb at the lungs (because of the flatness of the O_2 dissociation curve at high PO_2) but reduces the O_2 dissociation from Hb at the tissue, such that dissolved O_2 and $P\bar{v}O_2$ are disproportionally low on March 6.

Why was the Peak PAW Measured at the Ventilator Greater Than Normal?

The bronchial spasm, edema and mucous buildup in the small airways, characteristic of asthma, result in increased airway resistance, such that a greater than normal pressure gradient between the ventilator and the alveoli is required to inflate the lungs with a normal tidal volume at a normal rate. Furthermore, in this case the PEEP ventilation prevents the lungs from deflating to FRC, such that the breathing cycle is shifted to larger lung volumes. Since the larger the lung volume the lower the lung compliance (see lung compliance curve in mechanics chapter), the increased peak PAW also reflects the fact that the lungs are more stretched out (lower compliance).

Challenging Question

To improve tissue oxygenation, on March 6 three suggestions were proposed by the attending physicians:

A) To give the patient enough blood to increase Hb to 15 g/100ml blood

B) To reduce ventilation (and so increase $PaCO_2$) to bring pH_a to 7.3 (and $pH_{\bar{v}}$ to 7.25).

C) To reduce the PEEP pressure, but continue to provide a high FIO_2

Assuming no change in $\dot{Q}$ and $\dot{V}O_2$, would $P\bar{v}O_2$, $PaCO_2$, CaO_2, $C\bar{v}O_2$ and shunt fraction change with any of the three options? Can you provide a quantitative answer? Which one of the three methods would you expect to be most effective?

A) An increase in Hb concentration would obviously increase CaO_2 and $C\bar{v}O_2$. In the absence of changes in oxygen consumption and cardiac output, extraction will be the same. Thus, by extracting the same amount of oxygen from arterial blood with higher content, $\%S\bar{v}O_2$ and $P\bar{v}O_2$ will increase. Shunt would not change. Would PaO_2 change? Yes! Because by mixing the same fraction of shunted (venous) blood higher in saturation with ideal blood 100% O_2-saturated the O_2-saturation of arterial blood will increase (higher PaO_2).

$$CAiO_2 = 678 \times 0.0031 + (15 \times 1.34)1 = 22.202 \text{ vol\%}$$

$$\frac{\dot{Q}Cs}{\dot{Q}} = 0.446 = \frac{22.2 - CaO_2}{22.2 - (CaO_2 - 5)}$$

$$CaO_2 = 18.05 \text{ vol\%}$$

$$O_2 \text{ capacity} = 15 \times 1.34 = 20.1 \text{ vol\%}$$

$$\%SaO_2 = 18.05/20.1 = \sim 90\%$$

At $pHa = 7.47$, $PaO_2 = \sim 54$ mmHg. Diss. $O_2 = 54 \times 0.0031 = 0.167$ vol%

$$\%SaO_2 = O_2 \text{ content/capacity} = (18.05-0.167)/20.1 = 89\%$$

At $pHa=7.47$, **$PaO_2 = \sim 53$ mmHg**

$$C\bar{v}O_2 = 1.05 - 5 = 13.05 \text{ vol\%}$$

$$\%S\bar{v}O_2 = 13.05/20.1 = 65\%$$

At $pH\bar{v} = 7.42$, **$P\bar{v}O_2 = \sim 33$ mmHg**

Conclusion: small increase in arterial and mixed venous PO_2.

B) A reduction in pHa and $pH\bar{v}$ will cause the O_2 dissociation curve to shift to the right, resulting in higher $P\bar{v}O_2$ for the same extraction. $CAiO_2$ will decrease a little, not because of the pH-induced shift in the O_2 dissociation curve (this does not affect Hb loading capacity because at such a high PO_2 Hb is 100% saturated anyway) but because of the increase in PCO_2.

What would the new $PaCO_2$ be? To estimate it we need to calculate the $[HCO_3^-]$ at $pHa = 7.3$ and then $PaCO_2$ by the HH equation.

$$-9.5 = \frac{15.52 - [HCO_3^-]}{7.47 - 7.3}$$

$$[HCO_3^-]=17.135 \text{ mEq/l}$$

$$7.3 = 6.1 + \log 17.135 - \log(PaCO_2 - \log 0.0301)$$

$$\mathbf{PaCO_2 = \sim 36\ mmHg}$$

By knowing $PaCO_2$, we can calculate $PAiO_2$, $CAiO_2$, and both CaO_2 and $C\bar{v}O_2$ by the shunt equation, because extraction is the same and shunt fraction will not change.

$PAiO_2 = 664$ mmHg $CAiO_2 = 19.48$ vol%

$$0.446 = \frac{19.48 - CaO_2}{19.48 - (CaO_2 - 5)}$$

$CaO_2 = 15.45$ vol% $\%SaO_2 = \sim 88.7\%$

At pHa = 7.3, $PaO_2 = \sim 64$ mmHg, dissolved $O_2 = 0.198$ vol%, and $\%SaO_2 = 87.6\%$

At pHa = 7.3, **$PaO_2 = 63$ mmHg**

$C\bar{v}O_2 = 10.45$ vol% $\%S\bar{v}O_2 = 60\%$

At $pH\bar{v} = 7.25$, **$P\bar{v}O_2 = \sim 37$ mmHg**

C) This is ultimately the right thing to do.

In conclusion: option "B" provides a rapid reduction of hypoxemia and tissue hypoxia, but the acidosis will be a problem. Option "A" helps only minimally. Option "C" is ultimately the best option, because ventilation with a PEEP of 15 cmH_2O might have contributed to an increase in venous admixture through the foramen ovale, causing severe hypoxemia.

SEQUENCE OF EVENTS AND CONCLUSION

From the patient's history, the lab data, and our calculations we can deduce that this asthmatic patient, before admittance, suffered from a severe and prolonged asthma attack. The asthma was so persistent that the patient reached exhaustion and went into respiratory failure - a condition in which the patient is unable to perform sufficient respiratory work to take care of the metabolic needs, so that hypoxemia and hypercapnia develop.

On March 1, on the ventilator, the patient's status is reasonably good, although there is an abnormal physiological shunt fraction (11%) and metabolic acidosis. This physiological shunt fraction may result from maldistribution/diffusion shunt-like effect and/or conductive shunt because with 40% O_2 it is unlikely that all of shunt-like effects have been eliminated. In asthmatic patients breathing ambient air the shunt is mostly a maldistribution shunt-like effect, but very frequently during very severe asthma attacks a conductive shunt develops as a result of the opening of the foramen ovale. Usually, a patent foramen ovale, which is present in ~27% of the normal population [1], is asymptomatic as it results in small left-to-right shunt, since the left atrial pressure slightly exceeds right atrial pressure. However, severe asthma causes large changes in intra-alveolar and intra-pleural pressures during the breathing cycle. The very negative intra-pleural pressure in inspiration causes a large increase in venous return. The large influx of blood, most prominent from the inferior vena cava, floods the right atrium causing its pressure to exceed that of the left atrium; consequence of it is a right-to-left blood shunt resulting in hypoxemia [2]. PEEP ventilation reversed the sign of intra-alveolar and intra-pleural pressures, making them positive throughout the breathing cycle. In the presence of a patent foramen ovale, PEEP ventilation is likely to have caused an increase in the fraction of right-to-left shunt (see below) eventually increasing it over the next three days from 11% to ~45%.

On March 1, the base deficit is likely to represent metabolic compensation for chronic respiratory alkalosis, typical of asthma. However, it cannot be excluded that the base deficit was worsened by tissue hypoxia (lactic acid formation), due to severe hypoxemia. Over the next few days, in spite of unchanged ventilation and inspired O_2 fraction, severe hypoxemia developed such that PaO_2 dropped to dangerous levels (47 mmHg). We know that the hypoxemia is caused by a large shunt which is conductive because FIO_2 is 100%. With high FIO_2 alveolar collapse and consequential alveolar shunt could occur in poorly ventilated regions; however, in the present case alveolar collapse is unlikely because the patient is ventilated with a sizable tidal volume (580 ml) at larger than normal lung volumes (PEEP), such that the alveoli are more inflated at any phase of the breathing cycle. Therefore, in view of evidence for inter-atrial communication it is reasonable to believe that the increase in conductive shunt is due to increased venous admixture *via* the patent foramen ovale, as a consequence of the hemodynamic changes brought about by PEEP ventilation. Many theories have been proposed to explain the role of PEEP in exacerbating atrial venous admixture [3]. With PEEP ventilation the positive intra-thoracic pressure is believed to translate into an increase in the right atrial pressure [4], which is maintained higher than normal throughout the breathing cycle. This is believed to cause greater stretching of the inter-atrial septum and larger right-to-left blood shunt (venous admixture). Right-to-left inter-atrial shunt is known to be exacerbated when intra-thoracic pressure is increased by PEEP, during coughing, and with Valsalva maneuver. Indeed, PEEP ventilation has been shown to have deleterious, aggravating effects in patients with patent foramen ovale [5, 6].

Reduction of PEEP pressure eliminated hypoxemia over the following three days, indicating that the intra cardiac shunt had progressively decreased. It is unclear, however, why the shunt did not disappear sooner because, even though the stretched right atrium may recover its shape slowly, one might expect a reversal of blood flow through the foramen ovale, resulting in left-to-right blood shunt, as pressure in the left atrium is slightly greater that in the right atrium.

CASE #4 – TENSION PNEUMOTHORAX IN COPD PATIENT

(Adapted from Connolly, J.P., Hemodynamic measurements during a tension pneumothorax. Critical Care Med. 21, 294-296, 1993. Permission granted by Wolters Kluwer Health/ Lippincott Williams & Wilkins).

Table 5: Laboratory blood and gas data.

	6:00 PM	11:00 PM
pHa	7.34	7.24
$pH\bar{v}$	7.30	7.20
$PaCO_2$ (mmHg)	34	37
PaO_2 (mmHg)	76	47
Hb (g/ml blood)	14	14
VT (liters, BTPS)	0.75	0.75
F (breaths/min)	14	18
VCd (liters, BTPS)	0.16	0.16
PB (mmHg)	760	760
R	0.8	0.8
FIO_2 (%)	60	60
$\dot{V}O_2$ (liters/min, STPD)	0.33	0.3
Heart Rate (HR)	125	142
Stroke Volume (SV, ml)	56	27
Body Temperature (°C)	39	39
Peak Airway Pressure	22	53
Arterial Blood Pressure (mmHg)	138/63	120/60
Pulmonary artery pressure (mmHg)	38/19	50/34
Right Atrial Pressure (mmHg)	7	23

A 67 year old man with history of chronic obstructive pulmonary disease (COPD) was admitted in the morning of June 8 with dyspnea (shortness of breath) hemoptysis (coughing of mucous stained with blood) and fever, and was treated with antibiotics. In the early afternoon, because of increased respiratory difficulty, his trachea was intubated and he was placed on mechanical ventilation with 60% FIO_2. At 6:00 PM the values listed below (Table **5**) were obtained. His condition progressively deteriorated and at 11:00 PM another set of blood and gas samples was obtained (Table **5**). Administration of bronchodilators did not improve his conditions, whereas inter-costal needle insertion on the right side of the chest resulted in release of air under tension and rapidly improved the status.

Note: at Body Temperature = 39°C, the constant "863" becomes "868.6", and PH_2O is 51.6 mmHg at 100% saturation. Assume no added conductive dead

space by the ventilator. The normal value of peak PAW during mechanical ventilation ranges from 18 to 22 cm H_2O.

Based on the History and the Given Data, What Can One Say?

6:00 PM

- We know that the patient has COPD, so we would expect him to have abnormal right-to-left conductive shunt and/or maldistribution shunt-like effect, and some alveolar dead space ventilation. If this were the case, we would expect him to be chronically hypoxemic and hypercapnic, and to have a positive (compensatory) base excess before the acute episode.

- The symptoms described on admission (dyspnea, hemoptysis and fever) could be consistent with a pneumonia or other types of pulmonary infection. The increased respiratory difficulty of early afternoon indicates that he was rapidly approaching respiratory failure, such that PaO_2 would have dropped dramatically and $PaCO_2$ would have risen to dangerous levels. This is obvious because at 6:00 PM, even though he was ventilated with 60% O_2 at a rate sufficient to bring $PaCO_2$ to 34 mmHg, his PaO_2 was still low (76 mmHg).

- There is mild acidosis which is metabolic because $PaCO_2$ is lower than normal.

- PaO_2 is lower than normal, even though FIO_2 is 60% and $PaCO_2$ is lower than normal. This clearly indicates the presence of a sizable shunt, which is all conductive because with 60% FIO_2 maldistribution shunt-like effect and any potential diffusion problem are minimized or eliminated altogether.

- The ventilator settings for both VT and f are slightly higher than normal, but are still insufficient to bring PaO_2 and pHa to normal values. In this patient, aside from hypoxemia and acidosis, there is another reason for the need of increased ventilation: fever (39^0C) - increased metabolic rate ($\dot{V}O_2$ = 0.33 l/min).

- Since the patient has COPD, there might be some alveolar dead space ventilation that also would need to be compensated by increasing total minute ventilation ($\dot{V}E$). This is suggested by the fact that, in spite of a greater than normal $\dot{V}E$ (0.75 x 14 = 10.5 l/min), $PaCO_2$ is only slightly below normal.

- Heart rate is almost twice normal. Even though stroke volume is a bit low, this results in higher than normal cardiac output. Undoubtedly, the increase in metabolic rate (fever) is one of the reasons for the increase in $\dot{Q}$.

- Pulmonary artery and right atrial pressures are higher than normal due to the ventilator which, by inflating the lungs, makes the alveolar pressure positive and intra-pleural pressure less negative than normal. This increases the pulmonary vascular resistance, which results in an increase in both pulmonary artery and right atrial pressures, and impairs venous return.

<u>11:00 PM</u>

- More severe acidosis, which is metabolic because $PaCO_2$ is still below normal.

- Severe hypoxemia (PaO_2 = 47 mmHg) in spite of 60% O_2 breathing and lower than normal $PaCO_2$, indicating that there is a large shunt.

- VT was not changed since 6:00 PM, but frequency was increased from 14 to 18/min. This results in a much higher than normal minute ventilation ($\dot{V}E$ = 13.5 l/min). In spite of this, $PaCO_2$ is only slightly below normal, indicating that there is significant alveolar dead space ventilation, which is even greater than that present at 6:00 PM.

- Heart rate has increased even further and stroke volume has decreased a lot. This results in a low cardiac output which, combined with a slightly high $\dot{V}O_2$ (due to fever), results in large extraction. Large extraction combined with severe hypoxemia indicates points to tissue hypoxia and metabolic acidosis (anaerobic metabolism causing lactic acid production).

- Peak PAW is higher than normal, indicating increased airway resistance and/or decreased compliance. Since the administration of bronchodilators did not improve the patient's conditions, there is no increase in airway resistance due to bronchial spasm. Thus, a decrease in compliance is more likely. This is caused by the pneumothorax.
- Pulmonary artery and right atrial pressures are much higher than normal. This is consistent with the large increase in peak PAW. The large increase in alveolar and intra-pleural pressures that results from inflating the lungs with a high peak PAW (53 cm H_2O) increases pulmonary vascular resistance even more than at 6:00 PM. This increases both pulmonary artery and right atrial pressures, and reduces blood flow to the left atrium and ventricle (low SV and BP).

Is there an abnormal shunt fraction at 6:00 PM and at 11:00 PM? Is there a difference between the two values?

6:00 PM:

$CaO_2 = 17.49$ vol% $\dot{Q} = 7.0$ l/min $(CaO_2 - C\bar{v}O_2) = 4.7$ vol%

$$\frac{\dot{Q}Cs}{\dot{Q}} = 34.4\%$$

$C\bar{v}O_2 = 12.79$ vol% $(Ai\text{-}a)PO_2 = 312$ mmHg

11:00 PM:

$CaO2 = 12.715$ vol% $\dot{Q} = 3.83$ l/min $(CaO_2 - C\bar{v}O_2) = 7.8$ vol%

$$\frac{\dot{Q}Cs}{\dot{Q}} = 48\%$$

$C\bar{v}O_2 = 4.92$ vol% $(Ai\text{-}a)PO_2 = 337$ mmHg

Is there abnormal alveolar dead space ventilation at 6:00 PM and at 11:00 PM?

6:00 PM:

$$\frac{\dot{\mathbf{V}}\mathbf{Ad}}{\dot{\mathbf{V}}\bar{\mathbf{A}}} = \mathbf{18\%}$$

11:00 PM:

$$\frac{\dot{\mathbf{V}}\mathbf{Ad}}{\dot{\mathbf{V}}\bar{\mathbf{A}}} = \mathbf{47\%}$$

Is there a base excess (BE) at 6:00 PM and at 11:00 PM?

6:00 PM:

B.E. = -6.82 mEq/l

Metabolic acidosis partially compensate by increased ideal alveolar ventilation. The negative BE is likely to be the consequence of pre-existing tissue hypoxia due to severe hypoxemia before admission.

11:00 PM:

B.E. = -10.23 mEq/l

Severe metabolic acidosis without significant respiratory compensation, due to tissue hypoxia and lactic acid formation. Tissue hypoxia results from large extraction, due to low cardiac output and low CaO_2 caused by severe hypoxemia.

What can you say about the average tissue oxygenation ($P\bar{v}O_2$) at 6:00 PM and at 11:00 PM? Is there a difference between the two values? If so, what are the reasons?

6:00 PM:

$\%S\bar{v}O_2 = 68.2\%$

Due to Bohr shift, at $pH\bar{v}$ = 7.3 and T = 39^0 this $\%S\bar{v}O_2$ corresponds to:

$$P\bar{v}O_2 = \sim 45 \text{ mmHg}$$

<u>11:00 PM:</u>

$$\%S\bar{v}O_2 = 26.2\%$$

Due to Bohr shift, at $pH\bar{v}$ = 7.2 and T = 39^0 this $\%S\bar{v}O_2$ corresponds to:

$$P\bar{v}O_2 = \sim 25 \text{ mmHg}$$

Tissue oxygenation at 6:00 PM is better than normal in spite of hypoxemia (PaO_2 = 76 mmHg) and increase oxygen consumption, because of the significant increase in cardiac output (7 l/min) and consequential decrease in extraction (4.7 vol%). In part, it is also due to the right shift of the O_2 dissociation curve caused by higher body temperature and slight decrease in $pH\bar{v}$.

It isn't surprising to find poor tissue oxygenation at 11:00 PM, because there are several elements detrimental to normal oxygen delivery to tissue, such as: severe hypoxemia and consequential decreased arterial O_2 content, decreased cardiac output and increased oxygen consumption - increased extraction. $P\bar{v}O_2$, however, would be even lower than 25 mmHg if $pH\bar{v}$ were normal, due to the Bohr's shift. In fact, with a $\%S\bar{v}O_2$ of 26.2% $P\bar{v}O_2$ would be ~18 mmHg, with a normal $pH\bar{v}$ of 7.35 and 37^0C body temperature. Note that the low $P\bar{v}O_2$ at 11:00 PM increases the effect of shunt on hypoxemia, as the O_2-content of shunted (mixed venous) blood is lower than normal.

Why is Peak PAW Greater Than Normal at 11:00 PM?

Since peak PAW is measured at the ventilator during inflation, and so while air is flowing through the airways, its value is determined by two factors: the resistance of the airways and the change in compliance that results from expanding the lungs to larger volumes. Therefore, the increase in peak PAW seen at 11:00 PM could be attributed to increased airway resistance and/or decreased compliance. However, in this case it is stated that: administration of bronchodilators did not improve his conditions, whereas inter-costal needle insertion on the right side of the chest resulted in release of air under tension and rapidly improved the status. This tells us: first, that there was no increase in resistance due to a possible asthma attack, and second, that the intra-pleural space of the right lung is filled with gas at pressure greater than atmospheric. This condition occurs when a tension (valvular) pneumothorax develops. Tension pneumothorax results from a rupture in the lungs with valve-like action. This causes complete collapse of the right lung and large decrease in compliance, with a leftward shift of the mediastinum - hence, increased peak PAW (see Chapter 3: Clinical correlation – Pneumothorax; and Chapter 10: Restrictive Diseases – Pneumothorax).

Challenging Questions

Right atrial and pulmonary blood pressures are higher than normal at 6:00 PM, and they have increased even further by 11:00 PM. Why?

Right atrial and pulmonary blood pressures are higher than normal at 6:00 PM because the patient is on a ventilator. The ventilator inflates the lungs by pumping air into them. This results in positive intra-alveolar pressure which compresses the alveolar walls. Consequently, alveolar capillaries as well as pulmonary veins and arterioles are narrowed. This increases pulmonary vascular resistance and, consequently, pulmonary artery and right atrial pressures rise. As the tension pneumothorax develops and intra-pleural pressure progressively increases (becomes progressively more positive) more pressure is needed at the ventilator to inflate the system (large increase in peak PAW). This further increases the compression of the pulmonary vascular system, resulting in greater increase in vascular resistance and, consequently, further increase in pulmonary artery and right atrial pressures, as well as impairment of venous return to the right atrium.

Why is the systolic arterial blood pressure lower at 11:00 PM? Why is the SV lower than normal at 6:00 PM, and much lower than normal at 11:00 PM?

The increase in pulmonary vascular resistance, due to the high intra-thoracic pressure caused by the tension pneumothorax, reduces the blood flow to the left atrium and ventricle. This results in a large drop in stroke volume which is partly compensated by increased heart rate and presumably peripheral vascular resistance. The latter, would prevent a large drop in arterial blood pressure; indeed, systolic blood pressure only dropped by 18 mm Hg (see Chapter 10: Restrictive Diseases – Pneumothorax).

Did $\dot{V}Ad/\dot{V}\overline{A}$ Change Between 6:00 PM and 11:00 PM?

$\dot{V}Ad/\dot{V}\overline{A}$ increased from 18% to 47%, from 6:00 PM to 11:00 PM. Since alveolar dead space ventilation results from an increase in $\dot{V}/\dot{Q}$ ratio, the obvious reason for an increase in $\dot{V}Ad/\dot{V}\overline{A}$ is the reduced blood flow caused by the increase in intra-thoracic pressure. This is expected to further increase the $\dot{V}/\dot{Q}$ ratio of alveoli already poorly perfused because of emphysema.

SEQUENCE OF EVENTS AND CONCLUSION

Based on the given data and on calculated values, we can say that at 6:00 PM the patient was hypoxemic, in spite of hyperventilation and 60% O_2 breathing, because of a large shunt (34.4%). The shunt is entirely conductive because with 60% O_2 most if not all of the maldistribution and/or diffusion problems are eliminated. In view of the symptoms reported on admission (dyspnea, hemoptysis and fever), it is reasonable to believe that the conductive shunt was caused by pneumonia (alveoli filled with exudate resulting in $\dot{V}/\dot{Q} = 0$). The metabolic acidosis suggests that before being mechanically ventilated with 60% O_2 the patient was probably severely hypoxemic with significant tissue hypoxia. The resulting lactic acid production must have eliminated the usual compensatory base excess seen in COPD patients, and must have caused a base deficit that could not be compensated by respiration - the patient was in respiratory distress.

At 11:00 PM, the patient's status has considerably worsened. There is a sizable increase in shunt, more severe and virtually uncompensated metabolic acidosis, large increase in alveolar dead space ventilation, severe hypoxemia and tissue hypoxia. All of these changes are due to the tension (valvular) pneumothorax, which has caused the collapse of the right lung, and consequential increase in conductive shunt, and a large accumulation of gas in the right intra-pleural space at greater than atmospheric pressure which causes compression of pulmonary vessels, and shift to the left and compression of the mediastinum.

Pneumothorax is not an uncommon occurrence in patients mechanically ventilated, especially if emphysema is present. Tension pneumothorax is a very dangerous type of pneumothorax because the gas that diffuses from alveoli to intra-pleural space on inflation (by ventilator) cannot return back into the alveoli during lung deflation, the result being that greater and greater volumes of gas accumulate in the intra-pleural space compressing lungs and mediastinum more and more at each breathing cycle. Often, gas also accumulates within the alveolar walls, resulting in interstitial pneumothorax with further compression of the pulmonary vessels. (see Chapter 3: Clinical correlation – Pneumothorax; and Chapter 10: Restrictive Diseases – Pneumothorax).

CASE #5 – PNEUMONIA AND ARDS

A forty year-old male developed dry cough, fever and tachypnea (increased ventilation rate). He was hospitalized in a rural hospital and was given intravenous fluid and antibiotics. Soon after admission he developed rapidly progressing cyanosis, dyspnea (shortness of breath), severe hypoxemia and acidosis. He was intubated, connected to a ventilator with a Positive End Expiratory Pressure (PEEP) of 10 cm H_2O, and transferred to a University's Medical Center with the diagnosis of pneumonia and Adult Respiratory Distress Syndrome (ARDS) - ARDS is a very serious condition that develops as a result of lung injury or pneumonia and is characterized by pulmonary edema, increased pulmonary artery pressure and severe hypoxemia. During transfer, the data listed in Table **6** (June 8) were obtained.

Upon admission to the Section of Pulmonary and Critical Care Medicine, a right heart catheter was inserted and "wedged" into a small branch of the pulmonary artery, revealing a pulmonary capillary wedge pressure (P_{pcw}) of 22 mmHg (normal P_{pcw} = <10 mmHg). Based on these results and on the data gathered on transfer, the patient was given packed red blood cells and diuretics. Two days later, P_{pcw} had dropped to 5 mmHg and the data listed in Table **6** (June 10) were obtained while still on the ventilator.

Based on the history and the given values, what can one say?

<u>June 8</u>

- Since we know that the patient has pneumonia and ARDS, which involve the presence of exudate and plasma-like liquid both inside some of the alveoli and in the interstitial tissue, we expect a significant amount of shunt, which is conductive because with 100% O_2 breathing maldistribution and diffusion shunt-like effects are eliminated.

Table 6: Laboratory blood and gas data.

	June 8	June 10
pHa	7.3	7.45
$pH\bar{v}$	7.2	7.4
$PaCO_2$ (mmHg)	22	30
PaO_2 (mmHg)	38	65
Hb (g/ml blood)	10	15
$P\bar{v}O_2$ (mmHg)	-	36
VT (liters, BTPS)	0.6	0.5
PB (mmHg)	754	-
R	0.85	-
FIO_2 (%)	100	50
$\dot{V}O_2$ (liters/min, STPD)	0.22	0.26
$\dot{Q}$ (liters/min)	3.9	5
Heart Rate (HR)	120	80
Body Temperature (°C)	40	37
$\dot{Q}Cs/\dot{Q}$	-	17
B.E.	-	-3
At Body Temperature = 40°C, PH_2O is 54 mmHg at 100% saturation		

- There is mild acidosis ($pH_a = 7.3$), which is metabolic because $PaCO_2$ is 22 mmHg.

- Large conductive shunt, because PaO_2 is extremely low (in spite of 100% O_2 breathing) and $PaCO_2$ is much lower than normal (increased ventilation in an attempt to compensate for hypoxemia and metabolic acidosis).

- Anemia which complements hypoxemia and low cardiac output in causing severe tissue hypoxia and formation of lactic acid - the likely cause of metabolic acidosis.

- Oxygen consumption is lower than expected for a patient with a body temperature of 40^{0}C, indicating that a number of cells have switched to anaerobic metabolism due to inadequate oxygen delivery.

- Heart rate is high but cardiac output is low, indicating that stroke volume is lower than normal. The high P_{PCW} (22 mmHg) reflects a high pressure in the left atrium. This is consistent with low cardiac output – weak heart due to fluid overloading, coupled with severe hypoxemia and acidosis, causing blood backlog and stagnation in left atrium and pulmonary vessels.

June 10

- As a result of various treatments, in particular the reduction of blood volume by diuretic administration and the administration of blood cells (elimination of anemia), the patient has considerably improved.

- Minimal respiratory alkalosis which represents an overcompensation created by the ventilator to overcome hypoxemia and residual metabolic acidosis (B.E. of -3 mEq/l).

- Reduced hypoxemia (PaO_2 = 65 mmHg). However, $PaCO_2$ is lower than normal and the patient is given 50% O_2. Thus, a significant conductive shunt is still present ($\dot{Q}Cs/\dot{Q}$ = 17%).

- Almost normal tissue oxygenation ($P\bar{v}O_2$ = 36 mmHg). Oxygen delivery has increased because of increased Hb concentration and cardiac output, which almost fully compensate for the negative effect of hypoxemia.

- Since anaerobic metabolism has been eliminated, oxygen consumption is now normal and consistent with a body temperature of 37^{0}C.

Shunt fraction and (Ai-a)PO_2 gradient

June 8:

CaO_2 = 7.5 vol% $C\bar{v}O$ = 1.9 vol% (Ai-a)PO_2 = 640 mmHg

$$\frac{\dot{Q}Cs}{\dot{Q}} = 58.8\%$$

Very large conductive shunt, due to alveoli with $\dot{V}/\dot{Q} = 0$

Base Excess (B.E.)

B.E. = -14.3 mEq/l

Metabolic acidosis on June 8 partially compensated by increased ventilation ($PaCO_2$ = 22 mmHg). The negative BE is the consequence of severe tissue hypoxia due to severe hypoxemia, anemia, and low cardiac output, which results in increased extraction, and formation of lactic acid.

On June 10, B.E. is -3 mEq/l and pHa is 7.45. A decrease in B.E. of 14.3-3 = 11.3 mEq/l cannot occur physiologically in two days, as [HCO_3^-] generated by the kidneys will only increase by 1-2 mEq/l per day. Thus, the patient must have been given some buffers or H^+ was removed by naso-gastric suction.

Average Tissue Oxygenation (PO_2) on June 8

%$S\bar{v}O_2$ = 14.2%

Due to Bohr shift, at $pH\bar{v}$ = 7.2 and T = 40°C this %$S\bar{v}O_2$ corresponds to:

$P\bar{v}O_2$ = ~18 mmHg

Low $P\bar{v}O_2$ due to severe hypoxemia, anemia, and low cardiac output. Because of the low $pH\bar{v}$ and the high body temperature, however, $P\bar{v}O_2$ is not as low as one may expect it to be. This is due to the right shift of the O_2 dissociation curve. In contrast, on June 10, $P\bar{v}O_2$ = 36 mmHg is still slightly lower than normal, in spite of improved PaO_2 and $\dot{Q}$, and absence of anemia, due to higher pH and reduced body temperature, which shift the O_2 dissociation curve to the left.

Note that the very low $P\bar{v}O_2$ on June 8 increases even more the effect of shunt on hypoxemia, as the O_2-content of shunted (mixed venous) blood is much lower than normal.

On June 8, during ventilation with a PEEP of 10 cm H_2O, a static pressure of 20 cm H_2O was monitored at the end of each lung's inflation. On June 10, during ventilation with a PEEP of 5 cm H_2O, a static pressure of 10.5 cm H_2O was monitored at the end of each lung's inflation. Are these values abnormal? If so, what is the cause? Does this tell you anything about the compliance of this patient's respiratory system? Does this tell you anything about his airway resistance?

Compliance (C) = $\Delta V/\Delta P$

June 8:

$$C = \frac{600 \text{ ml}}{20 - 10 \text{ cmH}_2\text{O}} = \mathbf{60ml/cm\ H_2O}$$

June 10:

$$C = \frac{500 \text{ ml}}{10.5 - 5 \text{ cmH}_2\text{O}} = \mathbf{91ml/cm\ H_2O}$$

Compliance is low on June 8 and has increased to a near normal value on June 10. The low lung compliance on June 8 cannot result from a chronic condition (fibrosis) because it is near normal 48 hrs. later. Most likely, it is caused by interstitial and intra-alveolar edemas, which make the lungs stiffer and reduce the alveolar surface area coated with surfactant; another factor is the congestion of pulmonary vessels, which increases lung stiffness. To a lesser extent, low compliance is also due to the fact that with a PEEP of 10 cmH_2O the patient is ventilated at larger lung volumes, where the lung compliance curve is not as steep - the lungs get stiffer as they approach their maximum volume. The latter factor also applies to the compliance value recorded on June 10, although the reduction in PEEP from 10 to 5 cmH_2O brings ventilation to lung volumes closer to normal levels.

The improved compliance on June 10 is due to reduced interstitial and intra-alveolar pulmonary edemas, and to decreased vascular pressure, which reduce pulmonary stiffness. The reduced intra-alveolar edema increases the number of alveoli with normal surfactant lining, which lowers surface tension and decreases lung recoil. These values tell nothing about airway resistance because compliance is measures at static conditions (no gas movement).

What are the stroke volume values? (normal SV = 60-80 ml/beat).

June 8:

$$\mathbf{SV = 32.5\ ml}$$

June 10:

$$\mathbf{SV = 62.5\ ml}$$

The SV is very low on June 8 because the cardiac muscle (left ventricle) was weakened by fluid overloading, severe hypoxemia, and acidosis. On June 10, the increased blood oxygenation and pH, and reduced blood volume by diuretics, have improved left ventricular function, normalizing SV and cardiac output.

Challenging Questions

On June 8, a student suggested to administer a cardiac inotropic drug to increase cardiac output. Another student disagreed. Assuming no change in oxygen consumption, pHa, pH $\bar{v}$, and shunt fraction, would one expect hypoxemia and tissue oxygenation to improve with an increase in cardiac output from 3.9 to 5 L/min?

Yes! Hypoxemia and tissue oxygenation would improve, because extraction would decrease, and so $C\bar{v}O_2$, CaO_2, PaO_2 and $P\bar{v}O_2$ would increase.

$$\frac{\dot{V}O_2}{\dot{Q}} = \frac{0.22}{5} = 4.4 \text{ vol\%} \qquad \frac{\dot{Q}Cs}{\dot{Q}} = 0.588 = \frac{15.5 - CaO_2}{15.5 - (CaO_2 - 4.4)}$$

$CaO_2 = 9.22$ vol% $\qquad C\bar{v}O_2 = 9.22 - 4.4 = 4.82$ vol%

$\%SaO_2 = 9.22/(10 \times 1.34) = \sim 69\%$ At $pH_a = 7.3$, and $\%SaO_2 = \sim 69\%$

$$\mathbf{PaO_2 = \sim 48\ mmHg}$$

$\%S\bar{v}O_2 = 4.82/(10 \times 1.34) = \sim 36\%$ At $pH\bar{v} = 7.2$ and $\%S\bar{v}O_2 = \sim 36\%$

$$\mathbf{P\bar{v}O_2 = \sim 32\ mmHg}$$

Is it reasonable to assume no change in oxygen consumption and pH values with an increase in cardiac output?

No! With the increase in oxygen delivery that results from increased cardiac output, oxygen consumption will increase and anaerobic metabolism (lactic acid production) will decrease. pHa and $pH\bar{v}$ should not change right away with a reduction or elimination of tissue hypoxia, because it takes days for the kidneys to increase bicarbonate concentration (1-2 mEq/l per day). However, with an increase in $\dot{V}O_2$, $\dot{V}CO_2$ will also increase. This will cause an increase in $PaCO_2$ and a decrease in pHa and $pH\bar{v}$, if ventilation is not proportionally increased.

SEQUENCE OF EVENTS AND CONCLUSION

Before admission the patient had developed pneumonia. Upon hospitalization, excess i.v. fluid was administered. This, combined with the lung infection, caused ARDS which resulted in interstitial and intra-alveolar pulmonary edema, and cardiac overload. The pulmonary edema caused a large increase in the fraction of right-to-left blood shunt that must have preexisted due to pneumonia. The shunt was caused by reduced ventilation in alveoli filled with liquid (edema) and exudate (pneumonia). Some alveolar collapse may also have occurred due to loss of surfactant; however, the PEEP ventilation may have prevented it. The large shunt caused severe hypoxemia which, in conjunction with anemia and reduced cardiac output, resulted in severe tissue hypoxia and metabolic acidosis. Hypoxemia and acidosis further weakened the cardiac muscle, resulting in very low SV (32.5 ml) and causing a vicious circle involving increased pulmonary edema, increased shunt, decreased cardiac output, and worsened tissue hypoxia and metabolic acidosis. The high P_{PCW} indicates that the pressure in the left atrium, pulmonary veins and capillaries is much greater than normal, which is the reason for alveolar and interstitial edema. The alveolar and interstitial edema, the tissue infiltration by the pulmonary infection, the increased vascular congestion and the decreased surfactant in edematous alveoli, all contributed to decreasing lung compliance.

The treatments provided at the University's Medical Center reversed this very dangerous trend in a number of ways. The diuretic reduced pulmonary edema by decreasing blood volume and cardiac work. The administration of packed red blood cells corrected the anemia, improving oxygen delivery - reduced tissue hypoxia and metabolic acidosis. The PEEP ventilation helped reducing shunt by preventing end-expiratory alveolar collapse. Reduced hypoxemia and normalization of acid-base balance also contributed to improving cardiac function.

CASE #6 - RUPTURED CORONARY ARTERY DURING ANGIOPLASTY IN COPD PATIENT

(Adapted from: Sandifer, D.P. and Gonzalez, J.L. Refractory postoperative hypoxemia associated with regional cardiac tamponade and patent foramen ovale. Critical Care Med. 25, 1608-1611, 1997. Permission granted by Wolters Kluwer Health/ Lippincott Williams & Wilkins).

A sixty eight year old man without history of pulmonary disease underwent emergency coronary artery bypass surgery because of accidental rupture of the right coronary artery during an attempted percutaneous trans-luminal angioplasty. A few hours after angioplasty, the patient's arterial oxygen saturation had decreased from 99% (at FIO_2 = 50%) to 59% (at FIO_2 = 100%). The patient's trachea was intubated and he was placed on mechanical ventilation with 100% O_2 and positive-end-expiratory-pressure (PEEP). Soon after, the data listed below (Table 7) were obtained. A chest X-ray showed no sign of pulmonary edema or pulmonary embolism, but trans-esophageal echocardiography revealed compression of the right atrium and right ventricle by presumed thrombus with decreased right atrium and right ventricle cavity sizes, bowing of the inter-atrial septum into the left atrium, patent foramen ovale and lack of motility of the inferior septum and the posterior left ventricular wall. Based on these findings, the patient was brought back to the operating room for re-exploration. He was discovered to have a large mediastinal thrombus compressing the right atrium and ventricle. As a result of the surgical treatment, $\%SaO_2$ rapidly improved from 55% to 99% (at $FIO_2 = 100\%$).

Table 7: Laboratory blood and gas data.

pHa	7.3	**R**	0.8
$pH\bar{v}$	7.25	**FIO_2 (%)**	100
$PaCO_2$ (mmHg)	40	**$\dot{V}O_2$ (liters/min, STPD)**	0.25
PaO_2 (mmHg)	31	**Heart Rate (HR)**	120
Hb (g/ml blood)	14	**Systemic Blood pressure (mmHg)**	100/70
VT (liters, BTPS)	0.7	**Pulmonary Artery Pressure (mmHg)**	26/15
F (breaths/min)	15	**Right Atrial Pressure (mmHg)**	20
VCd (liters, BTPS)	0.165	**P_{PCW} (mmHg)**	14
PEEP (cm H_2O)	10	**Body Temperature (°C)**	37
PB (mmHg)	747	**$C\bar{v}O_2$**	4.6

Based on the History and the Given Values, What Can One Say?

- Following the bypass surgery there was a progressive decrease in arterial oxygen saturation (down to 59% with 100% O_2 breathing) which persisted ($PaO_2 = 31$) even after intubation and mechanical ventilation with 100% O_2 sufficient to maintain a normal $PaCO_2$ (40 mmHg). This clearly indicates that a large conductive shunt had developed.

- The shunt is unlikely to result from collapsed alveoli or alveoli filled with liquid (edema, *etc.*), because the chest X-ray was normal, and the patient is ventilated with PEEP which prevents alveolar collapse that might occur with $FIO_2 = 100\%$. Obviously, the shunt is not due to ventilation/perfusion maldistribution and/or diffusion impairment, because both of them are eliminated by 100% FIO_2 breathing.

- A clue to the origin of the shunt comes from echocardiography. The observation of a patent foramen ovale, bowing of the inter-atrial septum, and right atrial and ventricular compression, in conjunction with data for increased right atrial pressure (20 mmHg), which is greater than the left atrial pressure (P_{PCW} = 14 mmHg), clearly indicates the presence of a large flow of venous blood from the right atrium to the left atrium (right-to-left shunt, venous admixture).

- In spite of 100% FIO_2 breathing, and sufficient ventilation to maintain $PaCO_2$ at 40 mmHg, there is very severe hypoxemia. Thus, the hypoxemia is entirely caused by the large intra-cardiac shunt.
- There is also a significant acidosis, which is metabolic because $PaCO_2$ = 40 mmHg. The acidosis is not compensated by increased ventilation because $PaCO_2$ = 40 mmHg. The likely cause of the acidosis is tissue hypoxia and lactic acid formation.
- Tissue hypoxia appears to result primarily from hypoxemia because anemia is minimal; calculations (see below) will tell whether cardiac output is also a factor.
- The setting of the ventilator is such that ventilation is significantly higher than normal ($\dot{V}E$ = 0.7 x 15 = 10.5 l/min); in spite of this, $PaCO_2$ is normal. Since oxygen consumption is normal, this indicates that there is a significant increase in alveolar dead space ventilation.

Shunt fraction, $(Ai\text{-}a)PO_2$ gradient, cardiac output and stroke volume

CaO_2 = 9.85 vol% $CAiO_2$ = 20.8 vol% $C\bar{v}O_2 = 4.6$ vol%

$$\frac{\dot{Q}Cs}{\dot{Q}} = 67.4\%$$

$(Ai\text{-}a)PO_2$ = 629 mmHg

Extraction = CaO_2 - $C\bar{v}O_2$ = 5.25 vol%

$$\dot{Q} = 4.76\ l/min$$

SV = ~40 ml

The very large shunt fraction is entirely caused by venous admixture at the foramen ovale. There is no shunt from maldistribution and/or diffusion problems because, if present, both of them would have been eliminated by 100% O_2 breathing. Shunt due to alveolar collapse is very unlikely because PEEP ventilation maintains the lungs at larger than normal volumes. Moreover, the chest X-ray was normal. The cardiac output is near normal because the significantly increased heart rate (120/min) compensates for an abnormally low stroke volume (normal SV = 60-80 ml).

The left heart receives just about as much blood as normal, but while under normal circumstances virtually all of the blood flowing per minute comes to the left heart from the pulmonary veins, here the same amount of blood per minute comes for two sources: 67.4% from the right atrium, *via* the patent foramen ovale, and 32.6% from the lungs, *via* the pulmonary veins. The severe hypoxemia, caused by the right-to-left shunt at the foramen ovale, coupled with acidosis contributes to further weakening the left ventricle - small stroke volume. In addition, the luck of mobility of the inferior septum and left posterior ventricular wall indicates that the patient suffered a myocardial infarction due to rupture of the right coronary artery. This artery supplies blood to the lower posterior wall of the left ventricle, which is the principal reason for the myocardial weakness.

Alveolar Dead Space Ventilation

$\dot{V}E = 10.5$ l/min (BTPS) $\dot{V}Cd = 2.47$ l/min (BTPS) $\dot{V}\bar{A} = 8.03$ l/min (BTPS)

$\dot{V}CO_2 = 0.2$ l/min (STPD) $\dot{V}Ai = 4.3$ l/min (BTPS) $\dot{V}Ad = 3.73$ l/min (BTPS)

$$\frac{\dot{\mathbf{V}}\mathbf{Ad}}{\dot{\mathbf{V}}\bar{\mathbf{A}}} = \mathbf{46.5\%}$$

The large fraction of alveolar dead space ventilation is due to dramatically reduced lung perfusion, as ~67% of the blood bypasses the lungs, flowing from right to left atrium *via* the patent foramen ovale. This causes a large increase in $\dot{V}/\dot{Q}$ (increased ventilation and severely reduced blood perfusion). To a minor extent, the PEEP ventilation further reduces perfusion, as it increases alveolar pressure, causing compression of alveolar capillaries.

Acid/Base Status

B.E. = -6 mEq/l

Metabolic acidosis not compensated by increased ideal alveolar ventilation ($PaCO_2$ = 40 mmHg). The negative BE is the consequence of severe tissue hypoxia (formation of lactic acid), entirely due to severe hypoxemia.

Average Tissue Oxygenation

$$P\bar{v}O_2 = \sim 20 \text{ mmHg}$$

Low $P\bar{v}O_2$ due to severe hypoxemia, which results in reduced CaO_2. Since the cardiac output is relatively normal, as the increase in heart rate compensates for the low stroke volume, and anemia is absent, tissue hypoxia is due entirely to hypoxemia. Because of the low $pH\bar{v}$, $P\bar{v}O_2$ is not as low as one may expect it to be. This is due to the right shift of the O_2 dissociation curve. If $pH\bar{v}$ were normal (~7.35), $P\bar{v}O_2$ would be even lower (17-18 mmHg). Note that this extremely low $P\bar{v}O_2$ increases the effect of shunt on hypoxemia, as the O_2-content of shunted (mixed venous) blood is much lower than normal.

At the end of inspiration a static pressure of 18 cm H_2O was measured. What does this tell you about the patient in terms of respiratory mechanics?

$$C = \frac{700}{18 - 10} = \mathbf{87.5\ ml/cm\ H_2O}$$

Slight decrease in compliance (normal = 100 ml/cm H_2O). This is due primarily to the fact that with a PEEP of 10 cm H_2O the patient is ventilated at larger lung volumes, where the lung compliance curve is less steep (the lungs get stiffer as they approach their maximum volume). In part, it is also due to increased pressure (and so volume) in the mediastinum, indicated by evidence for cardiac compression. The static pressure value tells us nothing about airway resistance as it is measured without air movement.

What Could have Caused the Increase in Right Atrial Pressure?

A hemorrhage in the mediastinum following the emergency surgery is the cause of it. Indeed, in the operating room a large mediastinal thrombus was found to compress the right atrium and ventricle. This resulted in severely impaired venous return and consequential increased pressure in venae cave and right atrium, bowing of the inter-atrial septum into the left atrium, and opening of the foramen ovale. PEEP ventilation and consequential increase in pulmonary vascular resistance might have also contributed, although minimally, to increasing the right atrial pressure.

Challenging Question

What would increase PaO_2 more drastically: a doubling of ideal alveolar ventilation or a doubling of cardiac output? (Assume pHa = 7.44 with a doubling of ideal alveolar ventilation, and no change in oxygen consumption in either case).

Ventilation in this case is not a problem. Since there is 100% O_2 breathing, doubling $\dot{V}Ai$ will only increase minimally the oxygen content of ideal alveolar blood.

Doubling $\dot{V}Ai$ will cut in half $PaCO_2$ (20 mmHg).

$$PAiO_2 = 700 - 20 = 680$$

$$CAiO_2 = 680 \times 0.003 + (14 \times 1.34)1 = 20.87 \text{ vol\%}$$

The previously calculated $CAiO_2$ was 20.8 vol%. With the new ventilation $CAiO_2$ only increases by: 20.87 - 20.8 = 0.07 vol% (insignificant). Since the patient is ventilated with 100% O_2 the hemoglobin of blood coming from the ideal compartment is already fully saturated. Thus, the new ventilation will make only minimal differences in CaO_2 and $C\bar{v}O_2$, and so in PaO_2 and $P\bar{v}O_2$. Since there is no reason to believe that shunt fraction would change, we can estimate the new PaO_2:

$$\frac{\dot{Q}Cs}{\dot{Q}} = 0.674 = \frac{20.87 - CaO_2}{20.87 - (CaO_2 - 5.25)} \qquad CaO_2 = 10 \text{ vol\%},\ C\bar{v}O_2 = 4.75 \text{ vol\%}$$

$\%SaO_2 = 10/(14 \times 1{,}34) = \sim 53\%$ At pHa = 7.44, $\%SaO_2 = \sim 53\%$

$$\mathbf{PaO_2 = \sim 27\ mmHg}$$

Conclusion: decrease in PaO_2 by 4 mmHg. The drop in PaO_2 is due to the fact that with a drop in $PaCO_2$ from 40 to 20 mmHg, caused by a doubling of $\dot{V}Ai$, the increase in pHa results in a left shift of the O_2-dissociation curve.

In contrast, doubling cardiac output would increase PaO_2 from 31 to ~52 mmHg (see below). Again, since there is no reason to believe that shunt fraction will change, we can calculate the new CaO_2 from the shunt equation by first calculating the new extraction.

$\dot{Q} = 4.76 \times 2 = 9.52$ l/min O_2 extraction $= 0.25/9.52 = 2.6$ vol%

$$\frac{\dot{Q}Cs}{\dot{Q}} = 0.674 = \frac{20.8 - CaO_2}{20.8 - (CaO_2 - 2.6)}$$

$$CaO_2 = 15.22 \text{ vol\%}$$

$\%SaO_2 = \sim 82\%$. At pHa = 7.3, $\%SaO_2 = \sim 82\%$:

$$\mathbf{PaO_2 = \sim 52 \ mmHg}$$

Conclusion: increase in PaO_2 by 52 - 31 = 21 mmHg

The main reason why PaO_2 increases significantly with a doubling of cardiac output is that extraction is reduced to one half so that $C\bar{v}O_2$ increases from 4.6 to 12.62 vol%. Since CaO_2 reflect the mixing of ideal and mixed venous (shunted) blood (32.6% and 67.4%, respectively), any increase in $C\bar{v}O_2$ obviously results in an increase in both CaO_2 and PaO_2.

SEQUENCE OF EVENTS AND CONCLUSION

Two major problems have occurred in this patient. The rupture of the right coronary artery, during attempted percutaneous trans-luminal coronary angioplasty, caused ischemia of inferior septum and posterior left ventricular wall resulting in decreased stroke volume and compensatory increase in heart rate. The heart was additionally weakened by the severe hypoxemia and acidosis. The emergency bypass operation was complicated by a large hemorrhage in the mediastinum which compressed right atrium and ventricle. This caused a large increase in right atrial pressure, bulging of the inter-atrial septum to the left, opening of the foramen ovale and a large intra-cardiac right-to-left shunt. The shunt caused severe hypoxemia which resulted in tissue hypoxia and consequential metabolic acidosis, due to anaerobic metabolism and formation of lactic acid. The tissue hypoxia was not compensated by increased cardiac output (reduced extraction) because the heart was weakened by infarction, hypoxemia and acidosis.

The shifting of ~67% of the circulation away from the lungs *via* the intra-cardiac shunt severely reduced the lung perfusion resulting in large alveolar dead space ventilation. This prevented sufficient compensation of acidosis by increased VT and f, such that in spite of a large increase in minute ventilation, the $PaCO_2$ was only brought down to a normal value. A $PaCO_2$ of ~30 mmHg would have been needed for increasing pHa to 7.4.

PEEP ventilation prevented potential alveolar collapse that could have occurred with 100% FIO_2 breathing and that would have increased even further the shunt fraction. The small decrease in compliance was due to PEEP as the lungs were ventilated at larger volumes, where lung compliance is naturally reduced. The surgical re-intervention improved the $\%SaO_2$ because by removing the large hematoma from the mediastinum it eliminated the atrial compression and with that the large intra-cardiac shunt.

CASE #7 – HANTAVIRUS PULMONARY SYNDROME IN DIABETIC PATIENT

(Adapted from: Crowley, M.R., Katz, R,W., Kessler, R., Simpson, S.Q., Levy, H., Hallin, G.W., Cappon, J., Krahling, J.B. and Wernly, J. Successful treatment of adult with severe Hantavirus pulmonary syndrome with extracorporeal membrane oxygenation. Critical Care Med. 26, 409-414, 1998. Permission granted by Wolters Kluwer Health/ Lippincott Williams & Wilkins).

A forty one year old farmer suffering from diabetes presented at a rural hospital on May 1 with a 4-day history of cough, nausea, vomiting, polyuria, polydipsia, and a 30lb weight loss over the previous 3 months - the initial laboratory findings are shown in Table **8** (May 1). The next day he was transferred to a University's Medical Center where insulin and bicarbonate infusion was started. A day later (May 3) he developed symptoms consistent with severe Hantavirus Pulmonary Syndrome (HPS), including bilateral alveolar infiltrates on chest X-ray, increased oxygen requirement and hypotension. The patient's trachea was intubated and the lungs were mechanically ventilated with a Positive End Expiratory Pressure (PEEP) of 7 cm H_2O and 100% FIO_2. His circulatory support included: dopamine 20 μg/kg/min, norepinephrine 20 μg/min and intravenous epinephrine boluses to maintain a systolic pressure of ~75 mmHg. One hour later, the following laboratory data were collected (Table **8**, May 3).

Table 8: Laboratory blood and gas data.

	May 1	May 3
pHa	7.26	7.35
$pH\bar{v}$	7.2	7.2
$PaCO_2$ (mmHg)	16	20
PaO_2 (mmHg)	82	63
Hb (g/ml blood)	15	15
VT (liters, BTPS)	-	0.6
VCd (liters, BTPS)	-	0.17
F (breaths/min)	-	28
Blood Pressure (mm Hg)	-	76/43
Heart Rate (beats/min)	-	150
$\dot{Q}$ (l/min)	5	2.5
$\dot{Q}Ps/\dot{Q}$	17	-
PB (mmHg)	747	752
R	0.9	0.85
FIO_2 (%)	21	100
$\dot{V}O_2$ (liters/min, STPD)	0.25	0.3
Blood Glucose (mg/dl)	453	110
Body Temperature (°C)	37	39
At body temperature = 39°C, the constant 863 becomes 869 and the partial pressure of H_2O is ~52 mmHg.		

HPS is a very severe acute illness, caused by the Sin Nombre Virus. It is characterized by fulminating cardiopulmonary failure in adults with a history of rodent dropping contact. It was discovered in 1993, when an outbreak of this disease occurred in the South Western U.S.

In spite of the treatment the patient's cardiorespiratory condition continued to deteriorate and it was decided that he met the criteria for Extra-Corporeal Membrane Oxygenation (ECMO). The patient was cannulated for veno-arterial ECMO *via* the right femoral artery and vein. The ECMO apparatus takes venous blood from the right atrium and the inferior vena cava, it circulates it at a flow rate of 3 l/min through an O_2-CO_2 exchanger, which supplies O_2 and removes CO_2, and it re-injects oxygenated blood into the abdominal aorta and femoral artery. Over the next 48 hours the patient's lung function improved and the ECMO and ventilator support were weaned. He was discharged 25 days later neurologically intact and breathing room air.

Based on the history and the given values, what can you say?

May 1

- Significant acidosis ($pH_a = 7.26$), hypocapnia, hypoxemia and high blood sugar.

- Since hypocapnia indicates hyperventilation, it is obvious that the acidosis is metabolic (negative base excess) and that the hyperventilation is compensatory. This agrees with evidence for high blood glucose and indicates that there is diabetic acidosis. Obviously, the hyperventilation is insufficient to fully compensate for metabolic acidosis.

- The presence of mild hypoxemia in conjunction with hypocapnia is a clear indication of the presence of abnormal shunt fraction (venous admixture). The hyperventilation is caused by both metabolic acidosis and hypoxemia and is compensatory to both of them; in the absence of hyperventilation pH_a and PaO_2 would be lower than they are.

- The R value is higher than normal, whereas with diabetes we would expect it to be lower than normal due to altered glucose metabolism. Thus, most likely at the time of sampling respiration was not as steady state with metabolism (acute hyperventilation).

May 3

- Very mild acidosis ($pH_a = 7.35$) in spite of hypocapnia, indicative of negative base excess. Since blood glucose is now normal, ketoacidosis should have disappeared. A possibility is that there has not been enough time for the kidneys to regenerate enough bicarbonate. However, the patient was given bicarbonate infusion which should have normalized the bicarbonate concentration. Therefore, something else must explain the negative base excess.

- Severe hypoxemia in spite of hypocapnia and 100% O_2 breathing, which is a clear indication of the presence of a large conductive shunt.

- Very low cardiac output which, combined with slightly increased oxygen consumption, results in large extraction. This will obviously cause significant tissue hypoxia, anaerobic metabolism and formation of lactic acid. The consequence of this is metabolic acidosis (negative base excess).

- Fever, which is consistent with the pulmonary infection detected with the X-ray (pulmonary infiltrates). The infiltrates are likely to be the cause of the conductive shunt (alveoli with $\dot{V}/\dot{Q} = 0$).

- Blood pressure is quite low, indicative of cardiac failure caused by HPS - a very severe acute illness characterized by fulminating cardiopulmonary failure.

Shunt fraction and O_2 extraction on May 3

$CaO_2 = 17.68$ vol% $C\bar{v}O_2 = 5.68$ vol%

$$\frac{\dot{Q}Cs}{\dot{Q}} = 27\%$$

$$(Ai\text{-}a)PO_2 = 680\text{-}63 = 617 \text{ mmHg}$$

$$(Ca - C\bar{v}O_2) = 12 \text{ vol\%}$$

Significant conductive shunt fraction, and very large O_2 extraction due to low cardiac output.

Stroke Volume on May 3

$$SV = \dot{Q}/HR = 2.5/150 = \mathbf{16.7\ ml}$$

Very low stroke volume due to weak left ventricle. The myocardial weakness is caused by the HPS infection complicated by hypoxemia and mild acidosis. The heart rate is considerably increased. This provides some compensation for low stroke volume (with a normal HR of 72 beats/min a SV of 16.7 ml would result in $\dot{Q}$ = 1.2 l/min).

Alveolar Dead Space Ventilation on May 3

$\dot{V}E$ = 16.8 l/min $\dot{V}CO_2$ = 0.255 l/min $\dot{V}Ai$ = 11.8 l/min $\dot{V}Pd$ = 5.72 l/min

$\dot{V}Cd$ = 4.76 l/min $\dot{V}Ad$ = 0.96 l/min $\dot{V}\bar{A}$ = 12.04 l/min

$$\frac{\dot{\mathbf{V}}\mathbf{Ad}}{\dot{\mathbf{V}}\bar{\mathbf{A}}} = \mathbf{8\%}$$

Minimal increase in alveolar dead space ventilation due to PEEP ventilation. The positive alveolar pressure generated by the ventilator throughout the breathing cycle results in some compression of the alveolar capillaries. This reduces the blood perfusion in some areas of the lungs causing regional increase in $\dot{V}/\dot{Q}$ and so increased alveolar dead space ventilation.

On May 1, $C\bar{v}O_2$ = 14 vol%, what is the average tissue oxygenation?

$$\%S\bar{v}O_2 = C\bar{v}O_2/\text{capacity} = 14/(15\text{x}1.34) = 69.6\%$$

Due to Bohr shift, at $pH\bar{v}$ = 7.2 this $\%S\bar{v}O_2$ corresponds to:

$$\mathbf{P\bar{v}O_2 = \sim 46\ mmHg}$$

Is $P\bar{v}O_2$ consistent with the values of $C\bar{v}O_2$ and PaO_2?

$P\bar{v}O_2$ is higher than expected in spite of hypoxemia and lower than normal $C\bar{v}O_2$. The reason is that $pH\bar{v}$ is lower than normal. This causes a right shift in the O_2 dissociation curve which favors O_2 unloading from hemoglobin.

What is the average tissue oxygenation on May 3?

$\%S\bar{v}O_2 = 5.68/(15x1.34) = 28.3\%$. At $pH\bar{v} = 7.2$ and $T = 39^{\circ}C$, this $\%S\bar{v}O_2$ corresponds to:

$$\mathbf{P\bar{v}O_2 = \sim 26\ mmHg}$$

Significantly low $P\bar{v}O_2$ mainly due to very low $\dot{Q}$ (large O_2 extraction), and hypoxemia. Because of the low $pH\bar{v}$, $P\bar{v}O_2$ is not as low as one may expect it to be. This is due to the right shift of the O_2 dissociation curve. Note that the low $P\bar{v}O_2$ increases the effect of shunt on hypoxemia, as the O_2-content of shunted (mixed venous) blood is much lower than normal.

Acid/Base Status

May 1:

$$B.E. = -18.5\ mEq/l$$

May 3:

$$B.E. = -13.8\ mEq/l$$

Very negative base excess values. Since $PaCO_2$ is very low on both days, the patient has a severe metabolic acidosis partially compensated by hyperventilation. Because of the large decrease in cardiac output, due to weak cardiac muscle, blood stagnated in the tissue capillaries. This causes PCO_2 to increase in both tissue and mixed venous blood; consequentially, pH drops. We can estimate $P\bar{v}CO_2$ to increase by ~22 mmHg (from 20 to ~42 mmHg) on May 3 and by ~ 7 mmHg (from 16 to ~23 mmHg) on May 1.

Challenging Question

On May 3, a resident suggested that a significant increase in PaO_2 and tissue oxygenation could be obtained by lowering body temperature to 37°C. Another resident felt that this would make no difference. Who was right? What is your estimate of PaO_2 and $P\bar{v}O_2$ at 37°C? Assume pHa = 7.4, $pH\bar{v}$ = 7.25, $\dot{V}Ai$ = 10.9 l/min and no change in shunt fraction and $\dot{Q}$.

A reestablishment of the normal body temperature will cause $\dot{V}O_2$ and $\dot{V}CO_2$ to drop down to the values of May 1. Since $\dot{Q}$ does not change, with a drop in $\dot{V}O_2$ extraction will decrease and, at the same shunt fraction, both CaO_2 and $C\bar{v}O_2$ will increase. However, PaO_2 and $P\bar{v}O_2$ will not change significantly because the decrease in temperature and increase in pH will cause a left shift in the O_2 dissociation curve.

Quantitatively:

$\dot{V}CO_2 = 0.213$ l/min (STPD) $\quad PaCO_2 = \frac{863 \times 0.213}{10.9} = 16.9$ mmHg

$PAiO_2 = 688$ mmHg $\quad CAiO_2 = 22.16$ vol%

Extraction = 0.25/2.5 = 10 vol%

$$\frac{\dot{Q}Cs}{\dot{Q}} = 0.27 = \frac{22.16 - CaO_2}{22.16 - (CaO_2 - 10)}$$

$CaO_2 = 18.46$ vol%

$\%SaO_2$ ~92% $\quad$ At pHa = 7.4, $\%SaO_2$ = ~92% corresponds to

PaO_2 = ~62 mmHg

Iteratively (for more precision):

At PaO_2 = ~62 mmHg, dissolved O_2 = 0.186 vol%, $\%SaO_2$ = ~91%

At pHa = 7.4, $\%SaO_2$ = ~91% corresponds to

PaO_2 = ~60 mmHg

$C\bar{v}O_2 = 8.46$ vol% $\quad \%S\bar{v}O_2$ = ~42%

At pH$\bar{v}$ = 7.25, $\%S\bar{v}O_2$ = ~42% corresponds to

$P\bar{v}O_2$ = ~27 mmHg

Conclusion: virtually no change in PaO_2 and $P\bar{v}O_2$

SEQUENCE OF EVENTS

At the time of admission (May 1) the patient was found to have diabetes. This had caused ketoacidosis and compensatory hyperventilation. The pulmonary infection resulted in alveolar shunt (probably both maldistribution and conductive) causing hypoxemia and compensatory hyperventilation. On May 3, fever had developed – increase in metabolic rate. The pulmonary infection had worsened causing alveolar infiltrates. The infiltrates caused alveolar shunt and consequential hypoxemia, with some compensation by ventilator setting (hyperventilation) and by oxygen breathing, which eliminated potential maldistribution/diffusion shunt-like effects. The cardiac infection weakened the myocardium, resulting in reduced stroke volume, blood pressure and cardiac output; some compensation was provided by increased heart rate. The drop in cardiac output, in conjunction with hypoxemia and increased metabolic rate, resulted in severe tissue hypoxia (partly moderated by drop in pH and increased body temperature), formation of lactic acid and drop in pHa and $pH\bar{v}$, partially compensated by ventilator setting (reduced $PaCO_2$). PEEP breathing caused some compression of alveolar capillaries resulting in a small increase in alveolar dead space ventilation, compensated by the ventilator setting (increased VT and f).

CASE #8 – CANCER PATIENT WITH PARTIALLY COLLAPSED LUNG DEVELOPS HIGH FEVER AND SEVERE HYPERCAPNIA WHILE BEING MECHANICALLY VENTILATED

A 62 year old male suffering from lung cancer was admitted to a hospital because of severe shortness of breath. A chest x-ray determined the presence of a partially collapsed right lung. The patient was intubated and put on a respirator. At 10 p.m. an arterial blood sample was collected. In view of the lab results (Table **9**), the inspired O_2 fraction was increased. A few hours later the patient became semi-comatose and at 2 a.m. another blood sample was taken. Based on the lab data (Table C-9) the patient was given antibiotics, but the attending resident decided not to change the setting of the respirator and was puzzled as to what might have been the reason for such an increase in $PaCO_2$ (80.8 mmHg), referring it as ***"an unusual CO_2 retention"***.

Table 9: Laboratory blood and gas data.

	10:00 p.m.	2:00 a.m.
pHa	7.39	7.15
$pH\bar{v}$	7.34	7.10
$PaCO_2$ (mmHg)	43	80.8
PaO_2 (mmHg)	58	79.2
$\%SaO_2$	-	82.7
Hb (g/ml blood)	12	12
VT (liters, BTPS)	0.5	0.5
F (breaths/min)	30	30
VCd (liters, BTPS)	0.17	0.17
$\dot{Q}$ (l/min)	5	8.3
PB (mmHg)	750	750
R	0.85	0.85
FIO_2 (%)	50	100
$C\bar{v}O_2$ (vol%)	9.36	8.54
Body Temperature (°C)	37	41.5

Based on the History and the Given Values, What Can You Say?

10 p.m.

- Significant hypoxemia which combined with a fairly normal $PaCO_2$ is clearly indicative of abnormal right-to-left blood shunt. In this case, in fact, it points to large shunt because the patient is ventilated with 50% O_2 - a normal subject with a shunt fraction of ~4% would have a PaO_2 of ~230 mmHg when breathing 50% O_2. The large shunt is probably mostly conductive because 50% FIO_2 is likely to eliminate or minimize the maldistribution/diffusion shunt like effect.

- Moderate anemia.

- A ventilation of 15 l/min is roughly twice the normal but, in spite of that, $PaCO_2$ is slightly higher than normal. This indicates a large wastage of ventilation in dead spaces. In view of the high breathing frequency the wasted ventilation in the conductive dead space is greater than normal (0.170 x 30 = 5.1 l/min); however, when this is subtracted one finds a total alveolar ventilation of almost 10 l/min (approximately twice the normal), indicating the presence of a large alveolar dead space ventilation.

2 a.m.

- Very low pHa and $pH\bar{v}$ - acidosis.
- Very high $PaCO_2$, indicative of severe hypoventilation causing respiratory acidosis.
- Moderate hypoxemia in spite of 100% FIO_2 mainly due to a large conductive shunt. In this patient there is also severe hypoventilation, which is another important cause of hypoxemia. However, since the patient is ventilated with 100% FIO_2, the hypoxemia is due mostly to a large conductive shunt. Indeed, if this patient had a normal shunt fraction (2-4%) and the same degree of hypoventilation ($PaCO_2$ = 80.8 mmHg) his PaO_2 would be over 500 mmHg, with 100% FIO_2 breathing.
- Very high body temperature - significant increase in metabolic rate. The resulting increase in $\dot{V}CO_2$ requires an increase in ventilation. Since ventilation was not changed from 10 p.m. to 2 a.m., there is now severe hypoventilation - large increase in $PaCO_2$ due to insufficient $\dot{V}Ai$.

Shunt Fraction and O_2 Extraction

10 p.m.:

CaO_2 = 14.36 Vol % $C\bar{v}O_2$ = 9.36 Vol %

$$\frac{\dot{\mathbf{Q}}\mathbf{Cs}}{\dot{\mathbf{Q}}} = \mathbf{34.7\%}$$

(Ai-a) PO_2 = 248 mmHg O_2 extraction = 5 Vol %

2 a.m.:

CaO_2 = 13.54 Vol % $C\bar{v}O_2$ = 8.54 Vol %

$$\frac{\dot{\mathbf{Q}}\mathbf{Cs}}{\dot{\mathbf{Q}}} = \mathbf{47\%}$$

$(Ai\text{-}a)PO_2$ = 533 mmHg O_2 extraction = 5 Vol %

Very large conductive shunt fraction at both times.

Alveolar Dead Space Ventilation at 10:00 p.m.

$$\dot{V}E = 15\ l/\min(BTPS) \quad \dot{V}Cd = 5.1l/\min(BTPS) \quad \dot{V}\bar{A} = 9.9l/\min\ (BTPS)$$

$$\dot{V}Ai = 4.27l/\min\ (BTPS)\ \dot{V}Ad = 5.6l/\min\ (BTPS)$$

$$\frac{\dot{\mathbf{V}}\mathbf{Ad}}{\dot{\mathbf{V}}\bar{\mathbf{A}}} = \mathbf{57\%}$$

Very large alveolar dead space fraction

O_2 Consumption and CO_2 Production

$$CaO_2 - C\bar{v}O_2 = \text{extraction} = 5\text{vol}\%$$

$$\frac{\dot{V}O_2}{\dot{Q}} = CaO_2 - C\bar{v}O_2$$

$$\dot{V}O_2 = 0.05 \text{ x } 5$$

$$\dot{\mathbf{V}}\mathbf{O_2} = \mathbf{0.25\ l/min}$$

$$\dot{V}CO_2 = \dot{V}O_2 \text{ x } R = 0.25 \text{ x } 0.85$$

$$\dot{\mathbf{V}}\mathbf{CO_2} = \mathbf{0.212\ l/min}$$

Base Excess (BE)

<u>10 p.m.:</u>

BE = 1.14 mEq/l

Virtually normal acid-base balance (pHa = 7.39, $PaCO_2$ = 43, pHa = 7.39). Minimal based excess probably remnant of preceding renal compensation for mild respiratory acidosis.

2 a.m.:

$$BE = 1.05 \text{ mEq/l}$$

Severe acute respiratory acidosis (pHa = 7.15, $PaCO_2$ = 80.8) with minimal metabolic compensation.

$PaCO_2$ increased dramatically from 10:00 p.m. because ventilation was not increased to compensate for the increased metabolic rate (high body temperature). Metabolic rate increases by ~13% per each °C increase in body temperature. Thus, $\dot{V}O_2$ and $\dot{V}CO_2$ must have increased from 10 p.m. to 2 a.m. from 0.25 and 0.212 l/min to ~0.415 and ~0.353 l/min, respectively.

Since ventilation was not changed after 2 a.m., metabolic rate must have decreased (*i.e.* body temperature must have progressively dropped to normal), such that ventilation eventually matched metabolic rate as it did at 10 p.m. A decrease in alveolar dead space ventilation would also cause a decrease in $PaCO_2$ by increasing ideal alveolar ventilation. However, there are no reasons to believe that alveolar dead space ventilation would change and there is no indication that the resident attempted to re-expand the collapsed lung.

Average Tissue Oxygenation ($P\bar{v}O_2$)

Based on the values of $C\bar{v}O_2$ (see above), one would expect tissue oxygenation to be better at 10 p.m. then at 2 a.m. However, one must consider the effect of increased temperature and decreased $pH\bar{v}$ at 2 p.m., which would increase $P\bar{v}O_2$ for a given O_2 content due to the right shift of the O_2 dissociation curve.

In fact:

10 p.m.:

$$\mathbf{P\bar{v}O_2 \approx 32.3 \text{ mmHg}}$$

2 a.m.:

$$\mathbf{P\bar{v}O_2 \approx 48\ mmHg}$$

Note that in spite of the lower value of $C\bar{v}O_2$ at 2 a.m. $P\bar{v}O_2$ is ~16 mmHg higher at 2 a.m. than at 10 p.m. This is due to the right shift of the O_2 dissociation curve caused by the drop in pH and the large increase in body temperature.

Challenging Questions

At 2 a.m., what VT would bring $PaCO_2$ to 40 if frequency were reduced to 10 breaths per minute?

Since neither body temperature nor alveolar dead space fraction change:

$$\dot{V}CO_2 = \dot{V}CO_2^*, \dot{V}\bar{A} \text{ x } FAiCO_2 = \dot{V}\bar{A}^* \text{ x } FAiCO_2^*, \dot{V}\bar{A}^* = \frac{\dot{V}\bar{A} \text{ x } FAiCO_2}{FAiCO_2^*} = \frac{\dot{V}A \text{ x } PaCO_2}{PaCO_2^*}$$

$$\dot{V}\bar{A}^* = \frac{9.9 \text{ x } 80.8}{40} = 20\ \text{l/min}$$

$$V\bar{A}^* = \frac{\dot{V}\bar{A}^*}{10} = 2\ \text{l}$$

$$\mathbf{VT} = V\bar{A}^* + 0.17 = \mathbf{2.17\ liters}$$

At the same frequency (30/min):

$$V\bar{A}^* = \frac{\dot{V}\bar{A}^*}{30} = 0.67\ \text{l}$$

$$\mathbf{VT} = V\bar{A}^* + 0.17 = \mathbf{0.837\ liters}$$

Thus, at 2 a.m. either an increase in V_T from 0.5 l to 0.837 l at the same frequency, or from 0.5 l to 2.17 l at a frequency of 10/min, would have brought $PaCO_2$ down from 80.8 to 40 mmHg.

At 2 a.m., on the basis of the very low pHa value a student suggested injecting enough bicarbonate to raise the $[HCO_3^-]$ in plasma to 50 mEq/l. Another

student thought that this would be wrong, as this treatment could worsen the patient's condition. Who was right? Why?

With an increase in bicarbonate to 50 mEq/l, pHa will increase but the consequential left shift of the O_2 dissociation curve will result in a lower PaO_2 and $P\bar{v}O_2$ at the same CaO_2 and $C\bar{v}O_2$.

$$pHa = 6.1 + \log\frac{50}{80.8 \times 0.0301} = 7.41$$

Since an addition of $[HCO_3^-]$ is unlikely to change shunt fraction and extraction, and the increase in pHa from 7.15 to 7.41 does not affect $CAiO_2$, because at $PAiO_2$ = 622 mmHg Hb is fully saturated and a shift of the O_2 dissociation curve to the left brought about by the increase in pHa makes no difference to the O_2 content, CaO_2 would not change from the original value of 13.544 vol %. However, PaO_2 and $P\bar{v}O_2$ will decrease because of the left shift of the O_2 dissociation curve.

$$\%SaO_2 = \frac{CaO_2}{O_2\text{capacity}} = \frac{13.54}{12 \times 1.34} = 84.2\%$$

At $\%SaO_2 = 84.2$, pHa = 7.41, and T = 41.5EC

PaO_2 = ~61 mmHg

$$C\bar{v}O_2 = CaO_2 - \text{extraction}$$

$$C\bar{v}O_2 = 13.54 - 5 = 8.54 \text{ vol\%}$$

$$\%S\bar{v}O_2 = \frac{8.54}{12 \times 1.34} = 53\%$$

Assuming a $pH\bar{v}$ = 7.35 (reasonable because pHa = 7.41)

At $\%S\bar{v}O_2$ = 53%, $pH\bar{v}$ = 7.35, and T = 41.5EC

$P\bar{v}O_2$. ~39 mmHg

Thus, because of the left shift of the O_2 dissociation curve caused by the increase in pHa, the bicarbonate treatment would have worsened the hypoxemia (**PaO_2 down**

from 79.2 to ~61 mmHg), and tissue oxygenation would have dropped to a normal value (**$P\bar{v}O_2$ down from ~47 to ~39 mmHg**). Caveat! Note that in fact PaO_2 would be slightly lower than ~61 mmHg because the drop in $C\bar{v}O_2$ (lower $P\bar{v}O_2$), with the same shunt fraction, would have caused CaO_2, $\%SaO_2$ and PaO_2 to drop as well.

In conclusion, the bicarbonate treatment would have improved the acid base problem without seriously compromising tissue oxygenation, but would have significantly worsened the hypoxemia. The student obviously focused on the wrong parameter, because the acid/base problem was not metabolic but respiratory, and should have been taken care of by increasing ventilation and lowering the body temperature. In fact, once the ventilation problem had been fixed, the excess bicarbonate would have caused a long lasting metabolic alkalosis that would have taken days to correct.

SEQUENCE OF EVENTS AND CONCLUSIONS

The partial lung collapse caused a large right to left blood shunt, which resulted in severe hypoxemia that persisted in spite of high FIO_2 breathing. The patient had a large alveolar dead space ventilation (chronic lung disease) as well, which explains the fairly normal $PaCO_2$ value in spite of a greatly increased (approximately doubled) total alveolar ventilation ($\dot{V}E$ = 15 l/min). The shunt at 10:00 p.m. is probably all conductive because with 50% oxygen breathing shunt-like effects due to diffusion and/or maldistribution problems are minimized.

To correct the hypoxemia, after 10 p.m. FIO_2 was increased to 100%. This change in treatment in fact improved both arterial and tissue PO_2 but the benefits were partially offset by an increase in shunt fraction due to alveolar collapse ($\dot{V}/\dot{Q} = 0$), brought about by ventilating with 100% FIO_2 (without PEEP and with small VT) low $\dot{V}/\dot{Q}$ alveoli in the partially collapsed lung and other lung regions. In addition, the patient developed a high fever which increased considerably O_2 consumption and CO_2 production (significant increase in metabolic rate). The resident overlooked the effects of body temperature on gas exchange and in spite of obvious signs of severe hypoventilation ($PaCO_2$ = 80.8 mmHg) and respiratory acidosis (pHa = 7.15) he/she maintained the same minute ventilation. After 2 a.m., $PaCO_2$ gradually returned to normal, in spite of the unchanged minute ventilation, because body temperature and CO_2 production gradually returned to normal - due to treatment or because the patient went into shock. In other words, ventilation eventually matched CO_2 production such that $PaCO_2$ returned to normal.

Had you been the attending physician what would have been your first decision at 2 a.m.? The answer is: "**increase the ideal alveolar ventilation**". Since frequency is already very high, an increase in tidal volume would do it - an increase in VT by ~0.34 l (from 0.5 to 0.84) would have rapidly brought $PaCO_2$ down from 80.8 mmHg to 40 mmHg. An increase in ventilation would have also increased pHa and PaO_2. Furthermore, an increase in tidal volume and a reduction in FIO_2 might have also decreased the shunt fraction by re-establishing ventilation in some of the collapsed alveoli. Of course, lowering the body temperature would have also been an essential treatment.

In conclusion, the resident overlooked the effects of body temperature on gas exchange, as he/she disregarded relevance of the equation that relates $PaCO_2$ to metabolic rate ($\dot{V}CO_2$) and ideal alveolar ventilation ($\dot{V}Ai$; Eq. 1, see Chapter 4, Gas Exchange). More importantly, he/she did not understand that a **$PaCO_2$ of 80.8 mmHg unequivocally points to severe hypoventilation of the ideal alveolar compartment**.

$$PaCO_2 = \frac{K \times \dot{V}CO_2}{\dot{V}Ai} \quad ... \ (1)$$

Furthermore, the resident exceeded in increased FIO_2 to 100%, causing additional conductive shunt. The respirator setting (f = 30/min; VT = 0.5 l) was also not very helpful because low tidal volume and high frequency increases substantially the wasted ventilation in the conductive dead space. In this case, in spite of a total ventilation of 15 l/min the ideal alveolar ventilation was only ~4 l/min, due primarily to the large alveolar dead space ventilation and to a lesser extent to the unusual respirator setting.

CASE #9 – RESPIRATORY FAILURE IN COPD PATIENT OPERATED FOR ABDOMINAL ANEURYSM

A patient in her early 60's was scheduled for surgery for repair of an abdominal aortic aneurysm. During the operation for removal of the aneurysm, clamps are applied on the aorta above and below the aneurysm, which results in temporary ischemia of the lower extremities.

Before the operation no attention was paid to the patient's complaints of limited activity tolerance; no pulmonary function test was ordered; no base-line arterial blood gas measurements were done. Following induction of anesthesia, intubation of the trachea and placement of the patient on mechanical ventilation, an arterial blood sample was sent to the lab for gas analysis, and the values listed in Table **10** (11 a.m.) were obtained. Nobody taking care of the patient at that time paid any attention to a base excess (BE) of +5.76 mEq/l on that first specimen. The operation went well and nobody expected any trouble; in fact, at the end of the operation the observation of a BE = 0 mEq/l was taken as a good sign, "even better than usual".

Problems occurred in the recovery room when the patient, although able to breathe on her own, continued to run high $PaCO_2$ values and to oxygenate rather poorly (Table **10**, 2:00 p.m.). There were accusations of too much anesthesia, suspicions of pneumothorax and aspiration, and several other possible problems. As the problem eventually resolved, it became clear that some basic concepts of respiratory physiology had been overlooked.

Based on the History and the Given Values, What Can You Say?

<u>11:00 a.m.</u>

- pHa is slightly alkalotic, $PaCO_2$ is slightly elevated, and there is a base excess (normal BE = ~0). If we did not know the patient's history and the fact that she is on a ventilator, this could indicate either metabolic alkalosis partially compensated by hypoventilation or chronic respiratory acidosis compensated by increased bicarbonate (kidney compensation). Most likely before being artificially ventilated the patient had a higher $PaCO_2$, as she complained of limited activity tolerance, suggesting the possible existence of chronic cardio-respiratory problems. Thus, the ventilator might have provided acute respiratory overcompensation for chronic, metabolically compensated, respiratory acidosis.

Table 10: Laboratory blood and gas data.

	11:00 a.m. (in O.R., on a respirator)	2:00 p.m. (in ICU, breathing on her own)
pHa	7.42	7.18
$PaCO_2$ (mmHg)	47	74
PaO_2 (mmHg)	144	80
Hb (g/ml blood)	14	14
$\%SaO_2$	98.7	91
$\%SAiO_2$	99.3	98.9
VT (liters, BTPS)	0.78*	0.485
F (breaths/min)	16	16
VCd (liters, BTPS)	0.16	0.16
PB (mmHg)	747	747
R	0.85	0.85
FIO_2 (%)	35	40
Body Temperature (°C)	37	37
$\dot{V}O_2$ (l/min, STPD)	0.23	0.23
BE (mEq/l plasma)	+5.76	0
$\dot{Q}$ (liters/min)	4.5	4.5

*V_T at 11:00 a.m. includes an added VCd of 80 ml (BTPS) due to the respirator

- The minute ventilation ($\dot{V}E$ = 12.48 l/min) is very high for a normal $\dot{V}O_2$ even if we subtract the added dead space of the ventilator ($\dot{V}E$ = 11.2 l/min) – under normal conditions, with $\dot{V}O_2$ = 0.23 l/min, $\dot{V}E$ would be ~6 l/min. This is even more significant since there is slight hypoventilation ($PaCO_2$ = 47 mmHg). The high $\dot{V}E$, coupled to a slightly high $PaCO_2$, indicates that there is a large alveolar dead space ventilation.

- PaO_2 is higher than normal because of the high FIO_2.

- $\dot{Q}$ and $\dot{V}O_2$ are normal for a 60+ year old woman, and so extraction is also normal.

- There is no anemia

- Exchange ratio (R), cardiac output and oxygen consumption are normal.

2:00 p.m.

- pHa is very low, $PaCO_2$ is very high, and BE is zero. If we did not know the preceding circumstance we would classify this as acute respiratory acidosis. In fact, this is right; but, how could one explain the loss of 5.76 mEq/l of $[HCO_3^-]$ (BE = 0) in three hours? Certainly not *via* renal compensation, as it would take several days. A clue is provided by the surgical technique used for removal of the aneurysm, namely the application of aortic clamps. This produces ischemia of the lower extremities and consequential tissue hypoxia with formation of lactic acid. With the release of the clamps, the circulating lactic acid will be buffered by bicarbonate, reducing BE. In people without previous chronic respiratory acidosis this would generate a negative BE - metabolic acidosis. In this patient BE was high to begin with, and lactic acid brought BE down to a **deceptively** normal value (zero), wrongly welcomed by the attending physician who had paid no attention to the high BE value at 11:00 a.m. Therefore, based on the preceding events this condition is more accurately classified as a chronic respiratory acidosis complicated by an acute addition of lactic acid (acute metabolic acidosis).

- The minute ventilation ($\dot{V}E = 0.485 \times 16 = 7.76$ l/min) may appear only slightly greater than normal for a normal $\dot{V}O_2$ (normal $\dot{V}E$ for $\dot{V}O_2 = 0.23$ l/min would be ~6 l/min). In fact, even this greater than expected $\dot{V}E$ cannot maintain a normal gas exchange, as a $PaCO_2$ of 74 mmHg clearly points to severe hypoventilation (low $\dot{V}Ai$).

- PaO_2 is quite low in spite of a high FIO_2 (40%). This is due to hypoventilation, probably combined to an abnormal shunt fraction.

- Exchange ratio (R), cardiac output and oxygen consumption are normal.

Shunt Fraction

11:00 a.m.:

$CaO_2 = 18.96$ vol % $C\bar{v}O_2 = 13.86$

$$\frac{\dot{Q}Ps}{\dot{Q}} = 5\%$$

Slightly increased shunt fraction. The shunt is mostly conductive because FIO_2 is 35%

2:00 p.m.

$CaO_2 = 17.30$ vol % $C\bar{v}O_2 = 19.17$

$$\frac{\dot{Q}Ps}{\dot{Q}} = 26\%$$

Significant amount of conductive shunt

Alveolar Dead Space Ventilation

11 a.m.:

$\dot{V}E = 12.48$ l/min $\dot{V}Cd = 3.48$ l/min $\dot{V}\bar{A} = 8.64$ l/min $\dot{V}Ai = 3.6$ l/min

$$\frac{\dot{V}Ad}{\dot{V}\bar{A}} = 58\%$$

2:00 p.m.:

$\dot{V}E = 7.76$ l/min $\dot{V}Cd = 2.56$ l/min $\dot{V}\bar{A} = 5.2$ l/min $\dot{V}Ai = 2.3$ l/min

$$\frac{\dot{V}Ad}{\dot{V}\bar{A}} = 56\%$$

Very large alveolar dead space ventilation at both times

What do the values obtained at 11:00 a.m. tell about the patient's conditions before the operation?

In the absence of any reason for metabolic alkalosis, a BE of +5.76 mEq/l clearly points to chronic respiratory acidosis compensated by an increase in bicarbonate. This is supported by evidence of inadequate respiratory function - large alveolar dead space ventilation ($\dot{V}Ad/\dot{V}\overline{A}$ = 58%) and the patient's complaints of limited activity tolerance, consistent with COPD type A. Most likely the patient had chronic hypercapnia (partially compensated chronic respiratory acidosis) and hypoxemia. These abnormalities were eliminated by the ventilator settings, which brought pHa and PaO_2 to normal values, and $PaCO_2$ to a near normal value.

Why did BE becomes 0 mEq/l between 11:00 a.m. and 2:00 p.m.?

As mentioned above, with the removal of the aortic clamps the excess acid generated by the ischemic limbs was buffered by bicarbonate resulting in a decrease in extracellular bicarbonate and the elimination of the base excess (BE decreased from +5.76 to 0).

Mixed venous samples taken at 11:00 a.m. and at 2:00 p.m. gave $P\bar{v}O_2$'s of 40 and 44 mmHg, respectively.

This seems surprising at first because both PaO_2 and CaO_2 are higher at 11 a.m. than at 2 p.m. and even more so because even $C\bar{v}O_2$ is higher at 11 a.m. However, one must not forget the Bohr effect on the O_2-dissociation curve. At 2:00 p.m. pHa, and obviously $pH\bar{v}$, are much lower than at 11:00 a.m. (7.18 *versus* 7.42). Thus, the O_2-dissociation curve will be shifted to the right, such that $P\bar{v}O_2$ will be higher (44 *versus* 40 mmHg) – increased O_2 unloading at the tissue.

At 11 a.m. a static pressure of 2 cm H_2O was measured at the ventilator after inflating the lungs with 1/3 of VT from FRC. Does this tell anything about the patient's condition?

Compliance is a measure of the combined elastic properties of lungs and chest wall and is given by the ratio between an increment in lung volume and the increment in **static** pressure needed to keep that volume of gas in the lungs. In this case, when the patient's lungs were inflated with 1/3 of the tidal volume (780 ml / 3 = 260 ml) the static pressure (no air movement) measured at the ventilator was 2 cm of H_2O. Thus, the compliance of the patient's chest/lung system was 130 ml/cm H_2O. Since normal compliance is 100 ml/cm of H_2O, this patient's respiratory system has an increased compliance. A disease that causes an increased compliance is emphysema. Thus, this patient may have COPD type A.

SEQUENCE OF EVENTS AND CONCLUSIONS

Based on the patient's history, the given values and the calculations of shunt, alveolar dead space ventilation and compliance at 11:00 a.m., it is clear that the patient, before entering the hospital, was suffering from COPD Type A (emphysema). This caused a large amount of wasted ventilation in the alveolar dead space, which could not be adequately compensated because the patient was unable to maintain the ideal alveolar ventilation at pace with the metabolic requirements (chronic hypoventilation, complaints of limited activity tolerance). The result was a chronic respiratory acidosis metabolically compensated by an increase in bicarbonate concentration (BE = +5.76 mEq/l); one could guess that with this BE the patient might have had a $PaCO_2$ of ~55 mmHg, a pHa of ~7.36 and a PaO_2 of ~70 mmHg.

Upon intubation of the trachea and placement of the patient on mechanical ventilation with an FIO_2 of 35%, ventilation increased sufficiently to normalize the acid-base (pHa = 7.42). Thus, the ventilator provided an acute respiratory compensation to the chronic respiratory acidosis and hypoxemia.

During surgical procedure, the application of aortic clamps caused acute ischemia of the lower extremities, anaerobic metabolism and formation of lactic acid. Upon removal of the clamps, the circulating lactic acid was quickly buffered by bicarbonate, resulting in a decrease in BE to zero.

Following surgery, in the ICU unit, the patient returned to her chronic status of hypoventilation, in this case made even worse by the supply of O_2 (FIO_2 = 40%) and by the discomfort caused by laparotomy. An increase in bronchial secretion due to tracheal intubation and anesthesia might have obstructed some of the small airways, resulting in conductive shunt ($\dot{Q}Ps/\dot{Q}$ = 26%). Thus, the expected increase in PaO_2 due to O_2 therapy was offset by the increase in shunt fraction. The resulting hypoxemia (PaO_2 = 80 mmHg) was due to both hypoventilation and abnormal shunt fraction. The severe hypoventilation, combined with the loss of bicarbonate (BE = 0), resulted in severe acidosis (pHa = 7.18).

Case #10 – Pulmonary Embolism During Recovery from Surgery in a Diabetic Patient

Table 11: Laboratory blood and gas data.

	1:00 p.m.	2:00 p.m. (in ICU, on a respirator)
pHa	7.17	7.48
$pH\bar{v}$	7.12	7.43
$PaCO_2$ (mmHg)	74	39
PaO_2 (mmHg)	52	100
Hb (g/ml blood)	14.3	14.3
VT (liters, BTPS)	-	0.8
f (breaths/min)	-	14
VCd (liters, BTPS)	0.17	0.17
PB (mmHg)	749	749
R	0.7	0.85
FIO_2 (%)	100 (by mask)	100 (respirator)
Body Temperature (°C)	37	37
$\dot{V}O_2$ (l/min, STPD)	0.27	0.27
O_2 extraction (vol%)	-	5
Heart Rate (beats/min)	75	74
$\%S\bar{v}O_2$	50	-

A diabetic patient in his early 60's, who had been a moderate smoker for the past three decades, was recovering without complications a day after a hernia operation when suddenly at 12:30 p.m. he became short of breath. He was given 50% O_2 by mask and soon after an arterial blood sample was taken. The blood sample showed PaO_2 = 76 mmHg, $PaCO_2$ = 73 mmHg and pH_a 7.16; a right-to-left shunt fraction of 37% was calculated. In view of the lab report, FIO_2 was immediately increased to 100%. In spite of that, the patient's condition worsened and a half hour later samples of arterial and mixed venous blood were collected (Table **11**, 1:00 p.m.). In view of the latest lab data, the patient was transferred to ICU where he was intubated and mechanically ventilated (assume no additional conductive dead space). At 2:00 p.m. other samples of arterial and mixed venous blood were taken (Table **11**, 2:00 p.m.).

Based on the History and the Given Values, What Can You Say?

12:30 a.m. (60% O_2 by mask)

- Hypoxemia, hypercapnia, acidosis and a large right-to-left blood shunt. The hypoxemia is mild, but it is very significant since FIO_2 = 50%, indicating that hypoventilation only plays a minor role, the major cause being the large right-to-left blood shunt.

- Since with FIO_2 = 50% most of the shunt-effect caused by maldistribution and/or diffusion impairment is eliminated or minimized, the shunt is mostly conductive - possibly a combination of alveolar shunt (areas with $\dot{V}/\dot{Q} = 0$) and extra-alveolar shunts.

- The acidosis is caused mostly by hypercapnia (hypoventilation), but there is also a small metabolic component, as a quick calculation gives: $[HCO_3^-]_{actual}$= 25 mEq/l, $[HCO_3^-]_{predicted}$ = 26.54 mEq/l and a BE = -1.54 mEq/l. This tells us that the acidosis is both respiratory and metabolic, and that the respiratory component is due to acute hypoventilation.

1:00 p.m. (100% O_2 by mask)

- There is no change in $PaCO_2$ since 12:30 a.m. and little change in pH_a, but now we see a very low PaO_2. The severe hypoxemia may seem surprising since ventilation has not changed (same $PaCO_2$) and FIO_2 has been increased to 100%; the only possibility is that shunt fraction has significantly increased. The additional conductive shunt may result from alveolar collapse in low $\dot{V}/\dot{Q}$ areas, caused by breathing 100% O_2, and/or airway obstruction due to increased mucus secretion – areas with $\dot{V}/\dot{Q} = 0$.

- An R of 0.7 is abnormally low. There are two possible reasons for it. One is that the patient's diabetes was not under control, such that his ability to burn carbohydrates was markedly impaired resulting in lipids rather than carbohydrates being metabolized. However, this is unlikely because the patient was in the hospital for the hernia operation and the attending physicians would have kept the diabetes fully in control. The other, more likely, possibility is that the patient was not at steady state with the metabolic rate ($R \neq RQ$; acute hypoventilation); In this case, some of the CO_2 produced would be added to the body gas stores, such that the volume/min of CO_2 expired is lower than that produced by the tissue during that minute ($R < RQ$).

- $\%S\bar{v}O_2 = 50\%$ is quite below normal (~73%), but, since $pH\bar{v}$ is also way below normal, the average tissue oxygenation (reflected by $P\bar{v}O_2$) is not too far from normal ($P\bar{v}O_2 = \sim35$, *versus* normal $P\bar{v}O_2 = 40$), due to the Bohr right-shift of the O_2 dissociation curve. If $pH\bar{v}$ were normal ($pH\bar{v} = \sim7.37$) a $\%S\bar{v}O_2$ of 50% would correspond to a $P\bar{v}O_2$ of ~26 mmHg.

<u>2:00 p.m.</u> (on a respirator with 100% O_2)

- Both arterial and mixed venous pH's are higher than normal, but $PaCO_2$ is virtually normal, indicating that the alkalosis metabolic (BE is expected to have a positive sign).

- PaO_2 is now normal or a little greater than normal, but, since the patient is ventilated with 100% FIO_2 and is no longer hypoventilating ($PaCO_2 = 39$), a PaO_2 of 100 mmHg is much lower than expected and clearly indicates that there is still a large conductive shunt.

- A ventilation of 11.2 l/min (VT = 0.8 l, f = 14/min) is almost twice normal for a virtually normal oxygen consumption ($\dot{V}O_2 = 0.27$ l/min) but, in spite of that, $PaCO_2$ is virtually normal. This indicates a large wastage of ventilation in dead spaces. Since frequency is about normal, the wasted ventilation in the conductive dead space is not greater than normal (0.170 x 14 = 2.38 l/min); however, when it is subtracted from $\dot{V}E$, the resulting total alveolar ventilation $\dot{V}\bar{A}$ of 8.82 l/min (almost twice normal), indicating the presence of a large alveolar dead space ventilation.

- The R value is now normal, so the patient is at steady state (R = RQ).
- Since both $\dot{V}O_2$ and O_2 extraction are normal $\dot{Q}$ must also be normal (Fick equation).
- Since the heart rate (HR) is normal, the stroke volume must also be normal. Thus, there does not seem to be any obvious cardiac problem.

Shunt Fraction, (Ai-a)PO_2 Gradient, Cardiac Output and Stroke Volume

1:00 p.m.:

CaO_2 = 14.57 vol% $C\bar{v}O_2$ = 9.69 vol%

$$\frac{\dot{Q}Cs}{\dot{Q}} = 57.3\%$$

(Ai-a)PO_2 = 576 mmHg $\dot{Q}$ = 5.53 l/min SV = 73.8 ml

2:00 p.m.:

CaO_2 = 19.03 vol% $C\bar{v}O_2$ = 14.03 vol%

$$\frac{\dot{Q}Cs}{\dot{Q}} = 30\%$$

(Ai-a)PO_2 = 563 mmHg $\dot{Q}$ = 5.4 l/min SV = 73 ml

Alveolar Dead Space Ventilation at 2:00 p.m.

Since $P\bar{A}CO_2$ is not available, the alveolar dead space fraction can only be calculated by determining $\dot{V}\bar{A}$ and $\dot{V}Ai$

$\dot{V}E$= 11.2 l/min (BTPS) $\dot{V}Cd$ = 2.38 l/min (BTPS) $\dot{V}\bar{A}$ = 8.82 l/min (BTPS)

$\dot{V}CO_2$ = 0.23 l/min $\dot{V}Ai$ = 5.09 l/min $\dot{V}Ad$ = 3.73 l/min

$$\frac{\dot{V}Ad}{\dot{V}\bar{A}} = 42.3\%$$

Large alveolar dead space ventilation

Base Excess (BE)

1:00 p.m.:

BE = -0.14 mEq/l

Acute (uncompensated) respiratory acidosis

2:00 p.m.:

BE = 4.8 mEq/l

Metabolic alkalosis

Average Tissue Oxygenation ($P\bar{v}O_2$)

1:00 p.m.:

$P\bar{v}O_2$ = 35 mmHg

2:00 p.m.:

$P\bar{v}O_2$ = 37 mmHg

It might seem strange to have similar $P\bar{v}O_2$'s (35 and 37 mmHg) in spite of very different PaO_2's (52 and 100 mmHg), CaO_2's (14.5 and 19 vol%) and $C\bar{v}O_2$'s (9.7 and 14 vol%), and similar $\dot{V}O_2$ and $\dot{Q}$. The reason for it is the very different $pH\bar{v}$ values (7.12 *versus* 7.43), and resulting Bohr shifts: to the right at 1:00 p.m., favoring O_2 dissociation from Hb for any given $C\bar{v}O_2$, and to the left at 2:00 p.m., favoring O_2 association with Hb at the lungs but reducing the O_2 dissociation from Hb at the tissue.

At 2:00 PM a <u>static</u> pressure of 8 cm H_2O was measured at the ventilator at the end of each lung-inflation from functional residual capacity (FRC).

At FRC the chest wall tends to expand just as much as the lungs tend to collapse; in other words, the elastic force of the chest wall (pointing outward) is balanced by an equally strong elastic force generated by the lung recoil (pointing inward). The result is that the respiratory system is in equilibrium (it is at rest), such that the respirator does not need to apply any pressure (positive or negative) to prevent gases from moving in and out the lungs. Therefore, if the ventilator inflates the lungs from FRC with 800 ml of O_2, and at the end of the inflation shows a static pressure (pressure measured at zero air-flow) of 8 cm of H_2O, it means that the compliance of the lung-chest system is such that a pressure gradient of (+8 - 0) = +8 cm H_2O is needed create a volume gradient of [(800+FRC+RV) - (FRC+RV)] = 800 ml.

$$\mathbf{C} = \frac{\Delta V}{\Delta P} = \frac{800\ \text{ml}}{8\ \text{cmH}_2\text{O}} = \mathbf{100\ ml/cmH_2O}$$

This tells us that the compliance of this patient's lung-chest system is normal. This is quite surprising because, based on the observation of a large fraction of alveolar dead space ventilation ($\dot{V}Ad/\dot{V}\bar{A}$ = 42.3%) and on the long history of cigarette smoking, we were inclined to believe that the patient had severe emphysema. This observation tells us that the patient does not have significant emphysema; therefore, the alveolar dead space is due to something else.

<u>**Challenging Questions**</u>

Assuming that respiratory frequency is the same at 1:00 p.m. and at 2:00 p.m., what is your estimate of the tidal volume (VT^*) at 1:00 p.m.? Do you need to make other assumptions?

Since frequency is the same, VCd at 1:00 p.m. and at 2:00 p.m. are the same:

$$VCd = 0.170 \times 14 = 2.38\ l/min$$

The ideal alveolar ventilation can be easily calculated:

Since $\dot{V}CO_2 = 0.27 \times 0.7 = 0.189$ l/min and $PaCO_2 = 74$,

$$\dot{V}Ai^* = (863 \times 0.18)/74 = 2.24 \text{ l/min}$$

In the absence of alveolar dead space, we would just add $\dot{V}Ai^*$ to $\dot{V}Cd$ to obtain $\dot{V}E^*$ and calculate VT^* by dividing $\dot{V}E^*$ by frequency. However, in this case we know that at 2:00 p.m. the patient has a large alveolar dead space fraction. We also suspect that the alveolar dead space resulted from the acute episode that took place at 12:30 p.m. Thus, it is reasonable to believe that the dead space problem did not change significantly between 12:30 p.m. and 2:00 p.m. In any event, this is a reasonable assumption to make. However, we cannot just add the $\dot{V}Ad$ calculated at 2:00 p.m. (3.73 l/min) to $\dot{V}Ai^*$ and $\dot{V}Cd$ expecting to obtain the right $\dot{V}E^*$ at 1:00 p.m., because VAd, like other alveolar volumes, is an expandable volume that obviously will change with changes in VT, becoming greater or smaller the deeper or shallower the tidal volume – note that this does not mean at all that the alveolar dead space problem is more or less severe the larger or smaller VT becomes. In spite of relative changes in VAd, the fraction of wasted ventilation ($\dot{V}Ad/\dot{V}\overline{A}$) remains virtually the same as long as the number of alveoli affected does not change. In other words, VAd and $\dot{V}Ad$ will change while $\dot{V}Ad/\dot{V}\overline{A}$ and $\dot{V}Ai/\dot{V}\overline{A}$ will not.

Therefore:

$$\dot{V}Ai/\dot{V}\overline{A} = \dot{V}Ai^*/\dot{V}\overline{A}^*$$

$$\frac{5.09}{8.82} = \frac{2.24}{\dot{V}\overline{A}^*}$$

$$\dot{V}\overline{A}^* = 3.28 \text{ l/min}$$

$$\dot{V}E^* = \dot{V}\overline{A}^* + \dot{V}Cd = 3.82 + 2.38 = 6.2 \text{ l/min}$$

$$\mathbf{VT^*} = 6.2/14 = \mathbf{0.443\ liters}$$

If the patient's Hb concentration were 7g/100 ml blood, what heart rate (HR) would maintain the same tissue oxygenation ($P\bar{v}O_2$) at 1:00 PM, assuming a 30% increase in stroke volume and no change in the given values, except for

PaO_2? What would PaO_2 be? Why is it different? Is it reasonable to assume no change in pHa and pH$\bar{v}$?

New Heart Rate (HR*) and PaO_2*

To estimate the new heart rate, first we need to calculate the new cardiac output ($\dot{Q}^*$) by the Fick equation, after having calculated the new extraction. For calculating the new extraction first we need to calculate the new values of $C\bar{v}O_2$* and CaO_2*. $C\bar{v}O_2$* is easy to calculate by means of the O_2 content equation because we know that %$S\bar{v}O_2$ and pH$\bar{v}$ are the same, and so $P\bar{v}O_2$ is also the same (35 mmHg). In contrast, CaO_2* cannot be calculated by this equation because PaO_2 will change. However, we can be certain that the shunt fraction will not change because there is no reason why it would be affected by anemia. Thus, since we can calculate the new alveolar ideal content ($CAiO_2$*), we can calculate CaO_2* by the shunt equation.

$$CAiO_2^* = 628 \text{ x } 0.0031 + (7 \text{ x } 1.34)1 = 11.327 \text{ vol\%}$$

$$C\bar{v}O_2^* = 35 \text{ x } 0.00321 + (7 \text{ x } 1.34)0.5 = 4.79 \text{ Vol \%}$$

$$0.573 = \frac{11.33 - CaO_2}{11.33 - 4.79}$$

$CaO_2^* = 7.58$ vol% $\qquad \%SaO_2^* = \frac{7.58}{7 \text{ x } 1.34} = \sim 81\%$

At $\%SaO_2^* = \sim 81\%$, with pHa = 7.17, $PaO_2^* = \sim 58$ mmHg

At ~58 mmHg, dissolved $O_2 = 58 \text{ x } 0.0031 = 0.18$ vol%

$$\%SaO_2^* = \frac{7.58 - 0.18}{7 \text{ x } 1.34} = 79\%$$

At $\%SaO_2^* = 79\%$, with pHa = 7.17, **PaO2* = 56 mmHg**

New extraction = 7.58 - 4.79 = 2.8 vol%

$$\dot{Q}^* = 0.27/0.028 = 9.64 \text{ l/min}$$

$$SV^* = 73.8 + (73.8 \text{ x } 0.3) = 96 \text{ ml}$$

$$\mathbf{HR}^{*} = \frac{\dot{Q}}{SV} = \frac{9.64}{0.096} = \mathbf{\sim 100\ beats/min}$$

Why is PaO_2 Different?

The reason why PaO_2 would increase from 52 to 56 mmHg can be readily appreciated if we think of hemoglobin as an O_2-buffer. PaO_2 obviously reflects the amount of dissolved O_2 in the arterial blood, which is a mixture of ideal and mixed-venous blood. In this case we know that shunt fraction, pHa and $pH\bar{v}$ have not changed. In terms of O_2, HbO_2 has decreased dramatically in both alveolar ideal and mixed venous bloods because Hb has decreased from 14.3 to 7 g/100 ml of blood, but the dissolved O_2 is the same because $PAiO_2$ and $P\bar{v}O_2$ are the same (628 and 35 mmHg, respectively). This means that the ratio between hemoglobin (the O_2 buffer) and total O_2 content (CaO_2) has decreased significantly such that, **in arterial blood**, dissolved O_2, PO_2 and $\%SO_2$ will all be slightly higher than before.

Table 12: Laboratory blood and gas data (shunt fraction unchanged: 57.3%)

	Hb = 14.3g/100 ml	Hb = 7g/100 ml
	ALVEOLAR IDEAL (Ai) BLOOD	
$PAiO_2$ (mmHg)	628	628
Diss. O_2 (vol%)	1.95	1.95
HbO_2 (mmHg)	19.16	9.38
$CAiO_2$ (vol%)	21.11	11.33
	MIXED VENOUS ($\bar{v}$) BLOOD	
$P\bar{v}O_2$ (vol%)	35	35
Diss.O_2 (vol%)	0.11	0.11
HbO_2 (vol%)	9.58	4.69
$C\bar{v}O_2$ (vol%)	9.69	4.8
	ARTERIAL (a) BLOOD	
CaO_2 (vol%)	14.57	7.59
Hb/CaO_2	14.3/14.57 = 0.98	7/7.69 = 0.92
Diss. O_2 (vol%)	0.161	0.174
PaO_2 (mmHg)	52	56
$\%SaO_2$	75.2	79

To understand it quantitatively, see the values in alveolar ideal, mixed venous and arterial bloods (Table **12**). The difference in the Hb/CaO_2 ratio affects both the amount of O_2 associated with Hb and the dissolved O_2, such that, **in arterial blood**, the lower the relative amount of hemoglobin (O_2 buffer) available for buffering O_2 the greater the dissolved O_2, the percent of O_2 associated with Hb, and the PO_2.

Is it Reasonable to Assume no Change in pHa and pH$\bar{v}$?

No! The reason is that hemoglobin is also a pH buffer, such that the lower the Hb concentration the lower the buffering capacity (BC). With Hb = 14.3 g/100 ml, BC is -10.17, while with Hb = 7 g/100 ml BC is -6.4. This means that the slope of the acute buffering capacity line is much less steep, such that for the same change in PCO_2 at the tissue and at the lungs, the change in pH will be greater. In other words, the pHa - pH$\bar{v}$ gradient will increase slightly and both pH values will be slightly lower than with Hb = 14.3 g/100 ml blood.

SEQUENCE OF EVENTS AND CONCLUSIONS

A day after the operation the patient suffered an acute episode that caused him to be in respiratory distress. At that time (12:30 a.m.) there was a large shunt and hypoventilation, which caused hypoxemia in spite of 60% O_2 breathing, and there was acidosis caused almost entirely by hypoventilation (respiratory acidosis). In view of the hypoxemia, the attending physician decided to increase the inspired O_2 fraction to 100%. However, at 1:00 p.m. the substantial amount of bronchial mucus and the administration of 100% FIO_2 by mask might have caused poorly ventilated alveoli to collapse, resulting in a large increase in conductive shunt fraction and consequential worsening of the hypoxemia. In view of the severe hypoxemia and acidosis, it was decided to put the patient on a respirator, still with 100% FIO_2. We can guess some base might have been administered as well because a base excess of 4.8 mEq/l one hour later could not have occurred physiologically, and there is no evidence of excessive vomiting or use of naso-gastric suction that would have caused a loss of protons.

As a result of all this, the patient's condition considerably had improved at 2:00 p.m.: hypoxemia, hypercapnia and acidosis had disappeared and the shunt fraction had decreased significantly, although the presumed base treatment caused mild metabolic alkalosis. At this time we were also able to determine the presence of a large alveolar dead space fraction ($\dot{V}Ad/\dot{V}\bar{A} = 42.3\%$); obviously, this is not a chronic condition because there is no evidence for the presence of emphysema, as compliance is normal compliance.

In view of the data accumulated over the next hour and a half since the acute episode took place, one can guess that the patient suffered a pulmonary embolism. This is not uncommon, especially in older patients recovering in bed following an operation, and results from clogging of branches of the pulmonary artery by detached portions of venous thrombi which might have formed in deep veins of the lower extremities or in the abdomen. Pulmonary embolism causes a large decrease in blood perfusion of the affected lung region, resulting in large alveolar dead space and increased shunt. The shunt results from blood perfusing unventilated alveoli in infarcted regions (hemorrhagic atelectasis) and alveolar regions loss of surfactant leads to alveolar collapse ($\dot{V}/\dot{Q} = 0$).

At 12:30 p.m., the large alveolar dead space ventilation caused by the embolism severely reduced the size of the ideal (Ai) compartment (large $\dot{V}Ai$ drop at the same VT), such that a large compensatory increase in $\dot{V}E$ would have been necessary to prevent both respiratory acidosis and worsening of shunt-induced hypoxemia. Both hypoxemia and hypercapnia strongly stimulated breathing, and there is little doubt that the patient tried his best to increase his ventilation. However, the fact that $PaCO_2$ rose to 74 and pHa dropped to 7.17 at 1:00 p.m. indicates that for some reason (excessive mucus?) he was not able to compensate for the increase in wasted ventilation. At 2:00 p.m. the increase in VT set by the respirator, aside from providing sufficient ventilation of the alveolar ideal compartment, reduced the shunt fraction from 57.3 to 30%, as some of the collapsed alveoli reopened, and in conjunction with 100% FIO_2 eliminated the hypoxemia.

REFERENCES

[1] Hagen PT, Scholz DG, Edwards WD. Incidence and size of patent foramen ovale during the first ten decades of life: An autopsy study of 965 normal hearts. Mayo Clin Proc 1984;59:17-20.

[2] Mareedu RK, Mesa JE. Patent foramen ovale with right to left shunt as a cause of hypoxia. Wisconsin Med J 2008;107:331-334.

[3] Lynch JJ, Schuchard GH, Gross CM, Wann LS. Prevalence of right-to-left shunting in a healthy population: detection by Valsalva maneuver contrast echocardiography. Am J Cardiol 1984;53:1478–80.

[4] Shekerdemian L, Bohn D. Cardiovascular effects of mechanical ventilation. Arch Dis Child 1999:80:475-480.

[5] Moorthy SS, Losasso AM. Patency of foramen ovale in the critically ill patient. Anesthesiology 1974;41:405-407.

[6] Lemaire F, Richalet JP, Carlet J, Brun-Buisson C, MacLean C. Postoperative hypoxemia due to opening of patent foramen ovale confirmed by a right atrium-left atrium pressure gradient during mechanical ventilation. Anesthesiology 1982;57:233-236.

Tests

Camillo Peracchia

For Methods Used in Calculations (See Appendix 4)

For Symbols and Acronyms (See Appendix 3)

TEST #1

A forty year old man was admitted to the emergency department after CPR following drowning. At admission (3:00 p.m.), his condition was reasonably stable. He was treated with antibiotics, his trachea was intubated and he was connected to a PEEP (Positive End Expiratory Pressure) respirator with 100% FIO_2.

Later in the day his condition deteriorated dramatically (see Table **1**; 8:00 p.m.). Chest X-ray showed bilateral infiltrates and pleural effusion. Therefore, it was decided to introduce surfactant into the airway system. This treatment led to great improvement (Table **1**; 11:00 p.m.).

BASED ON THE HISTORY AND THE GIVEN VALUES AT 8:00 P.M., ANSWER THE FOLLOWING QUESTIONS:

1. What does PaO_2 = 43 mmHg indicate? (Select one)

   A. Hypercapnia

   B. Hypoxemia

   C. Anemia

   D. Increased FIO_2

   E. Increased $\dot{V}O_2$

2. What does $PaCO_2$ = 47 mmHg indicate? (Select one)

   A. Hyperventilation

B. Metabolic alkalosis

C. Hypoxemia

D. Hypoventilation

E. Metabolic acidosis

Table 1: Laboratory blood and gas data

BLOOD SAMPLES		
	8:00 p.m.	11:00 p.m.
PaO_2 (mmHg)	43	362
$PaCO_2$ (mmHg)	47	50
pHa	7.2	7.17
$pH\bar{v}$	7.15	7.10
Hb (g/100 ml blood)	9	9
Body Temperature (°C)	38	38
VENTILATION DATA		
VT (l/min, BTPS)	0.39	0.45
F (breaths/min)	18	13
FIO_2 (%)	100	80
R	0.8	0.8
$\dot{V}O_2$ (l/min, STPD)	0.28	0.28
VCd (l, BTPS)	0.13	0.13
PH_2O (mmHg)	49	49
PB (mm Hg)	749	749
Constant "863" at 38°C	866	866
PEEP (cm H_2O)	12	8
Peak inspiratory PAW* (cm H_2O)	42	36
Static PAW** (end of inspiration, cm H_2O)	30	22
CALCULATED DATA		
$\dot{Q}$ (l/min)	5.0	5.0
Extraction (vol%)	5.6	5.6
$\dot{Q}Cs/\dot{Q}$ (%)	53	7.6
$P\bar{v}O_2$ (mmHg)	19	47
BE (mEq/l plasma)	-7.73	-8.1
$\dot{V}Ad/\dot{V}\bar{A}$ (%)	11	7.2

* Peak inspiratory PAW = Peak inspiratory Pressure in Airways, during mechanical ventilation (normal value = 18-22 cm H_2O).

**Static PAW = Pressure in Airways measured under static (<u>no air movement</u>) conditions.

3. What do the combined values of PaO_2, $PaCO_2$, pHa and BE indicate? (Select one)

   A. Alveolar dead space ventilation

   B. Fever

   C. Shunt and metabolic acidosis

   D. Increased metabolic rate

   E. PEEP ventilation

   F. Hyperventilation and shunt

4. What do the combined values of $PaCO_2$, pHa and BE indicate? (Select one)

   A. Metabolic alkalosis

   B. Respiratory alkalosis

   C. Compensated respiratory acidosis

   D. Compensated metabolic acidosis

   E. Compensated respiratory alkalosis

   F. Combined respiratory and metabolic acidosis

   G. Combined respiratory and metabolic alkalosis

5. What could be the cause of BE = -7.73 mEq/l plasma? (Select one)

   A. Increased cardiac output

   B. Increased FIO_2

   C. Tissue hypoxia

D. PEEP breathing

E. Alveolar dead space ventilation

6. How would you define the state of tissue oxygenation? (Select one)

A. Normal

B. Hyperoxic

C. Hypoxic

7. Which of the following values allows you to define the state of tissue oxygenation? (Select one)

A. $PaO_2 = 43$ mmHg

B. $PaCO_2 = 47$ mmHg

C. $pH\bar{v} = 7.15$

D. $P\bar{v}O_2 = 19$ mmHg

E. $\dot{V}O_2 = 0.28$ vol%

F. Extraction = 5.6 vol%

G. $\dot{Q} = 5$ l/min

H. Hb = 9 g/100 ml blood

I. $FIO_2 = 100\%$

8. Indicate with plus (+), minus (-) or zero (0) whether each of the following factors has positive, negative or no effect, respectively, on tissue oxygenation.

A) $PaO_2 = 43$ mmHg

B) Hb = 9g/100 ml blood

C) $pH\bar{v} = 7.15$

D) $\dot{V}O_2 = 0.28$ l/min

E) PB = 749 mmHg

9. What is your estimate of respiratory compliance? Provide a quantitative answer.

10. If compliance is abnormal, what might have caused it to change? (Select one)

    A) Bronchial spasm

    B) Abnormal alveolar dead space

    C) Increased FIO_2

    D) Increased respiratory frequency

    E) Loss of surfactant

11. What kind of shunt the patient has? (Select one)

    A) Maldistribution shunt-like effect

    B) Conductive shunt

    C) Diffusion impairment related

12. What is the most likely cause of the shunt? (Select one)

    A) Hypoventilated alveoli

    B) Collapsed alveoli

    C) Interstitial edema

    D) Intra-cardiac right-to-left blood flow

E) Patent ductus arteriosus

13. What is causing $\dot{V}Ad/\dot{V}\bar{A}$ to be 11%? (Select one)

A) Shunt

B) Alveolar collapse

C) Hypoxemia

D) Acidosis

E) PEEP ventilation

WHAT CAN YOU TELL ABOUT THE PATIENT'S CONDITION AT 11:00 P.M.?

Read carefully the history and think of what the lab values gathered at 11:00 p.m. mean by themselves and in relation to other relevant values. In the process, answer the following questions:

14. What is the major reason why PaO_2 increases between 8:00 and 11:00 p.m.? (Select one)

A) Reduced FIO_2

B) Increased VT

C) Decreased shunt fraction

D) More negative BE

E) Reduced alveolar dead space

15. Is the ideal alveolar ventilation ($\dot{V}Ai$) at 11:00 p.m. better, the same or worse than at 8:00 p.m.? Provide a quantitative answer.

16. Why did $PaCO_2$ increase from 47 to 50 mmHg, in spite of the fact that VT increased and alveolar dead space decreased? (Select one)

    A) More negative BE

    B) Decreased PEEP ventilation

    C) Decreased peak PAW value

    D) Decreased respiratory frequency

17. How would you define the condition of tissue oxygenation at 11:00 p.m. with respect to 8:00 p.m.? (Select one)

    A) Better

    B) Worse

    C) The same

18. Which are the major factors that changed tissue oxygenation from 8:00 to 11:00 p.m.? (Select all correct statements)

    A) Increased PaO_2

    B) Decreased $pH\bar{v}$

    C) Decreased alveolar dead space ventilation

    D) Decreased FIO_2

    E) Increased VT

19. What caused the decrease in shunt fraction at 11:00 p.m.? (Select one)

    A) Reduced alveolar dead space ventilation

    B) Introduction of surfactant

C) Decreased pHa

D) Increased VT

20. What is the most likely mechanism by which the shunt fraction was reduced? (Select one)

A) Improved O_2 diffusion

B) Increased $\dot{V}Ad/\dot{V}\bar{A}$ ratio

C) Decreased $\dot{V}Ad/\dot{V}\bar{A}$ ratio

D) Re-expansion of collapsed alveoli

E) Change in BE

21. Describe the sequence of events.

ANSWERS

1: B. 2: D. 3: C. 4: F. 5: C. 6: C. 7: D. 8: A(-), B(-), C(+), D(-), E(0).

9: Compliance = 390/(30-12) = 22 ml/cm H_2O (very low! Normal value = 100 ml/cm H_2O)

10: E. 11: B. 12: B. 13: E. 14: C.

15: Worse. Since $\dot{V}Ai = (866 \times \dot{V}CO_2)/PaCO_2$ and $\dot{V}CO_2 = \dot{V}O_2 \times 0.8$, $\dot{V}Ai = 4.13$ l/min at 8:00 p.m. and 3.88 l/min at 11:00 p.m.

16: D. 17: A. 18: A and B. 19: B. 20: D.

21: At 8:00 p.m., there is severe hypoxemia due to a very large shunt (53%) which is entirely conductive because with 100% FIO_2-breathing maldistribution shunt-like effect and/or diffusion impairment are eliminated. The mild hypercapnia ($PaCO_2$ = 47 mmHg) plays minimal role in the hypoxemia. The shunt is due to collapsed alveoli, which is confirmed by the chest X-ray report of “bilateral infiltrates and pleural effusion". There is also severe acidosis which is mostly metabolic (BE = -7.73 mEq/l plasma) as $PaCO_2$ is only moderately elevated. There is a relatively small amount of alveolar dead space ventilation, most likely due the PEEP ventilation (mild compression of pulmonary vessels). There is significant tissue hypoxia ($P\bar{v}O_2$ = 19 mmHg), caused mostly by severe hypoxemia as extraction is only moderately elevated (5.6 vol%). Tissue hypoxia would even be greater if there weren't acidosis ($pH\bar{v}$ = 7.15) and fever, both of which shift the HbO_2 dissociation curve to the right. Tissue hypoxia causes some cells to shift to anaerobic metabolism; the resulting formation of lactic acid is the cause of the severe metabolic acidosis. Compliance is very low (22 ml/cm H_2O) due to loss of surfactant, which resulted in large increase in surface tension, collapsed alveoli and pleural effusion. All of these factors render the lungs stiffer than normal. Pleural effusion is likely to result from the low osmolarity of alveolar fluid (drowning), which results in water diffusion from alveoli to pleural space.

At 11:00 p.m. the patient's status is much improved. The hypoxemia has been eliminated; PaO_2 is now greater than normal due to 80% FIO_2 breathing and the large drop in conductive shunt (from 53% to 7.6%) caused by re-expansion of collapsed alveoli, as the introduction of surfactant dramatically decreased the alveolar surface tension. Hypercapnia is slightly greater than at 8:00 p.m. ($PaCO_2$ = 50 mmHg) due to the respirator's setting - metabolic rate is unchanged and the fraction of alveolar dead space ventilation has dropped, but the setting of the respirator caused $\dot{V}Ai$ to decrease by ~6%. There is still severe acidosis, which again is mostly metabolic as BE = -8.1 mEq/l plasma (lactic acid). Tissue hypoxia has vanished. In fact, $P\bar{v}O_2$ is greater than normal (47 mmHg), as PaO_2 is high and both acidosis and fever shift the HbO_2 dissociation curve to the right. In spite of normal tissue oxygenation metabolic acidosis persists, because it takes several days for the organism to sufficiently increase the blood bicarbonate and bring BE to zero. A rapid return to normal pHa could be achieved by increasing $\dot{V}Ai$. In order to bring pHa to the normal value (7.4), $PaCO_2$ needs to be decreased from 50 to ~24 mmHg. This can be done by increasing $\dot{V}Ai$ from 3.9 to ~8 l/min; if respiratory frequency remains unchanged (13 breaths/min.), VT needs to be increased from 450 to ~800 ml.

TEST #2

(Adapted from: Ortega-Carnicer, J., Ambrós, A. and Alcazar, R. Obstructive shock due to labor-related diaphragmatic hernia. Crit. Care Med. 26, 616-618, 1998. Permission granted by Wolters Kluwer Health/ Lippincott Williams & Wilkins).

A 23 year old primipara weighing 106 pounds had a spontaneous full-term vaginal delivery in a rural hospital. In the immediate post-partum period, she became tachycardic, dyspneic, cyanotic and hypotensive. Severe blood loss and a low hemoglobin value of 6.8 g/100 ml blood were detected. She was treated with methylergonovine maleate infusion, plasma and packed red blood cell transfusion. A uterine curettage disclosed retained placental tissue. Despite the treatment, uterine bleeding continued. A hysterectomy was performed, but the patient's condition did not improve. Since a chest radiograph showed entire opacity of the left lung, a 8-French thoracotomy tube was inserted through the fourth intercostal space, and 800 ml of serosanguineous fluid was drained.

After the procedure, the patient was transferred to the intensive care unit of a university hospital. On arrival, she was in coma. She was immediately intubated and mechanically ventilated with 100% FIO_2 and a positive-end-expiratory-pressure (PEEP) of 5 cm H_2O. She was cyanotic and diaphoretic (perspiring). There was distension of the neck veins and fullness of the supraclavicular fossa and neck. Examination of the chest demonstrated absence of breath sounds in the left hemithorax. Heart sounds were heard to the right of the sternum. A chest X-ray showed non-homogeneous opacity and gas bubbles in the entire left hemithorax, shift of the heart and the mediastinum to the right and loss of the sharp left hemidiaphragm line. Laboratory data were obtained (Table **2**) and both base excess (BE) and alveolar dead space fraction ($\dot{V}Ad/\dot{V}\overline{A}$) were calculated (Table **2**).

Table 2: Laboratory blood and gas data

BLOOD SAMPLES			
PaO_2 (mmHg)	43	**Arterial $[HCO_3^-]$ (mEq/l plasma)**	16

$PaCO_2$ (mmHg)	41	**%SaO_2**	71
pHa	7.21	**$P\bar{v}O_2$ (mmHg)**	21
BP (mmHg)	745	**$P\bar{v}CO_2$ (mmHg)**	65
Hb (g/100 ml blood)	12	**Body Temperature (°C)**	36
		CIRCULATION DATA	
$\dot{Q}$ (l/min)	2.6	**Arterial Blood Pressure (mmHg)**	60/0
HR (beats/min)	130	**Right Atrial Pressure (mmHg)**	12
		VENTILATION DATA	
VT (l/min, BTPS)	0.29	**$\dot{V}O_2$ (l/min, STPD)**	0.22
F (breaths/min)	20	**PEEP (cm H_2O)**	5
FIO_2 (%)	100	**PH_2O (mmHg, 100% sat. at 36°C)**	45
		CALCULATED DATA	
BE (mEq/l plasma)	-10.7	**$\dot{V}Ad/\dot{V}\bar{A}$ (%)**	2

In view of the data, the patient was rushed to the operating room. After surgery, the patient's blood pressure increased from 60/0 to 125/80 mmHg, the right atrial pressure decreased from +12 to +1 mmHg, and PaO_2 increased to 154 mmHg while receiving mechanical ventilation with FIO_2 = 50%. The postoperative course was uneventful and the patient was discharged two weeks after surgery.

BASED ON THE HISTORY AND THE GIVEN VALUES ANSWER THE FOLLOWING QUESTIONS:

1. What does PaO_2 = 43 indicate? (Select one)

   A) Acidosis

   B) Anemia

   C) Hypocapnia

   D) Hypoxemia

   E) Normal tissue oxygenation

2. What does $PaCO_2$ = 41 indicate? (Select one)

   A) Alveolar dead space

B) Hyperventilation

C) Hypoxemia

D) Metabolic acidosis

E) Normal ideal alveolar ventilation

F) Normal tissue oxygenation

3. Judging from the values of PaO_2, $PaCO_2$, and FIO_2, which of the following conditions is present? (Select one)

   A) Abnormal alveolar dead space fraction

   B) Anemia

   C) Conductive shunt

   D) Respiratory alkalosis

   E) $\dot{V}/\dot{Q}$ maldistribution shunt-like effect

4. Which of the following is the most important factor causing the $\%SaO_2$ to be 71%? (Select one)

   A) Body Temperature = 36°C

   B) Hb = 12 g/100 ml blood

   C) PaO_2 = 43 mmHg

   D) $\dot{Q}$ = 2.6 l/min

   E) $\dot{V}O_2$ = 0.22 l/min

5. Calculate the shunt fraction. In the process, answer the following questions:

What are the values of $PAiO_2$, $CAiO_2$ and CaO_2?

What are the values of O_2 extraction and $C\bar{v}O_2$?

6. Which of the following contributed to the shunt? (Select one)

   A) Body temperature = 36°C

   B) Patent ductus arteriosus

   C) Unventilated alveoli

   D) $\dot{V}Ad/\dot{V}\bar{A}$ = 2%

   E) $\dot{V}/\dot{Q}$ maldistribution (shunt-like effect)

7. Which of the following values is partially the result of having Hb = 12 g/100 ml blood? (Select one)

   A) $PaCO_2$ = 41 mmHg

   B) $P\bar{v}O_2$ = 21 mmHg

   C) Right Atrial Pressure = 12 mmHg

   D) $\%SaO_2$ = 71%

   E) $\dot{V}O_2$ = 0.22 l/min

8. What do the combined values of $PaCO_2$, pHa and BE indicate? (Select one)

   A) Compensated metabolic acidosis

   B) Compensated respiratory acidosis

   C) Metabolic acidosis

   D) Metabolic alkalosis

E) Partially compensated metabolic acidosis

F) Partially compensated respiratory alkalosis

G) Respiratory alkalosis

9. What is the most likely cause of BE = -10.7 mEq/l plasma? (Select one)

A) HR = 130 beats/min

B) Lactic acid

C) $PaCO_2$ = 41 mmHg

D) pHa = 7.21

E) $\dot{V}O_2$ = 0.22 l/min

10. What does $P\bar{v}O_2$ = 21 mmHg indicate (Select one)

A) High heart rate

B) Hypercapnia

C) Low body temperature

D) Metabolic alkalosis

E) Tissue hypoxia

F) $\dot{V}/\dot{Q}$ maldistribution shunt-like effect

11. What causes $P\bar{v}O_2$ to be 21 mmHg? (Select one)

A) Body temperature = 36°C and FIO_2 = 100%

B) PaO_2 = 43 mmHg, $\dot{Q}$ = 2.6 l/min and Hb = 12 g/100 ml blood

C) pHa = 7.21 and $PaCO_2$ = 41 mmHg

D) $P\bar{v}CO_2 = 65$ mmHg

E) $\dot{V}O_2 = 0.22$ l/min, F = 20 and body temperature = 36°C

12. Normally the gradient between $P\bar{v}CO_2$ and $PaCO_2$ is ~8 mmHg. Here it is 14 mmHg. What is the major reason for it? (Select one)

A) Body temperature = 36°C

B) $PaO_2 = 43$ mmHg

C) pHa = 7.1

D) $\dot{Q} = 2.6$ l/min

E) VT = 0.29 l

13. At the end of inspiration a static pressure of 11 cm H_2O was measured at the respirator. What is the value of compliance (in ml/cm H_2O)? (Select one)

A) 26

B) 48

C) 55

D) 83

E) 100

F) 132

14. What kind of changes in respiratory mechanics are likely to have occurred in this patient? (Select one)

A) Decreased airway resistance

B) Decreased compliance

C) Increased compliance

D) Increased total lung capacity

E) Increased vital capacity

15. What is the value of stroke volume?

16. Before the second surgical intervention, the tentative diagnoses listed below were considered. Based on the patient's history, the physical examination, the lab data and the X-ray evidence, which do you think is be the most likely diagnosis? (Select one)

    A) Cardiogenic shock from unknown heart disease

    B) Herniated intestine through ruptured diaphragm

    C) Massive pulmonary embolism

    D) Peripartum cardio-myopathy

    E) Tension pneumothorax

17. If the patient were not on a respirator, based on the given lab data which factor(s) would stimulate breathing? (Select one)

    A) Hb = 12 g/100 ml blood and BE = -10.7

    B) $[HCO_3^-]$ = 16 mEq/l plasma and $P\bar{v}O_2$ = 21 mmHg

    C) $PaCO_2$ = 41 mmHg

    D) PaO_2 = 43 mmHg and pH = 7.21

    E) $P\bar{v}CO_2$ = 65 mmHg

    F) $P\bar{v}O_2$ = 21 mmHg

18. Describe the sequence of events that took place from delivery to the recovery from the second surgery.

ANSWERS

1: D. 2:E. 3: C. 4: C.

5A.

$PAiO_2 = (745 - 45)1 - 41 = 659$ mmHg

$CAiO_2 = 659 \times 0.003 + (12 \times 1.34) \times 1 = 18.06$ vol%

$CaO_2 = 43 \times 0.003 + (12 \times 1.34) \times 0.71 = 11.55$ vol%

5B.

$$\text{Extraction} = \frac{\dot{V}O_2}{\dot{Q}} = \frac{0.22\ \text{vol\%}}{2.6\ \text{l/min}} = 8.5\ \text{vol\%}$$

$C\bar{v}O_2 = 11.55 - 8.5 = 3.05$ vol%

5C.

$$\frac{\dot{Q}Cs}{\dot{Q}} = \frac{18.06 - 11.55}{18.06 - 3.05} = 43.4\%$$

6: C. 7: B. 8: C. 9: B. 10: E. 11: B. 12: D. 13: B. 14: B.

15:

$$SV = \frac{\dot{Q}}{HR} = \frac{2.6\ \text{l/min}}{130} = 20\ \text{ml}$$

16: B. 17: D.

18: Soon after delivery the patient was tachycardic, dyspneic and hypotensive. Since we know that she had lost a lot of blood, tachycardia, dyspnea and hypotension are consistent with the severe anemia (Hb = 6.8 g/100 ml blood). The fact that the administration of packed red blood cells and hysterectomy did not improve her condition indicates that someting else has occurred, in addition to hemorrhage. A clue is given by X-ray evidence for complete opacification of the left lung, caused by accumulation of sero-sanguineous fluid in the left pleural space. Fluid in the pleural space caused collapse of the left lung resulting in alveoli with $\dot{V}/\dot{Q} = 0$ and consequential conductive shunt. Additional conductive shunt might have occurred if the foramen ovale had opened due to high pressure in the right atrium. The shunt caused hypoxemia.

Upon transfer to the university hospital, the physicians observed distension of the neck veins, fullness of the supraclavicular fossa and neck, which point to impairment of venous return to the heart. X-ray evidence for left hemithorax opacity and shift of heart and mediastinum to the right are consistent with the large accumulation of blood in the left pleural space and the absence of breath sounds in the left hemithorax.

The lab data show:

Severe hypoxemia, which is entirely due to conductive shunt, as there is no hypoventilation ($PaCO_2$ = 41 mmHg). The hypoxemia is impressive, especially since the patient is ventilated with 100% O_2; the reason is the large conductive shunt fraction (43.4%).

Uncompensated metabolic acidosis, due to formation of lactic acid because of tissue hypoxia ($P\bar{v}O_2$ = 21 mmHg). Mechanical ventilation does not compensate at all, because $PaCO_2$ is maintained to a normal value (41 mmHg). The collapsed left lung and shift of the mediastinum to the right does not allow the physicians to compensate for the acidosis by increasing VT.

Tissue hypoxia is due to hyoxemia, anemia and low cardiac output, which result in large extraction (~8.5 l/min). The right shift of the O_2 dissociation curve, significant due to large drop in pH, helps in raising $P\bar{v}O_2$ - the lower than normal body temperature (36°C) moderates only minimally the right shift.

Blood pressure is extremely low due to impaired venous return and heart compression, which result in a large drop in stroke volume (20 ml). The very high heart rate (130/min) provides some compensation for the very low stroke volume.

Right atrial pressure is quite high (12 mmHg; mean normal value = <5 mmHg), consistent with increased intra-thoracic pressure and impaired venous return; since the mean left atrial pressure is 9 mmHg, the increased pressure gradient between right and left atrium might have caused the opening of the foramen ovale adding to the conductive shunt. Note that ~30% of the normal population have a patent foramen ovale that may result in a small left-to-right shunt.

All of the above make sense, but many questions remain ananswered. Why are there gas bubbles mixed with nonhomogeneous opacity in the left hemithorax? What caused the usually sharp hemidiaphragm line to disappear? Both of these observations gave important clues, which were confirmed in the operating room. During labor, the high intra-abdominal pressure resulted in a rupture of the diaphragm and displacement of bowl into the left thorax, causing all of the cardio-respiratory complications mentioned above.

Problem Based Learning

Camillo Peracchia

For Methods Used in Calculations See Appendix 4

For Symbols, Acronyms and Normal Values see Appendix 3

WHAT SMOKING DID TO MR. McDONALD'S LUNGS

For Students

Part One

Mr. McDonald is a 67 year-old, 165 lb., man who has lived in Florida for the past ten years since his early retirement taken for health reasons. He smoked two packs of cigarettes per day for over 40 years, but quit five years ago because of increasing respiratory problems. On May 10 he was examined by his internist because of increased difficulty breathing.

Table 1: Laboratory blood and gas data

May 10		
VC (liters)	3.2	68% of predicted
FEV1 sec (liters)	1	38% of predicted
Peak Expiratory Flow (l/min)	100	29% of predicted
Maximum Inspiratory Flow (l/min)	360	90% of predicted
PaO_2 (mmHg)	65	Normal = 98
$PaCO_2$ (mmHg)	50	Normal = 40
$PACO_2$ (mmHg)	40	Normal = 40
pHa	7.35	Normal = 7.4
HCO_3^- (mEq/l plasma)	27	Normal = 24
BE (mEq/l plasma)	+2.5	Normal = 0

Physical exam (vital signs) and appearance: weight loss, sits forward in hunched position attempting to squeeze air out of the lungs with each respiratory effort, appears barrel-chested and complains of dyspnea (shortness of breath). During this visit a pulmonary function test was performed, and blood and gas samples were taken while breathing room air (Table **1**).

Based on these values, a 14% physiological right-to-left blood shunt fraction ($\dot{Q}Ps/\dot{Q}$) was calculated (normal value = <7%), which decreased to 7% when the blood samples were taken while the patient was breathing 100% O_2.

A resident asked the students whether the abnormal pulmonary-function-test values (VC, FEV1 and Peak Expiratory Pressure) could be due to smoking, and, if so, which disease process could be involved. She advised the students to carefully evaluate the patient's history and lab values and, in an attempt of making a differential diagnosis, to consider a number of pulmonary diseases such as Chronic Obstructive Pulmonary Disease (COPD), chronic asthma, fibrosis, *etc.*

Learning Objectives - Part One

Define the most relevant lung volumes, such as vital capacity, tidal volume, residual volume, *etc.*, and think of how these volumes are measured. Review the pulmonary function test used clinically and explain their significance for the differential diagnosis of pulmonary diseases.

Think of how smoking may affect lung elasticity, airway resistance, and ventilation-perfusion relationship, and relate the abnormal values of the pulmonary function test to pulmonary diseases.

Part Two

A student was puzzled by the fact that PaO_2 is quite low whereas $PaCO_2$ is only moderately increased. Another student thought that there should not be a difference between $PACO_2$ and $PaCO_2$ and felt that there might be an error in the data sheet. The resident said that there was no error; in turn, she asked the students if they knew of pathological processes that cause $PACO_2$ to differ from $PaCO_2$, and whether the data were sufficient to evaluate the situation quantitatively. As a rule, the resident advised the students to train themselves to recognize normal and abnormal values and to understand what they mean by themselves and in relation to other values.

Based on the value of pHa, a nurse asked the resident whether she should administer bicarbonate. The resident turned to the students and asked them to define the acid-base status and indicate whether compensation had taken place.

There was considerable discussion among the students about the effect of 100% FIO_2 breathing on shunt fraction. The resident told them to think of how a large increase in alveolar PO_2 might reduce the effect of ventilation/perfusion maldistribution (mismatch) on PaO_2.

Learning Objectives - Part Two

Just looking at the data what can one say?

Train yourself to recognize abnormal values and to understand what they mean by themselves and in relation to other values. Define the conditions that can cause these values to be abnormal. In the process, think of the causes of hypoxemia and hypercapnia. In addition, think of how ventilation affects blood pH and ask yourself the following questions: 1. Are the values of $PaCO_2$, pH_a and BE consistent with an acute or chronic acid/base problem? 2. How would you define the acid/base condition of this patient?

Understand how the presence of alveolar dead space ventilation is quantitatively evaluated. To do so, learn how to calculate the fraction $\dot{V}Ad/\dot{V}\bar{A}$ and think of how the presence of alveolar dead space ventilation alters the composition of expired gases. In particular, why does $PACO_2$ differ from $PaCO_2$? Does alveolar dead space ventilation cause hypoxemia and/or hypercapnia?

Understand the concept of right-to-left blood shunt (venous admixture) and think of how 100% FIO_2 breathing might affect PaO_2 and shunt fraction. Note that in this patient the shunt fraction decreased from 14% to 7% with 100% FIO_2 breathing.

Part Three

The patient was sent home with supplemental oxygen therapy. He was stable for a few days, but eventually his conditions deteriorated and in the morning of June 8 he was admitted to the hospital with dyspnea (shortness of breath) hemoptysis (coughing of mucous stained with blood) and fever, and was treated with antibiotics. In the early afternoon, because of increased respiratory difficulty, his trachea was intubated and he was placed on mechanical ventilation with 60% O_2. At 6:00 p.m. the values listed in Table **2** were obtained.

Table 2: Laboratory blood and gas data –June 8, 6:00 p.m.

		Normal values
PaO_2	76	98
$PaCO_2$ (mmHg)	34	40
pHa	7.34	7.4
$P\bar{v}O_2$ (mmHg)	45	40
$pH\bar{v}$ (mmHg)	7.30	7.35
HB (g/100 ml blood)	14	16
VT (liters, BTPS)	0.75	0.5
F (breaths/min)	14	12
VCd (liters)	0.16	0.15
R	0.8	0.8-0.85
FIO_2 (%)	60	-
Peak PAW (cm H2O)*	22	18-22
$\dot{V}Ad/\dot{V}\bar{A}$ (%)	18	0
$\dot{V}O_2$ (liters/min, STPD)	0.33	0.25
HR (Heart Rate, beats/min)	125	70
SV (stroke volume, ml)	56	70
Body Temperature (°C)	39	37
H_2O Partial Pressure at 39 °C (mmHg)	51.6	-
PB (mmHg)	760	-

* Peak inspiratory airway pressure during mechanical ventilation. Assume no added conductive dead space by the ventilator. The constant A863" in the alveolar air equation becomes A869" at 39°C.

The students had different opinions on what disease would cause dyspnea, hemoptysis and fever. Diseases like lung cancer, bronchitis, tuberculosis and pneumonia were mentioned. The resident suggested to make a working hypothesis and to test it by evaluating the problem qualitatively as well as quantitatively based on the available lab values and the patient's history.

A student had a hard time understanding how ventilator-mediated breathing and independent breathing differ in their effect on pulmonary circulation. The resident suggested him to think of how mechanical ventilation might affect intra-pleural and intra-alveolar pressures during the breathing cycle.

Some students started calculating right away shunt fraction, base excess, *etc.*, rather than spending time to figure out what could be extracted qualitatively from lab values and patient's history. The resident pointed out that this is definitely the wrong approach. Instead, she advised the students to evaluate carefully the lab values, recognize normal *versus* abnormal values, relate one value to another, and differentiate primary from compensatory changes in value, before performing calculations.

Based on PaO_2 and $PaCO_2$ values, while breathing with 60% FIO_2, a student felt that the shunt fraction might have increased significantly from May 10 to June 8. Another student strongly disagreed. The resident suggested them to settle their dispute by calculating the shunt fraction.

Once again, a nurse asked the resident whether the administration of bicarbonate would be appropriate based on the pHa value. The resident felt that she would decide based on the base excess (BE) value. A student volunteered to calculate BE and to evaluate the acid-base status.

Most students were puzzled by evidence that tissue oxygenation appeared to be better than normal in spite of the fact that PaO_2 was quite low. The resident told them to think of all the factors that play a role in oxygen delivery to tissue.

Learning Objectives - Part Three

Understand the difference between independent, spontaneous, breathing and ventilator breathing. Think of how intra-alveolar and intra-pleural pressures are affected by the ventilator and how they may alter pulmonary circulation.

Think of which acute pulmonary disease can cause dyspnea (shortness of breath), hemoptysis (coughing of mucous stained with blood) and fever, and what would be its consequences to arterial blood oxygenation.

Understand how blood shunt is evaluated quantitatively. To do so, learn how to calculate: partial pressure of ideal alveolar blood ($PAiO_2$), O_2 content in ideal alveolar ($CAiO_2$) and arterial (CaO_2) blood, O_2 extraction, $(Ai\text{-}a)PO_2$ gradient, and shunt fraction. In the process understand how blood pH and body temperature affect the O_2 dissociation curve; think of what would be the value of $\%SaO_2$ if pHa and body temperature were normal.

Table 3: Laboratory blood and gas data - June 8, 11:00 p.m.

		Normal values
PaO_2 (mmHg)	47	98
$PaCO_2$ (mmHg)	37	40
pHa	7.24	7.4
$pH\bar{v}$	7.20	7.35
Hb (g/100 ml blood)	14	16
VT (liters, BTPS)	0.75	0.5
f (breaths/min)	18	12
R	0.8	0.8-0.85
FIO_2 (%)	60	-
Peak PAW (cm H_2O)*	53	18-22
$\dot{V}O_2$ (liters/min, STPD)	0.3	0.25
HR (heart rate, beats/min)	142	70
SV (stroke volume, ml)	27	70
$C\bar{v}O_2$ (vol%)	4.9	14.6
Body Temperature (°C)	39	37
$\dot{Q}Cs/\dot{Q}$ (%)	48	<7
B.E. (mEq/l plasma)	-10.3	0

* Peak inspiratory airway pressure during mechanical ventilation.

Understand how the acid-base status of a patient is evaluated quantitatively, how the presence of a metabolic component is determined and, if present, how one can decide whether it is a compensatory or complicating factor. In the process, learn how to calculate the actual bicarbonate concentration, buffer capacity and base excess (BE), and think of how hemoglobin concentration affects blood pH.

Understand the factors involved in O_2 delivery to tissue. In particular, think of the interplay among arterial PO_2, hemoglobin concentration, cardiac output, O_2 consumption, O_2 extraction, mixed venous pH, and body temperature. In the process ask yourself why $P\bar{v}O_2$ (45 mmHg) is greater than normal in spite of the fact that PaO_2 (76 mmHg) is below normal.

Part Four

The patient's conditions progressively deteriorated and at 11:00 p.m. another set of blood and gas samples was obtained (Table **3**). Administration of bronchodilators did not improve his conditions, whereas inter-costal needle insertion on the right side of the chest resulted in release of air under tension and rapidly improved the status.

The students were confused about what could have caused gas to accumulate under pressure in the intra-pleural space. A student thought that the increased PAW value might have resulted from an acute asthma attack. Most students disagreed based on other available data. The resident advised the students to gather information on the mechanism that causes "tension pneumothorax" and the consequences of this process to ventilation and circulation.

A student was puzzled by the fact that in spite of an increase of total ventilation ($\dot{V}E = VT \times f$), $PaCO_2$ was higher than at 6:00 p.m. The resident suggested to consider the possibility of an increase in wasted alveolar ventilation and to test this hypothesis by performing the necessary calculations.

The resident asked the students to look at all of the factors that determine oxygen delivery to tissue, and to tell her whether they felt that tissue oxygenation had changed since 6:00. After a long discussion the students were advised to confirm or disprove their conclusion by calculating mixed venous PO_2. The resident also ordered a biopsy of the apical region of the lung and asked the students to predict, based on their knowledge of lung structure, what the biopsy might show.

Finally, the resident asked for a volunteered to present to the other students his/her perspective of the sequence of events, and their causes, that had taken place between May 10 and June 8 (11:00 p.m.).

Learning Objectives - Part Four

Think of what could be the reasons why the intercostal needle insertion on the right side of the chest resulted in release of air under tension. What do you think happens when the surface of the lung ruptures and the alveolar compartment opens into the intra-pleural space? Why was the air under tension?

Just looking at the data what can one tell? Train yourself to recognize normal *versus* abnormal values and to understand what these values mean by themselves and, above all, as they relate to the values of other relevant parameters.

Understand how the average tissue oxygenation is estimated and think of the factor involved in O_2 delivery to tissue. In particular, think of the interplay among arterial PO_2, hemoglobin concentration, cardiac output, O_2 consumption, O_2 extraction, mixed venous pH, and body temperature. Understand the reasons why tissue oxygenation has deteriorated drastically between 6:00 and 11:00 p.m., in spite of significant decrease in mixed venous pH.

Understand what determines peak inspiratory airway pressure (PAW) during mechanical ventilation and think of what could have caused it to dramatically increase between 6:00 and 11:00 p.m.

Understand how the alveolar dead space ventilation can be quantitatively evaluated in the absence of mixed alveolar gas ($PACO_2$) values. In the process, learn how to calculate the fraction $\dot{V}Ad/\dot{V}\overline{A}$ by knowing $\dot{V}O_2$, R, $PaCO_2$, VT, f and VCd.

Understand the sequence of events and the complications that have occurred.

Problem Based Learning

Camillo Peracchia

For Methods Used in Calculations (See Appendix 4)

For Symbols, Acronyms and Normal Values (See Appendix 3)

WHAT SMOKING DID TO MR. MCDONALD'S LUNGS

Answers

Part One

From autopsy reports, almost 95% of people who smoked one or more packs of cigarettes per day for several decades show some degree of emphysema, while over 90% of non-smokers have little or no emphysema. Smoking affects both the airways and the lung tissue causing emphysema and/or chronic bronchitis. In most patients both of these diseases are present.

Airways show inflammation, edema and excess mucous secretion, and occasionally become completely obstructed. Airway obstruction increases air flow resistance and reduces or eliminates ventilation in the affected areas causing maldistribution shunt-like effect (low $\dot{V}/\dot{Q}$ ratio) or shunt ($\dot{V}/\dot{Q} = 0$), respectively.

The lung tissue loses elasticity as alveolar walls become disrupted, generating large cavities. The loss of alveolar walls reduces the capillary bed and so the vascular perfusion, causing large increase in $\dot{V}/\dot{Q}$ ratio (alveolar dead space). The loss of elasticity (reduced lung recoil) causes airway collapse in expiration leading to large increase in expiratory flow resistance.

Reduced FEV1 sec and peak expiratory flow indicate increased expiratory flow resistance, which is observed in both asthma and emphysema. However, what allows one to distinguish between the two diseases are the values of maximum inspiratory flow (MIF) and vital capacity (VC). In emphysema, MIF is close to normal and VC is significantly reduced. In asthma, MIF is significantly reduced and VC is normal.

Part Two

Low PaO_2 (65 mmHg) means hypoxemia. There are two major causes of hypoxemia: shunt and hypoventilation. Here, hypoventilation is certainly a factor, as $PaCO_2$ (50 mmHg) is greater than normal, but it is so by only 10 mmHg, whereas PaO_2 is lower than normal by at least 30 mmHg. So the hypoxemia is caused by both shunt and hypoventilation. Hypercapnia is caused by hypoventilation. Due to the large increase in work of breathing that results from increased airway resistance and wasted ventilation in alveolar dead space, these patients tend to chronically hypoventilate (reduced ideal alveolar ventilation) and build up CO_2 (chronic respiratory acidosis); pH_a, however, is not that low due to metabolic compensation (increased HCO_3^-). Hypoventilation increases $PaCO_2$ and so it lowers pH_a. In time the kidneys compensate by increasing bicarbonate concentration, so that pH_a increases toward normal values. In this patient, there is a chronic respiratory acidosis partially compensated (positive base excess).

The mixed (total) alveolar ventilation ($\dot{V}\bar{A}$) is the sum of ideal alveolar ventilation ($\dot{V}Ai$) and alveolar dead space ventilation ($\dot{V}Ad$). The fraction of $\dot{V}\bar{A}$ wasted as $\dot{V}Ad$ ($\dot{V}Ad/\dot{V}\bar{A}$) is easily calculated by determining the drop PCO_2 undergoes as ideal gas ($PaCO_2$) mixes with room air ($PCO_2 = 0$) coming from the alveolar dead space. Note that in normal people this fraction is virtually zero. In this patient:

$$\frac{\dot{V}Ad}{\dot{V}\bar{A}} = \frac{PaCO_2 - P\bar{A}CO_2}{PaCO_2} = \frac{50 - 40}{50} = 20\%$$

The presence of **alveolar dead space does not affect blood gas composition** unless the patient cannot compensate for it. This is done by increasing the total ventilation ($\dot{V}E$) to maintain a normal ideal alveolar ventilation ($\dot{V}Ai$) - increased $\dot{V}E$ by greater VT and/or f, to maintain a normal $\dot{V}Ai$ in spite of the increase in wasted ventilation ($\dot{V}Ad$).

Right-to-left blood shunt (venous admixture) is the result of an influx of venous (deoxygenated) blood into arterial (oxygenated) blood. Shunt can have many causes and is either reversible with oxygen breathing (maldistribution/diffusion shunt-like effect) or irreversible (conductive shunt). In this patient the shunt fraction is 14% while breathing air (physiological shunt) and 7% when breathing 100% FIO_2 (conductive shunt). This means that the maldistribution shunt fraction (alveoli with very low $\dot{V}/\dot{Q}$) is: 14 - 7 = 7%, and the rest (7%) is conductive shunt (alveoli with $\dot{V}/\dot{Q} = 0$ and/or extra-alveolar shunt).

Part Three

With mechanical ventilation the lungs expand (inspiration) as air is pumped into them by pressure generated by the ventilator, and return passively to their resting volume (expiration to FRC) by means of the lung recoil.

In spontaneous breathing (at rest), the alveolar pressure becomes negative in inspiration and positive in expiration, and it is zero in the absence of air movement (end of inspiration and end of expiration); the intra-pleural pressure is always negative, and more so at the end of inspiration due to stretching of lung tissue

With mechanical ventilation, the alveolar pressure is positive both during inspiration and expiration and becomes zero at the end of expiration (FRC), unless the ventilator is a PEEP (positive end expiratory pressure) ventilator. The intra-pleural pressure is negative throughout the breathing cycle, but less negative than in spontaneous breathing during inspiration.

The more positive (or less negative) pressures in both intra-pleural and alveolar compartments increase slightly the vascular resistance as arterioles, veins and alveolar capillaries become slightly compressed. The less negative intra-pleural pressure also slightly reduces the venous return to the right atrium.

Dyspnea (shortness of breath, awareness of breathing, need to breathe more) is observed in most cardio-respiratory diseases. Hemoptysis is observed most commonly in lung cancer, bronchiectasis (inflammatory, localized dilatations of the airways), bronchitis, tuberculosis and bacterial pneumonia. In the present case, since it is an acute condition with fever, the most likely disease is bacterial pneumonia. Pneumonia would lower PaO_2 (hypoxemia) as the filling of alveoli with liquid and cell debris (exudate) causes shunt ($\dot{V}/\dot{Q} = 0$).

We know that the patient has chronic obstructive pulmonary disease (COPD), which caused abnormal right-to-left shunts, maldistribution shunt-like effects, and alveolar dead space. Before the acute episode, this has caused hypoxemia and hypercapnia, with a positive (compensatory) base excess. The symptoms described on admission (dyspnea, hemoptysis and fever) are consistent with bacterial pneumonia. The increased respiratory difficulty of early afternoon indicates that he was rapidly approaching respiratory failure. In this case, PaO_2 would have dropped dramatically and $PaCO_2$ would have risen to dangerous levels. This is obvious because at 6:00 p.m., even though he was ventilated with 60% O_2 at a rate sufficient to bring $PaCO_2$ to 34 mmHg, his PaO_2 was still low (76 mmHg).

In addition, we notice the following abnormal values:

- Mild acidosis which is metabolic because $PaCO_2$ is lower than normal.

- PaO_2 is lower than normal, even though FIO_2 is 60% and $PaCO_2$ is lower than normal. This clearly indicates the presence of a sizable shunt, which is probably all conductive because with 60% FIO_2 maldistribution shunt and any potential diffusion problem are minimized or eliminated altogether.

- The ventilator settings for both VT and f are slightly higher than normal, but still insufficient to bring PaO_2 and pHa to normal values. In this patient, aside from hypoxemia and acidosis, there is another reason for the need to increase ventilation: fever (39^{0}C) and consequential increase in metabolic rate ($\dot{V}O_2$ = 0.33 l/min). Since the patient has COPD, there might be some alveolar dead space ventilation, which also would need to be compensated by increasing total ventilation; this is the case because, in spite of greater than normal $\dot{V}E$ (0.75 x 14 = 10.5 l/min), $PaCO_2$ is only slightly below normal.

- Heart rate is almost twice normal. Even though stroke volume is a bit low, this results in higher than normal cardiac output. The increase in cardiac output is due to increased metabolic rate.

Shunt:

$$PAiO_2 = (760 - 51.6)0.6 - \frac{1 - 0.6(1 - 0.8)}{0.8}34 = 388 \text{ mmHg}$$

At $PAiO_2 = 388$, $\%SAiO_2$. 100%

$CAiO_2 = 388 \times 0.0031 + (14 \times 1.34)1 = 19.96$ vol%

At $PaO_2 = 76$ and pHa = 7.34, $\%SaO_2 = \sim 92\%$

$CaO_2 = 76 \times 0.0031 + (14 \times 1.34)0.92 = 17.49$ vol%

$\dot{Q} = SV \times HR = 0.056 \times 125 = 7.0$ l/min

O_2 extraction = $\dot{V}O_2/\dot{Q} = 0.33/7.0 = 0.047 = 4.7$ vol%

$$C\bar{v}O_2 = CaO_2 - 4.7 = 17.49 - 4.7 = 12.79 \text{ vol\%}$$

$$\frac{\dot{\mathbf{Q}}\mathbf{Cs}}{\dot{\mathbf{Q}}} = \frac{\mathbf{9.96 - 17.49}}{\mathbf{19.96 - 12.79}} = \mathbf{34.4\%}$$

$(Ai\text{-}a)PO_2 = 388 - 76 = 312$ mmHg

Base Excess:

$$\text{pH} = 6.1 + \log\frac{[HCO_3^-]}{\alpha \times PaCO_2}$$

$$10^{\text{pH}-6.1} = \frac{[HCO_3^-]}{\alpha \times PaCO_2}$$

$$10^{7.34-6.1} = \frac{[HCO_3^-]_{Actual}}{0.0301 \times 34}$$

$$[HCO_3^-]_{Actual} = 17.78 \text{ mEq/l (plasma)}$$

$$BC = \frac{8.2 + (1.56 \times 14)}{3} = 10$$

$$-10 = \frac{24 - [HCO_3^-]_{Predicted}}{7.4 - 7.34}$$

$$[HCO_3^-]_{Predicted} = 24.6 \text{ mEq/l}$$

$$BE = [HCO_3^-]_{Actual} - [HCO_3^-]_{Predicted}$$

$$BE = 17.78 - 24.6 = -6.82 \text{ mEq/l}$$

Conclusion: metabolic acidosis partially compensated by increased ideal alveolar ventilation. The negative BE is likely to be the consequence of pre-existing tissue hypoxia (lactic acid) due to severe hypoxemia before admission.

Tissue oxygenation at 6:00 p.m.is better than normal in spite of hypoxemia (PaO_2 = 76 mmHg) and increased oxygen consumption because of the right shift of the O_2 dissociation curve, due to fever, slight decrease in $pH\bar{v}$, and in part to increased cardiac output (7 l/min), with consequential slight decrease in extraction (4.7 vol%).

Part Four

The most obvious reason why the intercostal needle insertion resulted in release of air under tension is the presence of "tension pneumothorax". Smoking causes a nine fold increase in the risk of pneumothorax in females and 22% increase in males. In this case, the ventilator breathing, which results in positive alveolar pressure during most of the breathing cycle, increased even more the chance that an emphysematous bleb or bulla might burst (usually at apical lung regions where alveolar compliance is lower) and let air flowing into the intra-pleural compartment (lung collapse).

At 11:00 p.m. one notices the following:

- More severe acidosis, which is metabolic because $PaCO_2$ is still below normal. Indeed, BE = -10.3 mEq/l plasma.
- Severe hypoxemia (PaO_2 = 47 mmHg) in spite of 60% O_2 breathing and lower than normal $PaCO_2$, indicating that there is a large shunt.

- VT was not changed since 6:00 p.m., but frequency was increased from 14 to 18/min. This resulted in much greater than normal minute ventilation ($\dot{V}E$ = 13.5 l/min). In spite of this, $PaCO_2$ is only slightly below normal, indicating that there is a large alveolar dead space ventilation, which is even greater than that present at 6:00 p.m.

- Heart rate has increased even further and stroke volume has decreased a lot. This results in a low cardiac output. This, combined with a slightly high $\dot{V}O_2$ (due to fever), results in large extraction. Large extraction, combined with severe hypoxemia, is likely to result in tissue hypoxia and metabolic acidosis (anaerobic metabolism causing lactic acid production).

- Peak PAW is higher than normal, indicating increased airway resistance and/or decreased compliance. Since the administration of bronchodilators did not improve the patient's conditions, there is no increase in airway resistance due to bronchial spasm. Thus, a decrease in compliance is more likely. This is caused by the pneumothorax.

Tissue oxygenation:

$$\%S\bar{v}O_2 = C\bar{v}O_2/\text{capacity} = 4.9/(14 \times 1.34) = 26\%$$

Due to Bohr shift, at $pH\bar{v}$ = 7.2 and T = 39^0C this $\%S\bar{v}O_2$ corresponds to:

$$P\bar{v}O_2 = \sim 25 \text{ mmHg}$$

It's not surprising to find poor tissue oxygenation at 11:00 p.m. because there are several elements detrimental to normal oxygen delivery to tissue such as: severe hypoxemia and consequential decreased arterial O_2 content, decreased cardiac output and increased oxygen consumption, resulting in increased extraction. However, due to the Bohr's shift, $P\bar{v}O_2$, would be even lower than 25 mmHg if $pH\bar{v}$ were normal. Indeed, with a $\%S\bar{v}O_2$ = 26%, at normal $pH\bar{v}$ (7.35) and 37^0C, $P\bar{v}O_2$ would be ~18 mmHg.

Since peak PAW is measured at the ventilator during inflation, and so while air is flowing through the airways, its value is determined by two factors: the resistance of the airways and the change in compliance that results from stretching the lungs to larger volumes. Therefore, the increase in peak airway pressure seen at 11:00 p.m. could be attributed to increased airway resistance and/or decreased compliance. However, in this case it is stated that "administration of bronchodilators did not improve his conditions, whereas intercostal needle insertion on the right side of the chest resulted in release of air under tension and rapidly improved the status". This tells us: first, that there was no increase in airway resistance due to a possible asthma attack, and, second, that the intra-pleural space of the right lung is filled with gas at a pressure greater than atmospheric. This condition occurs when a tension (valvular) pneumothorax develops. Tension pneumothorax causes increasing volumes of gas to accumulate in the intra-pleural space, and pleural pressure to progressively grow to dangerous levels. The result is complete collapse of the right lung and large decrease in compliance - hence, increased peak PAW (see Chapter 3: Clinical correlation – Pneumothorax; and Chapter 10: Restrictive Diseases – Pneumothorax).

Alveolar dead space:

$$\dot{V}Ai = \frac{869 \text{ x } \dot{V}CO_2}{PaCO_2}$$

$$\dot{V}CO_2 = \dot{V}O_2 \text{ x } R = 0.3 \text{ x } 0.8 = 0.24 \text{ l/min}$$

$$\dot{V}Ai = \frac{869 \text{ x } 0.24}{37} = 5.64 \text{ l/min}$$

Since body weight is 160 lb., VCd is ~160 ml (BTPS)

$\dot{V}Cd = 0.160 \text{ x } 18 = 2.88$ l/min

$\dot{V}E = 0.75 \text{ x } 18 = 13.5$ l/min

$\dot{V}\bar{A} = 13.5 - 2.88 = 10.62$ l/min

$\dot{V}Ad = 10.62 - 5.64 = 4.98$ l/min

$$\frac{\mathbf{\dot{V}Ad}}{\mathbf{\dot{V}\bar{A}}} = \frac{\mathbf{4.98}}{\mathbf{10.62}} = \mathbf{47\%}$$

Based on the given data and the calculated values, we can tell that at 6:00 p.m. the patient was hypoxemic, in spite of hyperventilation and 60% O_2 breathing, because of a large shunt (34.4%). The shunt is probably entirely conductive because with 60% FIO_2 most if not all of the maldistribution and/or diffusion components must have been eliminated. In view of the symptoms reported on admission (dyspnea, hemoptysis and fever), it is reasonable to believe that the shunt was caused by pneumonia (alveoli filled with exudate resulting in $\dot{V}/\dot{Q} = 0$). The metabolic acidosis suggests that before being mechanically ventilated with 60% FIO_2 the patient was probably severely hypoxemic with significant tissue hypoxia. The resulting lactic acid production must have eliminated the usual compensatory base excess seen in COPD patients, and must have caused a base deficit, that could not be compensated by respiration because the patient was in respiratory distress.

At 11:00 p.m., the patient's status has considerably worsened. There is a sizable increase in shunt, a more severe and virtually uncompensated metabolic acidosis, a large increase in alveolar dead space, and severe hypoxemia and tissue hypoxia. All of these changes are due to the tension pneumothorax, which has caused the collapse of the right lung - and consequential increase in conductive shunt - and a large accumulation of gas in the right intra-pleural space at greater than atmospheric pressure. This caused compression of pulmonary vessels, and both a shift to the left and compression of the mediastinum.

Pneumothorax is not uncommon in patients mechanically ventilated, especially if emphysema is present. In this case the pneumothorax is of the tension (valvular) type. Tension pneumothorax is very dangerous because the gas that goes from the alveoli to the intra-pleural space on inflation (by ventilator) cannot return into the alveoli during lung deflation. Often, gas also accumulates within the alveolar walls, resulting in interstitial pneumothorax and further compression the pulmonary vessels (see Chapter 3: Clinical correlation – Pneumothorax; and Chapter 10: Restrictive Diseases – Pneumothorax).

Problem Based Learning

Camillo Peracchia

What Smoking Did to Mr. McDonald's Lungs

TUTOR'S GUIDE

On day-1, the students should spend the first half hour to 45 min evaluating and discussing the relevant data of the history and the pulmonary function test given in Part One. Then they should be given Part Two and should be advised to evaluate the blood gas data and relate them to shunt, alveolar dead space and acid-base balance. They should calculate the fraction of the alveolar ventilation wasted in alveolar dead space and should start discussing how 100% FIO_2-breathing might affect the shunt due to ventilation/perfusion maldistribution. At the end of day-1 the students should be given Part Three, to be discussed on day-2.

On day-2 the students should discuss the data given in Part Three. They should evaluate the history and the blood gas data, discuss the differences between independent and ventilator-assisted breathing and consider diseases that could cause the described symptoms and affect blood gas values. During this PBL the students should calculate shunt fraction and base excess. At the end of day-2 the students should be given Part Four, to be discussed on day-3.

On day-3, the students should discuss the data given in Part Four. They should discuss the mechanism and consequences of tension pneumothorax and potential causes of increased peak PAW. Once more they should evaluate blood gas data individually and in relation to other data and discuss their relevance to shunt, alveolar dead space, acid-base balance and O_2 delivery to tissue. The students should calculate mixed venous PO_2 (indicative of tissue oxygenation) and the fraction of the alveolar ventilation wasted in alveolar dead space.

APPENDIX 1

Gas Exchange

A. VOLUME CONVERSIONS

Volume conversion among ATPS, BTPS and STPD conditions are accomplished by means of the ideal gas law, a combination of Boyle-Marriotte's and Charles' (Gay-Lussac's) laws. Ideal gases by definition do not condense, evaporate or sublime at the operating range. O_2 and N_2 are ideal gases; CO_2 is not, but for the purposes of respiratory physiology can be considered an ideal gas as well. In contrast, water vapor does not follow the ideal gas laws; therefore its partial pressure needs to be subtracted away in the volume conversion equation (see later).

The Boyle-Marriotte's law states that at constant temperature changes of volume (V) are inversely related to changes in pressure (P; Eq. 1):

$$P \times V = K \text{ (constant)} \ldots \quad (1)$$

The Charles' law (Eq. 2) states that a gas kept at constant pressure (P) changes in volume (V) proportionally to temperature (T). Conversely, at constant V the gas changes in P proportionally to T (absolute temperature, °K):

$$\frac{V_1}{V_2} = \frac{T_1}{T_2} \frac{P_1}{P_2} = \frac{T_1}{T_2} \ldots \quad (2)$$

Example: 1l of dry air (V_1) at 37°C (310°K; T_1) becomes 0.88l (V_2) at 0°C (273°K; T_2), see Eq. 3:

$$V_2 = V_1 \frac{T_2}{T_1} = 1 \times \frac{273}{310} = 0.88 \text{ l} \ldots \quad (3)$$

Since under physiological conditions temperature, volume and pressure must be considered concurrently, the most useful relationship is expressed in the "ideal gas law" (Eq. 4):

$$P \times V = nR^{*}T \ldots \quad (4)$$

where P is the gas pressure expressed in atmospheres, V the gas volume expressed in liters, "n" the number of gram-moles of gas, and R* a constant = 0.082 (l x atm/mole x °K). T is the absolute temperature of the gas (°K).

When one converts a volume of gas from one condition to another (for example from ATPS to BTPS), the number of moles (n) of the ideal gases (O_2, CO_2, and N_2) remains constant; thus: n x R^* = K (constant). Since H_2O vapor is not an ideal gas (in fact, from ATPS to BTPS the n of H_2O will increase due to evaporation), as mentioned above its partial pressure has to be subtracted from the barometric pressure. By doing so both for ATPS and for BTPS, we introduce in the equation the correction factor for the increase in volume caused by the increase in the number of H_2O molecules, as temperature increases from T_A to T_B (Eqs. 5-8; at 37°C, PH_2O = 47 mmHg):

$$\frac{(P_{ATPS}-P_{H_2O})V_{ATPS}}{T_{ATPS}} = K \ldots \quad (5)$$

$$\frac{(P_{BTPS}-47)V_{BTPS}}{T_{BTPS}} = K \ldots \quad (6)$$

$$\frac{(P_{ATPS}-P_{H_2O})V_{ATPS}}{T_{ATPS}} = \frac{(P_{BTPS}-47)V_{BTPS}}{T_{BTPS}} \ldots \quad (7)$$

$$V_{BTPS} = \frac{(P_{ATPS}-P_{H_2O})V_{ATPS}\times T_{BTPS}}{(P_{BTPS}-47)T_{ATPS}} \ldots \quad (8)$$

Examples:

a) To convert 1l of air from ATPS (T = 273°K + 20°K; P_B = 760 mmHg; PH_2O = 17.5 mmHg) to BTPS, see Eq. 9:

$$V_{BTPS} = \frac{(760-17.5)1(273+37)}{(760-47)(273+20)} = 1.202\,l \ldots \quad (9)$$

b) To convert 1l of O_2 from ATPS (same as above) to STPD, see Eq. 10:

$$V_{STPD} = \frac{(760-17.5)1x273}{760(273+20)} = 0.91\,l \ldots \quad (10)$$

B. DERIVATION OF O_2 CONSUMPTION AND CO_2 PRODUCTION EQUATIONS (AT STPD):

O_2 Consumption Equation (Eq. 14)

For calculating the O_2-consumption per minute ($\dot{V}O_2$) one could use a simple equation (Eq. 11), but it would require measuring both inspired ($\dot{V}I$) and expired ($\dot{V}E$) minute ventilations.

$$\dot{V}O_2 = \dot{V}I \text{ x } FIO_2 - \dot{V}E \text{ x } FEO_2 \;\ldots \qquad (11)$$

$\dot{V}I$, however, can easily be removed from the equation (see Eqs. 12-14) because, since there is no N_2 exchange, the number of inspired and expired N_2 molecules is the same. Therefore:

$$\dot{V}I \text{ x } FIN_2 = \dot{V}E \text{ x } FEN_2 \;\ldots \qquad (12)$$

$$\dot{V}I = \dot{V}E\frac{FEN_2}{FIN_2} \;\ldots \qquad (13)$$

$$\dot{V}O_2 = \dot{V}E\left(FIO_2\frac{FEN_2}{FIN_2} - FEO_2\right) \;\ldots \qquad (14)$$

$FIO_2 = 0.21$, $FIN_2 = 0.79$, and $FEN_2 = 1 - (FEO_2 + FECO_2)$. FEO_2 and $FECO_2$ are determined from gas samples taken from the expiratory collection bag, by means of O_2 and CO_2 meters.

Similarly, using ideal alveolar gases (see Eqs. 15-18):

$$\dot{V}O_2 = \dot{V}I \text{ x } FIO_2 - (\dot{V}Ai \text{ x } FAiO_2 + \dot{V}Pd \text{ x } FIO_2) \;\ldots \qquad (15)$$

$$\dot{V}I \text{ x } FIN_2 = \dot{V}Ai \text{ x } FAiN_2 + \dot{V}Pd \text{ x } FIN_2 \;\ldots \qquad (16)$$

$$\dot{V}O_2 = \left(\dot{V}Ai\frac{FAiN_2}{FIN_2} + \dot{V}Pd\right)FIO_2 - (\dot{V}Ai \text{ x } FAiO_2 + \dot{V}Pd \text{ x } FIO_2) \;\ldots \qquad (17)$$

$$\dot{V}O_2 = \dot{V}Ai\left(FIO_2\frac{FAiN_2}{FIN_2} - FAiO_2\right) \;\ldots \qquad (18)$$

The reason for showing the O_2 consumption equation using ideal gas values is that this equation is needed for deriving the alveolar gas equation (see below: **E**). The alveolar gas equation is relevant only for ideal (Ai) gases, because $PAiO_2$ can only calculated by this equation, while $P\bar{A}O_2$ (average alveolar PO_2) can be measured from end-tidal gas samples – the Ai compartment gas cannot be sampled.

CO_2 Production Equations (at STPD, Eq. 19):

$$\dot{V}CO_2 = \dot{V}E \text{ x } FECO_2 = \dot{V}\bar{A} \text{ x } F\bar{A}CO_2 = \dot{V}Ai \text{ x } FAiCO_2 \;... \qquad (19)$$

C. DERIVATION OF DEAD SPACE EQUATIONS

Conductive Dead Space Ventilation ($\dot{V}Cd$)

In normal circumstances $FICO_2 = 0$. Therefore, all the expired CO_2 comes from the alveoli ($\dot{V}\bar{A}$). In the expired ($\dot{V}E$) and alveolar ($\dot{V}\bar{A}$) ventilations the number of CO_2 molecules is the same, only their concentration is different ($F\bar{A}CO_2 > FECO_2$ because $\dot{V}\bar{A} < \dot{V}E$); thus, the conductive dead space ventilation is calculated as follows (see Eqs. 20-24):

$$\dot{V}E \text{ x } FECO_2 = \dot{V}\bar{A} \text{ x } F\bar{A}CO_2 \;... \qquad (20)$$

$$\dot{V}\bar{A} = \dot{V}E - \dot{V}Cd \;... \qquad (21)$$

$$\dot{V}E \text{ x } FECO_2 = (\dot{V}E - \dot{V}Cd)F\bar{A}CO_2 \;... \qquad (22)$$

$$\dot{V}Cd = \dot{V}E\frac{F\bar{A}CO_2 - FECO_2}{F\bar{A}CO_2} \;... \qquad (23)$$

If the gases are all measured at the same conditions, fractional concentrations (F) can be replaced by partial pressures (P). See Eq. 24:

$$\dot{V}Cd = \dot{V}E\frac{P\bar{A}CO_2 - PECO_2}{P\bar{A}CO_2} \;... \qquad (24)$$

$$\dot{V}Ai \text{ x } PaCO_2 = \dot{V}E \text{ x } PECO_2 = \dot{V}\bar{A} \text{ x } P\bar{A}CO_2$$

Physiological Dead Space Ventilation ($\dot{V}Pd$)

In subjects with alveolar dead space ventilation ($\dot{V}Ad$), when $FICO_2 = 0$ all of the CO_2 comes from the alveolar ideal compartment ($\dot{V}Ai$); thus, the physiological dead space ventilation is calculated as follows (see Eqs. 25-29):

$$\dot{V}E \times FECO_2 = \dot{V}Ai \times FAiCO_2 \ldots \quad (25)$$

$$\dot{V}Ai = \dot{V}E - \dot{V}Pd \ldots \quad (26)$$

$$\dot{V}E \times FECO_2 = (\dot{V}E - \dot{V}Pd)FAiCO_2 \ldots \quad (27)$$

$$\dot{V}Pd = \dot{V}E\frac{FAiCO_2 - FECO_2}{FAiCO_2} \ldots \quad (28)$$

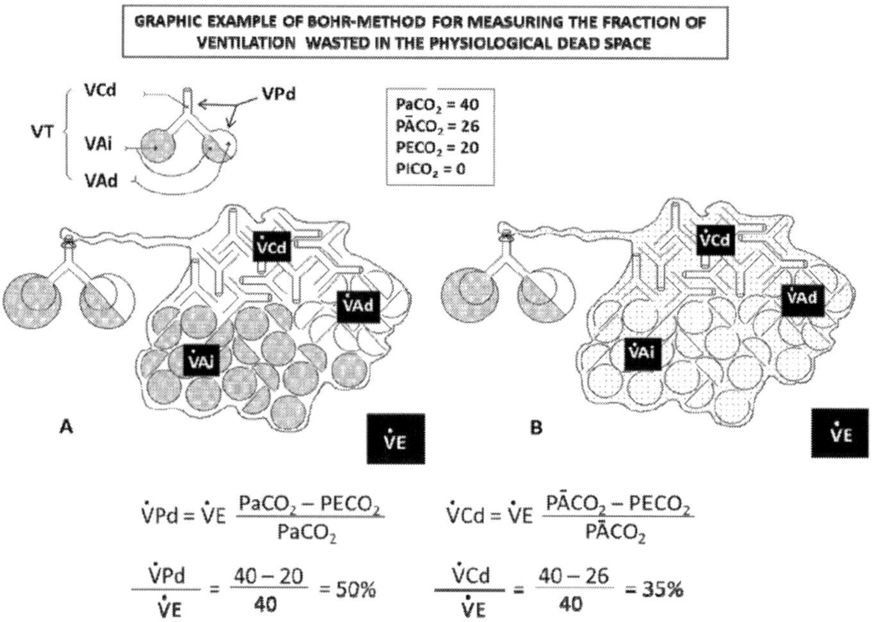

Figure 1: Graphic example of the functional equivalent of lungs with large alveolar dead space ventilation (**$\dot{V}$Ad**). The gases expired in the collecting bag per minute (**$\dot{V}$E**), which are a mixture of alveolar ideal (**$\dot{V}$A**i), alveolar dead space (**$\dot{V}$A**d, room air) and conductive dead space (**$\dot{V}$Cd**, room air) gases, are assumed to be either compartmentalized (A) or mixed (B) in the collecting bag.

Replacing F with P, and remembering that $PAiCO_2 \approx PaCO_2$, one calculates $\dot{V}Pd$ (Eq. 29):

$$\dot{V}Pd = \dot{V}E\frac{PaCO_2 - PECO_2}{PaCO_2} \ldots \quad (29)$$

Fig. **1** shows a graphic example of gas composition in different lung compartments ($\dot{V}E$, $\dot{V}Ai$, $\dot{V}Ad$ and $\dot{V}Cd$).

D. ALVEOLAR-IDEAL *VERSUS* ARTERIAL PO_2 AND PCO_2

Alveolar ideal and arterial PCO_2 values are virtually the same ($PAiCO_2 \approx PaCO_2$) even in cases of sizable right-to-left blood shunts, because the curve relating PCO_2 to total CO_2-content in blood is quite steep (Fig. **2**) - changes in CO_2-content are reflected by relatively small changes in PCO_2. In contrast, the alveolar ideal PO_2 ($PAiO_2$) cannot be equated to the arterial PO_2 (PaO_2) because, as Hb approaches O_2 saturation the curve relating PO_2 to the O_2 content in blood becomes progressively flatter (Fig. **2**) - even a small decrease in blood O_2 content due to admixture of shunted blood (right-to-left shunt) causes a sizable drop in PaO_2. In the example of Fig. **2**, a shunt fraction as large as 50% would result in a (a-Ai)PCO_2 gradient of only ~2 mmHg (negligible), while the (Ai-a)PO_2 gradient would be about 47 mmHg.

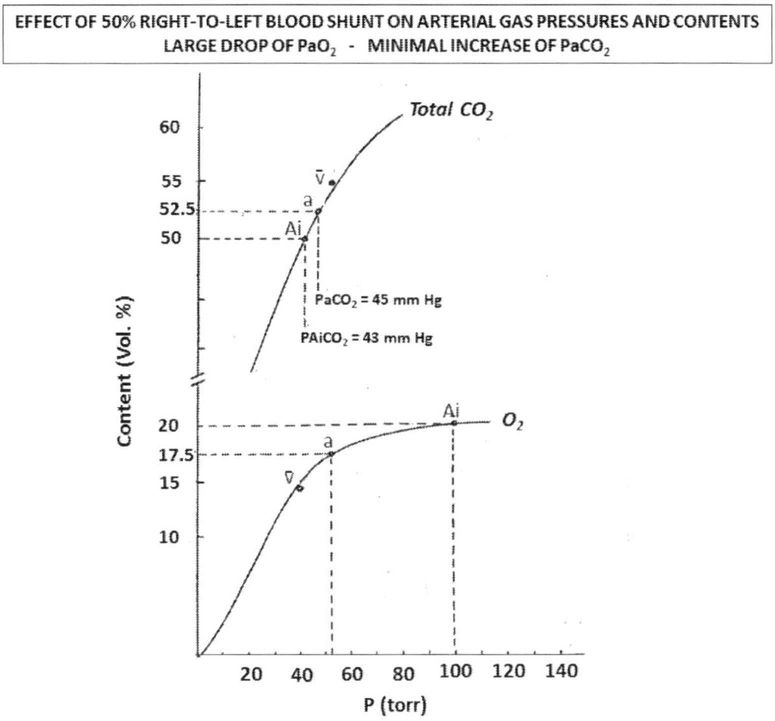

Figure 2: Plots of the relationship between partial pressures and contents of O_2 and CO_2 in blood in a patient with a 50% right-to-left blood shunt fraction (note that the O_2 content is HbO_2, while the CO_2 content represents the total CO_2). O_2 and CO_2 contents change by the same amount (2.5 vol%,

from Ai to a), but PO_2 drops dramatically from 100 to 52 torr (mmHg) while PCO_2 only increases by ~2 torr (mmHg). The mixed venous ($\bar{v}$) points are placed slightly off the curves because pH$\bar{v}$ causes a shift in the curves, as it is lower than pHAi and pHa (see Chapter 7). Note! In this example we have assumed that no compensation to hypoxemia (by hyperventilation) has taken place - compensatory hyperventilation would drastically reduce $PaCO_2$ and increase PaO_2.

E. DERIVATION OF ALVEOLAR GAS EQUATION

The alveolar gas equation (Eq. 33), is derived as follows (Eqs. 30-33):

$$R = \frac{\dot{V}CO_2}{\dot{V}O_2} = \frac{\dot{V}Ai \text{ x } FAiCO_2}{\dot{V}Ai(FIO_2\frac{FAiN_2}{FIN_2} - FAiO_2)} \ldots \quad (30)$$

$$FAiN_2 = 1 - (FAiO_2 + FAiCO_2) \ldots \quad (31)$$

$$FIN_2 = 1 - FIO_2 \ldots \quad (32)$$

Substituting, converting F to P, remembering that $FAiCO_2 \approx FaCO_2$ (and so $PAiCO_2 \approx PaCO_2$), and solving for $PAiO_2$:

$$PAiO_2 = PIO_2 - \frac{1-FIO_2(1-R)}{R} PaCO_2 \ldots \quad (33)$$

When R = 1, or when breathing 100% O_2 (FIO_2 = 1), the equation becomes (Eq. 34):

$$PAiO_2 = PIO_2 - PaCO_2 \ldots \quad (34)$$

because in both cases (Eq. 35):

$$\frac{1-FIO_2(1-R)}{R} = 1 \ldots \quad (35)$$

F. DERIVATION OF EQUATION RELATING $PaCO_2$ TO $\dot{V}Ai$ AND METABOLIC RATE ($\dot{V}CO_2$)

This equation (Eq. 41) is derived as follows (see Eqs. 36-41). Since all of the alveolar CO_2 comes from the alveolar ideal compartment:

$$\dot{V}CO_2(BTPS) = \dot{V}Ai(BTPS) \text{x } FAiCO_2 \ldots \quad (36)$$

$$FAiCO_2 = \frac{PaCO_2}{PB-47} \quad ... \qquad (37)$$

$$\dot{V}CO_2(BTPS) = \dot{V}Ai(BTPS)\frac{PaCO_2}{PB-47} \quad ... \qquad (38)$$

Since $\dot{V}CO_2$ is usually expressed in STPD, the STPD to BTPS conversion factor needs to be incorporated in the final equation:

$$\dot{V}CO_2(BTPS) = \dot{V}CO_2(STPD)\frac{310 \times 760}{273(PB-47)} = \dot{V}CO_2(STPD)\frac{863}{PB-47} \quad ... \qquad (39)$$

Substituting:

$$\dot{V}CO_2(STPD)\frac{863}{PB-47} = \dot{V}Ai(BTPS)\frac{PaCO_2}{PB-47} \quad ... \qquad (40)$$

$$PaCO_2 = \frac{863 \times \dot{V}CO_2(STPD)}{\dot{V}Ai(BTPS)} \quad ... \qquad (41)$$

Note: the constant "863" only varies with changes in body temperature (Table **1**)

Table 1: Effect of temperature on the "863" value (Eq. 41)

Body Temperature (°C)	37	38	39	40	41
Constant	863	865.8	868.6	871	874

APPENDIX 2

Ventilation-Perfusion

A. CALCULATION OF RIGHT-TO-LEFT BLOOD SHUNT AND ALVEOLAR DEAD SPACE FRACTIONS FOR THE NORMAL SUBJECT PRESENTED IN CHAPTER 7 (FIGURE 10). PB = 760 mmHg; HB = 15 g/100ml blood; R = 0.8; O_2 extraction: $(CaO_2 - C\bar{v}O_2)$ = 5 vol%.

End Capillary Blood O_2 Content in Each of the Three Lung Regions (Eqs. 1-3):

BASE: At $PO_2 = 90$ mmHg, pH 7.38, $\%SO_2 = 96\%$

$$O_2 \text{ content} = 90 \times 0.0031 + (15 \times 1.34)0.96 = 19.58 \text{ vol\%} \ldots \quad (1)$$

MIDDLE: At $PO_2 = 100$ mmHg, pH 7.4, $\%SO_2 = 97.1\%$

$$O_2 \text{ content} = 100 \times 0.0031 + (15 \times 1.34)0.971 = 19.83 \text{ vol\%} \ldots \quad (2)$$

UPPER: At $PO_2 = 130$ mmHg, pH 7.44, $\%SO_2 = 98.6\%$

$$O_2 \text{ content} = 130 \times 0.0031 + (15 \times 1.34)0.986 = 20.22 \text{ vol\%} \ldots \quad (3)$$

Arterial O_2 Content (Eqs. 4-5) and PaO_2 (Note: In This Example We Assume That There is No Conductive Shunt):

$$CaO_2 = 19.58 \times 3/6 + 19.83 \times 2/6 + 20.22 \times 1/6 \ldots \quad (4)$$

$$CaO_2 = 19.77 \text{ vol \%} \ldots \quad (5)$$

A content of 19.77 vol% at pH = 7.4 corresponds to $PaO_2 = \sim 98$ mmHg

Ideal Compartment $PAiO_2$ (Eq. 6) and O_2 Content (Eq. 7):

$$PAiO_2 = 149.3 - \frac{1-0.2094(1-0.8)}{0.8}40 = 101.4 \text{ mmHg} \ldots \quad (6)$$

At $PAiO_2 = 101.4$ mmHg, $\%SAiO_2 = 97.2\%$

$CAiO_2 = 101.4 \times 0.0031 + (15 \times 1.34)0.971 = 19.85$ vol% … (7)

O_2 content of Mixed Venous Blood (Eq. 8):

$C\bar{v}O_2 = CaO_2$ - extraction = 19.77 - 5 = 14.77 vol% … (8)

$(Ai\text{-}a)PO_2$ Gradient (Eq. 9):

$(Ai\text{-}a)PO_2 = 101.4 - 98 = 3.4$ mmHg … (9)

This gradient indicates that there is a very small amount of maldistribution/diffusion shunt-like effect.

Physiological Shunt Fraction (Eq. 10):

$$\frac{\dot{Q}Ps}{\dot{Q}} = \frac{19.85 - 19.77}{19.85 - 14.77} = 1.6\% \; ... \qquad (10)$$

1.6% of the total cardiac output is made of shunted (venous) blood.

Mixed Alveolar (End Tidal) PO_2 (Eq. 11) and PCO_2 (Eq. 12):

$P\bar{A}O_2 = 90 \times 2.5/6 + 100 \times 2/6 + 130 \times 1.5/6 = 103.3$ mmHg … (11)

$P\bar{A}CO_2 = 42 \times 2.5/6 + 40 \times 2/6 + 35 \times 1.5/6 = 39.6$ mmHg … (12)

$(\bar{A}\text{-}Ai)PO_2$ (Eq. 13) and $(Ai\text{-}\bar{A})PCO_2$ (Eq. 14) Gradients:

$(\bar{A}\text{-}Ai)PO_2 = 103.3 - 101.4 = \sim 2$ mmHg … (13)

$(Ai\text{-}\bar{A})PCO_2 = 40 - 39.6 = 0.4$ mmHg … (14)

Indicative of Minimal Alveolar Dead Space Ventilation

Alveolar Dead Space Fraction (Eq. 15):

$$\frac{\dot{V}Ad}{\dot{V}\bar{A}} = \frac{PaCO_2 - P\bar{A}CO_2}{PaCO_2} = \frac{40 - 39.6}{40} = 1\% \; ... \qquad (15)$$

B. CALCULATIONS OF RIGHT-TO-LEFT BLOOD SHUNT AND ALVEOLAR DEAD SPACE FRACTIONS FOR THE PATIENT DESCRIBED IN CHAPTER 7 (SEE DATA REPEATED IN TABLE 1)

Table 1: Laboratory blood and gas data (air breathing)

PB (mmHg)	760	**Hb (g/100 ml blood)**	15
PaO_2 (mmHg)	80	**pHa**	7.42
$PaCO_2$ (mmHg)	35	**R**	0.8
$P\bar{A}CO_2$ (mmHg)	30	**$(Ca - C\bar{v})O_2$ (vol%)**	5

Physiological Shunt Fraction (Eq. 22):

$$PIO_2 = (760\text{-}47)0.2094 = 149.3 \text{ mmHg} \ldots \quad (16)$$

$$PAiO_2 = 149.3 - \frac{1-0.2094(1-0.8)}{0.8}35 = 107.4 \text{ mmHg} \ldots \quad (17)$$

At $PAiO_2$ = 107.4 mmHg, pHAi = 7.42, $\%SAiO_2$ = 97.7%

$$CAiO_2 = 107.4 \times 0.0031 + (15 \times 1.34)0.977 = 19.97 \text{ vol\%} \ldots \quad (18)$$

At PaO_2 = 80 mmHg, pHa = 7.42, $\%SaO_2$ = 95.1%

$$CaO_2 = 80 \times 0.0031 + (15 \times 1.34)0.951 = 19.36 \ldots \quad (19)$$

$$C\bar{v}O_2 = 19.36 - 5 = 14.36 \text{ vol\%} \ldots \quad (20)$$

$$(Ai\text{-}a)Po_2 = 107.4 - 80 = 27.4 \text{ mmHg} \ldots \quad (21)$$

$$\frac{\dot{Q}Ps}{\dot{Q}} = \frac{19.97-19.36}{19.97-14.36} = 10.8\% \ldots \quad (22)$$

Alveolar Dead Space Fraction (Eq. 23):

$$\frac{\dot{V}Ad}{\dot{V}\bar{A}} = \frac{PaCO_2 - P\bar{A}CO_2}{PaCO_2} = \frac{35-30}{35} = 14\% \ldots \quad (23)$$

14% of the total alveolar ventilation is wasted in alveolar dead space.

C. CALCULATION OF ANATOMICAL (CONDUCTIVE, Eq. 30) AND MALDISTRIBUTION-DIFFUSION (Eq. 31) COMPONENTS OF PHYSIOLOGICAL SHUNT (Eq. 22) FOR THE PATIENT DESCRIBED IN CHAPTER 7 (SEE DATA REPEATED IN TABLE 2)

The patient has the following values while breathing 100% O_2:

Table 2: Laboratory blood and gas data (100% FIO_2 breathing)

PB (mmHg)	760	**Hb g/100 ml blood**	15
PaO_2 (mmHg)	600	**pHa**	7.38
$PaCO_2$ (mmHg)	40	**R**	0.8
$P\bar{A}CO_2$ (mmHg)	34	**$(Ca - C\bar{v})O_2$ (vol%)**	5

Conductive (Anatomical) Shunt Fraction:

$PIO_2 = (760 - 47)1 = 713$ mmHg … (24)

$PAiO_2 = 713 - 40 = 673$ mmHg … (25)

At $PAiO_2 = 673$ mmHg, $\%SAiO_2 = 100\%$

$CAiO_2 = 673 \times 0.0031 + (15 \times 1.34)1 = 22.19$ vo% … (26)

At $PaO_2 = 600$ mmHg, $\%SaO_2 = 100\%$

$CaO_2 = 600 \times 0.0031 + (15 \times 1.34)1 = 21.96$ vol% … (27)

$C\bar{v}O_2 = 22 - 5 = 16.96$ vol% … (28)

$(Ai\text{-}a)Po_2 = 673 - 600 = 73$ mmHg … (29)

$$\frac{\dot{Q}Cs}{\dot{Q}} = \frac{22.19-21.96}{22.19-16.96} = 4.4\% \ \ldots \quad (30)$$

Maldistribution Shunt:

$$\frac{\dot{Q}Ms}{\dot{Q}} = \frac{\dot{Q}Ps}{\dot{Q}} - \frac{\dot{Q}Cs}{\dot{Q}} = 10.8 - 4.4 = 6.4\% \ \ldots \quad (31)$$

> **Note!** With 100% O_2 breathing $(Ai\text{-}a)PO_2$ increases from 27.4 to 73 mmHg in spite of the fact that the shunt fraction decreases from ~11% to ~4%. The reasons are explained in Chapter **7**, Figs. **15** and **16**.

APPENDIX 3

Symbols, Normal Values, Equations and Oxygen Dissociation Curves

A. SYMBOLS (TABLE 1)

Table 1: Most common symbols used in respiratory physiology

Primary Symbols	Definition	Secondary Symbols	Definition
C	Concentration of gas in blood	A	Alveolar
D	Diffusing capacity	$\bar{A}$	Alveolar average gas (mixed, end-tidal)
F	Fractional concentration of dry gas	Ad	Alveolar dead space gas
f	frequency of breathing (breaths per minute)	Ai	Alveolar ideal gas
P	Pressure of gas	Ae	Alveolar effective gas
Q	Blood volume	B	Barometric
$\dot{Q}$	Blood volume per unit time – flow rate	Cd	Conductive dead space gas
R	Respiratory Exchange Ratio ($\dot{V}CO_2/\dot{V}O_2$). At steady state, R = RQ (Respiratory Quotient)	Cs	Conductive blood shunt
S	Saturation of hemoglobin with O_2 or CO_2	E	Expired
V	Volume of gas	I	Inspired
$\dot{V}$	Volume of gas per unit time - usually referred to as "minute ventilation"	Ms	Maldistribution shunt-like effect
		Ps	Physiological blood shunt

B. NORMAL VALUES USEFUL IN RESPIRATORY PHYSIOLOGY

Oxygen

$(Ai\text{-}a)PO_2$ (gradient between alveolar ideal and arterial PO_2, also symbolized as $AaDO_2$; air breathing) = 2-4 mmHg (up to 10 mmHg in old people)

$(Ai\text{-}a)PO_2$ gradient (100% O_2 breathing) = 35 mmHg

CaO_2 (total) = 19.8 vol% = 19.8 ml O_2/100 ml blood (Hb = 15 g/100 ml blood, pHa = 7.4, PaO_2 = 98 mmHg)

Camillo Peracchia and Nasr H. Anaizi

CaO_2 (dissolved) = 0.30 vol% (PaO_2 = 98 mmHg)

CO_2 (total) = 14.6 vol% ($P\bar{v}O_2$ = 40 mmHg, Hb = 15 g/100 ml blood, $pH\bar{v}$ = 7.35)

$C\bar{v}O_2$ (dissolved) = 0.124 vol% ($P\bar{v}O_2$ = 40 mmHg)

$FAiO_2$ = 14% ($PAiO_2$ = 100 mmHg)

FIO_2 = 20.94%

HbO_2 capacity = 1.34 ml O_2/g Hb (it should be 1.39, but some Hb is likely to be associated with carbon monoxide)

Hb-P_{50} = 26.5 mmHg (37°C, pH = 7.4, PCO_2 = 40 mmHg)

O_2 debt (max) = 20 l (70 kg, adult male)

(CaO_2 - $C\bar{v}O_2$) = 5 vol% (O_2 extraction at rest, normal $\dot{V}O_2$ and $\dot{Q}$)

$(CaO_2 - C\bar{v}O_2)_{cerebral}$ = 6.4 vol%

$(CaO_2 - C\bar{v}O_2)_{coronaric}$ = 11.5 vol%

$(CaO_2 - C\bar{v}O_2)_{renal}$ = 1.3 vol%

$(CaO_2 - C\bar{v}O_2)_{splancnic}$ = 4.1 vol%

O_2 solubility factor = 0.0031 vol%/mmHg

O_2 stores ≈1.3 l (STPD)

PaO_2 = 98 mmHg

$PAiO_2$ = 100 mmHg (alveolar ideal PO_2)

$P\bar{v}O_2$ = 40 mmHg (mixed venous PO_2)

%SaO_2 = 97.1% (% Hb's O_2 saturation in arterial blood at 37°C, pH 7.4, PO_2 = 100 mmHg)

$\dot{V}O_2$ (at rest, STPD) = 250 ml/min (males), 200 ml/min (females)

$\dot{V}O_2$ (max/kg, in a young male) = 58 - 0.4 x age (years), ml/kg x min

Carbon Dioxide

$CaCO_2$ (total) = 21 mEq/l blood (Hct = 0.45, $PaCO_2$ = 40 mmHg) ≈ 47 Vol.%

$CaCO_2$ (dissolved) = 1.2 mEq/l ($PaCO_2$ = 40 mmHg)

$C\bar{v}CO_2$ (total) = 22.5 mEq/l blood (Hct = 0.45, $P\bar{v}CO_2$ = 47 mmHg) ≈ 50.4 Vol.%

($C\bar{v}CO_2$ - $CaCO_2$) = 4 vol%

CO_2 solubility factor = 0.0301 mEq/l x mmHg. CO_2 stores ≈ 6 l (STPD)

$FAiCO_2$ = 5.6% (Fraction of mixed alveolar or end tidal, CO_2)($P_{Ai}CO_2$ = 40 mmHg, P_B = 760 mmHg)

$FICO_2$ = 0 mmHg (Fraction of inspired CO_2)

$P\bar{A}CO_2$ = 40 mmHg (Pressure of mixed alveolar or end tidal, CO_2)

$PAiCO_2$ = 40 mmHg (Pressure of ideal alveolar CO_2)

$PaCO_2$ = 40 mmHg (Pressure of arterial CO_2)

$P\bar{v}CO_2$ = 47 mmHg (Pressure of mixed venous CO_2)

$\dot{V}CO_2$(at rest, STPD) = 200 ml/min

Nitrogen

$F\bar{A}N_2$ = 80.4% ($F\bar{A}O_2$ = 14%, $F\bar{A}CO_2$ = 5.6%)

FIN_2 = 79.06%

$P\bar{A}N_2$ = 573 mmHg (PB = 760 mmHg, T = 37°C, $P\bar{A}O_2$ = 100 mmHg, $P\bar{A}CO_2$ = 40 mmHg)

PIN_2 = 564 mmHg (PB = 760 mmHg, T = 37°C)

Table 2: Partial Pressures of Water Vapor

T, °C	PH_2O (mmHg)	T, °C	PH_2O (mmHg)
20	17.5	27	26.7
21	18.7	28	28.5
22	19.8	29	30.0
23	21.1	37	47.0
24	22.4	38	49.3
25	23.8	39	51.6
26	25.2	40	53.9

Water (Table 2)

PH_2O (37°C) = 47 mmHg

PAH_2O = 47 mmHg (37°C)

PIH_2O = 47 mmHg (37°C)

For other temperatures, PH_2O can be approximated by the following empirical relationship:

$$PH_2O = \text{antiln}[(1.717 \text{ x} \ln T) - 2.3475]$$

Lung Volumes (For a young adult male)

ERV = 1200 ml

FRC = 2400 ml

IC = 3600 ml

RV = 1200 ml

TLC = 6000 ml

VC = 4800 ml

RV/TLC = 20%

VC/TLC = 80%

FRC/TLC = 40%

Ventilation

F = 12 breaths/min

$\dot{V}\bar{A}$ = 4500 ml/min

VCd = 150 ml

$\dot{V}E$ = 6000 ml/min

VT = 500 ml

$\dot{V}/\dot{Q}$ = 0.8 - 1

$\dot{V}Pd/\dot{V}\bar{A}$ = 0.3

$\dot{V}Cd/\dot{V}E$ = 0.3

Mechanics of Breathing

Airway resistance = 1.6 cm H_2O/ l x sec

Compliance of lungs and chest wall (C) = 100 ml/cm H_2O

1 mmHg = 1 torr = 13.6 mm H_2O = 1.36 cm H_2O

10 cm H_2O = 1 kilopascal (K_{PA})

FEV_1/FVC (forced expiratory volume over forced vital capacity, 1 sec) = 83%

FEV_3/FVC (forced expiratory volume over forced vital capacity, 3 sec) = 97%

$FEF_{25-75\%}$ (middle volume expired per second) = 3.5 l/sec

$\dot{V}max_{50\%}$ (maximum flow after expiration of 50% VC) = 4 l/sec

$\dot{V}max_{75\%}$ (maximum flow after expiration of 75% VC) = 2.5 l/sec

Maximal work of breathing = 10 kg x m/breath

PEFR (peak expiratory flow rate, ATPS) = >400 l/min

PIFR (peak inspiratory flow rate, ATPS) = >300 l/min

Peak Air Way pressure (PAW, during mechanical ventilation) = 18 - 22 cm H_2O

MVV (maximal voluntary ventilation, at ATPS) = 170 l/min

Work of quiet breathing = 0.5 kg x m/min

Acid Base

Buffering capacity of blood (BC): *in vitro* = 8.2 + 1.56 x [Hb]; *in vivo* ≈ 1/3 of the *in vivo* value

$[HCO_3^-]$ = 24 mEq/l plasma (pH = 7.4)

$\Delta[HCO_3^-]/\Delta pH$ (blood *in vitro*) = -30 slykes (Hb = 15 g/100 ml blood)

$\Delta[HCO_3^-]/\Delta pH$ (blood *in vivo*) = -10 slykes (Hb = 15 g/100ml blood)

pHa = 7.4

$pH\bar{v}$ = 7.35

Circulation

Arterial blood pressure (BP) = 125/75 mmHg

Pulmonary artery pressure = 21/9 mmHg

Right atrial pressure (mean) = <5 mmHg

Pulmonary capillary wedge pressure (P_{pcw}, mean) = 9 mmHg (indicative of left atrial pressure)

[Hb] = 16 g/100 ml blood (male); 14 g/100 ml blood (female)

Hematocrit = 47% (male); 43% (female)

Heart Rate (HR) = 70/min

HR (max) = 210 – (0.7 x age) (in years)

Ejection fraction = 67%

Cardiac output ($\dot{Q}$) = 5-6 l/min

Cardiac index = $\dot{Q}/m^2$. Body surface area (m^2) = 0.0097(Height in cm + Weight in Kg)

$\dot{Q}Ps/\dot{Q}$ =<7%

Plasma volume = 42 ml/Kg weight

Plasma proteins = 7.3 gm/100 ml

Serum albumine = 4.6 gm/100 ml

Metabolism

1 liter O_2 = 4.83 kcal/min

R (exchange ratio) = 0.8 - 0.85 (at rest, at steady state, mixed diet)

RQ = 0.8 - 0.85 (mixed diet)

RQ = 0.7 (fat oxidation)

RQ = 1.0 (carbohydrate oxidation)

C. EQUATIONS MOST COMMONLY USED

- Oxygen consumption (atmospheric exchange, Eq. 1)

$$\dot{V}O_2 = \dot{V}E(FIO_2 \frac{FEN_2}{FIN_2} - FEO_2 \text{ (STPD) } \ldots \qquad (1)$$

- Fick equation for measuring oxygen consumption (circulatory exchange, Eq. 2) - $(CaO_2 - C\bar{v}O_2)$ is usually referred as O_2 extraction $(\dot{V}O_2/\dot{Q}$ ratio)

$$\dot{V}O_2 = \dot{Q}(CaO_2 - C\bar{v}O_2)\ (STPD)\ \ldots \quad (2)$$

- CO_2 production (atmospheric exchange, Eq. 3), assuming $FICO_2 = 0$

$$\dot{V}CO_2 = \dot{V}E \times FECO_2 = \dot{V}\bar{A} \times F\bar{A}CO_2 = \dot{V}Ai \times FAiCO_2\ (STPD)\ \ldots \quad (3)$$

- Fick equation for CO_2 consumption (circulatory exchange, Eq. 4)

$$\dot{V}CO_2 = \dot{Q}(C\bar{v}CO_2 - CaCO_2)\ (STPD)\ \ldots \quad (4)$$

- Exchange ratio (R; Eq. 5) At steady state R = RQ (respiratory quotient)

$$R = \frac{\dot{V}CO_2}{\dot{V}O_2}\ \ldots \quad (5)$$

- Conductive dead space ventilation, assuming $FICO_2 = 0$ (Eq. 6)

$$\dot{V}Cd = \dot{V}E\frac{P\bar{A}CO_2 - PECO_2}{P\bar{A}CO_2}\ (BTPS)\ \ldots \quad (6)$$

- Physiological dead space ventilation, assuming $FICO_2 = 0$ (Eq. 7). In normal subjects $\dot{V}Cd = \dot{V}Pd$ because the alveolar dead space ventilation $(\dot{V}Ad)$ is close to zero.

$$\dot{V}Pd = \dot{V}E\frac{PaCO_2 - PECO_2}{PaCO_2}\ (BTPS)\ \ldots \quad (7)$$

- Alveolar dead space ventilation (Eq. 8)

$$\dot{V}Ad = \dot{V}E\frac{PaCO_2 - P\bar{A}CO_2}{PaCO_2}\ (BTPS)\ \ldots \quad (8)$$

- Alveolar gas equation (Eq. 9). Note: by using $P\bar{A}CO_2$ rather than $PaCO_2$ one calculates $P\bar{A}O_2$ (mixed alveolar PO_2)

$$PAiO_2 = PIO_2 - \frac{1 - FIO_2(1-R)}{R}PaCO_2\ \ldots \quad (9)$$

- Relation among ideal alveolar ventilation, $PaCO_2$ and metabolic rate, at 37°C (Eq. 10).

$$PaCO_2 = \frac{863 \text{ x } \dot{V}CO_2}{\dot{V}Ai} \frac{(STPD)}{(BTPS)} \ldots \quad (10)$$

- Oxygen content equation (sum of dissolved O_2 and Hb associated O_2, Eq. 11)

$$C\,O_2 = PO_2 \text{ x } 0.0031 + (Hb \text{ x } 1.34)\%SO_2 \ldots \quad (11)$$

- Henderson-Hasselbalch equation (relationship among pH, plasma $[HCO_3^-]$ and PCO_2, Eq. 12)

$$pH = 6.1 + \log \frac{[HCO_3^-]}{0.0301 \text{ x } PCO_2} \ldots \quad (12)$$

- Buffering capacity (BC) of blood (Eqs. 13 and 14; for a normal Hb = 14.5 – 15 g/100 ml blood, the *in vivo* BC ≈ 10).

$$BC\ (in\ vitro) = 8.2 + 1.56 \text{ x } [Hb] \ldots \quad (13)$$

$$BC\ (in\ vivo) = \frac{8.2 + 1.56 \text{ x } [Hb]}{3} \ldots \quad (14)$$

- Equation used to calculate the **"predicted"** bicarbonate concentration ($[HCO_3^-]_{predicted}$), if pHa were achieved as a result of a pure, uncompensated, respiratory condition (Eq. 15).

$$-BC = \frac{[HCO_3^-]_{standard} - [HCO_3^-]_{predicted}}{pHa_{standard} - pHa} \ldots \quad (15)$$

where $[HCO_3^-]_{standard} = 24$ mEq/l (plasma) and $pHa_{standard} = 7.4$, and BC is the Buffer Capacity. Note that BC has a negative sign because in the plot of $[HCO_3^-]$ *versus* pH because the BC line has a negative slope (see the Davenport diagram in **Chapter 6, Figure 5**).

- Base excess (BE; Eq. 16) is the difference between actual and predicted $[HCO_3^-]$

$$BE = [HCO_3^-]_{actual} - [HCO_3^-]_{predicted} \cdots \quad (16)$$

- Equation used to calculate the change in $[HCO_3^-]$ with a change in pH due to a pure, uncompensated, respiratory disorder (Eq. 17; $[HCO_3^-]_{standard} = 24$, $pH_{standard} = 7.4$).

$$-BC = \frac{\Delta HCO_3^-}{\Delta pH} = \frac{[HCO_3^-]_{standard} - [HCO_3^-]_x}{pH_{standard} - pH_x} = \frac{24 - [HCO_3^-]_x}{7.4 - pH_x} \ldots \quad (17)$$

- Physiological blood shunt fraction equation (Eq. 18)

$$\frac{\dot{Q}Ps}{\dot{Q}} = \frac{CAiO_2 - CaO_2}{CAiO_2 - C\bar{v}O_2} \ldots \quad (18)$$

- Ideal blood-flow fraction equation (Eq. 19)

$$\frac{\dot{Q}Ai}{\dot{Q}} = \frac{CaO_2 - C\bar{v}O_2}{CAiO_2 - C\bar{v}O_2} \ldots \quad (19)$$

- Equation for volume conversion of gas or gas mixture (Eq. 20; a change in gas volume results from changes in P, T and humidity):

$$\frac{(P_1 - PH_2O_1)V_1}{T_1} = \frac{(P_2 - PH_2O_2)V_2}{T_2} = K \ldots \quad (20)$$

- Equation for conversion of fractional concentration to partial pressure and *vice versa* (Dalton's law; Eq. 21):

$$P_x = F_x(PB - PH_2O) \ldots \quad (21)$$

- Equation for calculating compliance (C, Eq. 22) - pressure/volume curve.

$$C = \frac{\Delta\,Volume}{\Delta\,Pressure} \ldots \quad (22)$$

D. OXYGEN DISSOCIATION CURVES

The following HbO_2 dissociation curves (Figures. 1-4), corrected for pH and temperature, can be used to approximate the hemoglobin's O_2 saturation (%) knowing PO_2 and *vice versa*. A more precise value can be obtained from the blood oxygen dissociation line chart, published by Kleman, G.R. and Nunn, J.F. (J. Appl. Physiol., 21, 1484, 1966), which allows one to determine O_2 saturation (or PO_2) corrected for pH, temperature and base excess (BE).

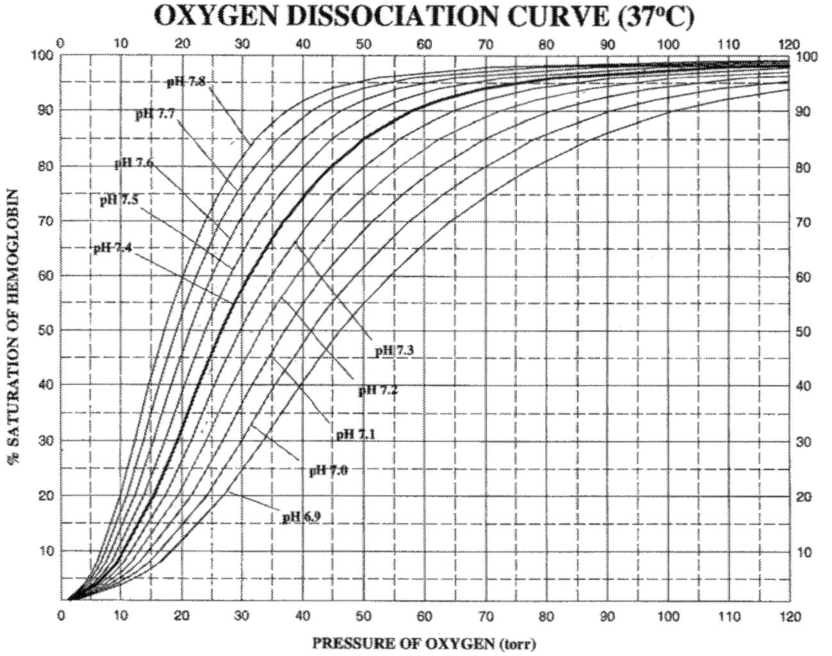

Figure 1: Effect of pH on the hemoglobin's oxygen-dissociation curve at 37°C

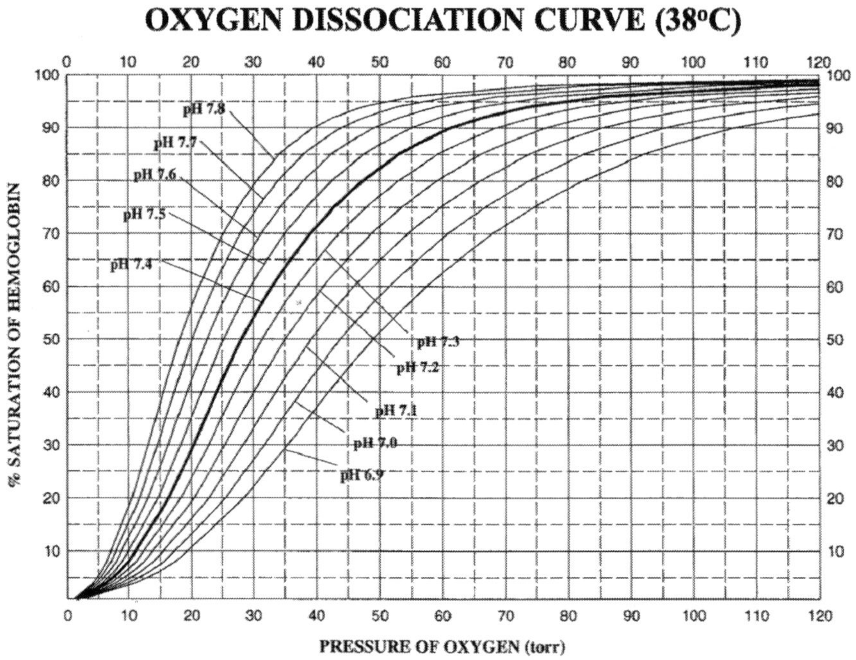

Figure 2: Effect of pH on the hemoglobin's oxygen-dissociation curve at 38°C

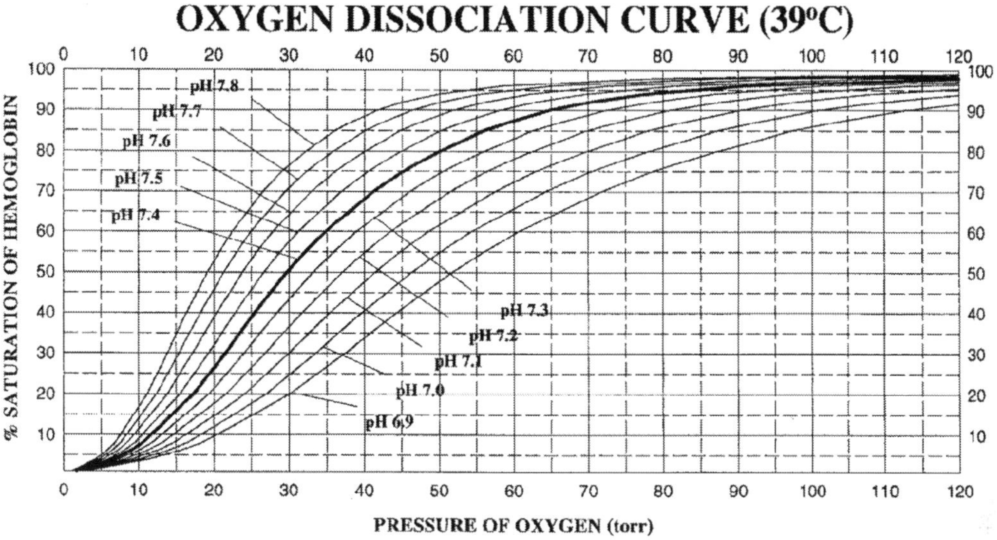

Figure 3: Effect of pH on the hemoglobin's oxygen-dissociation curve at 39°C

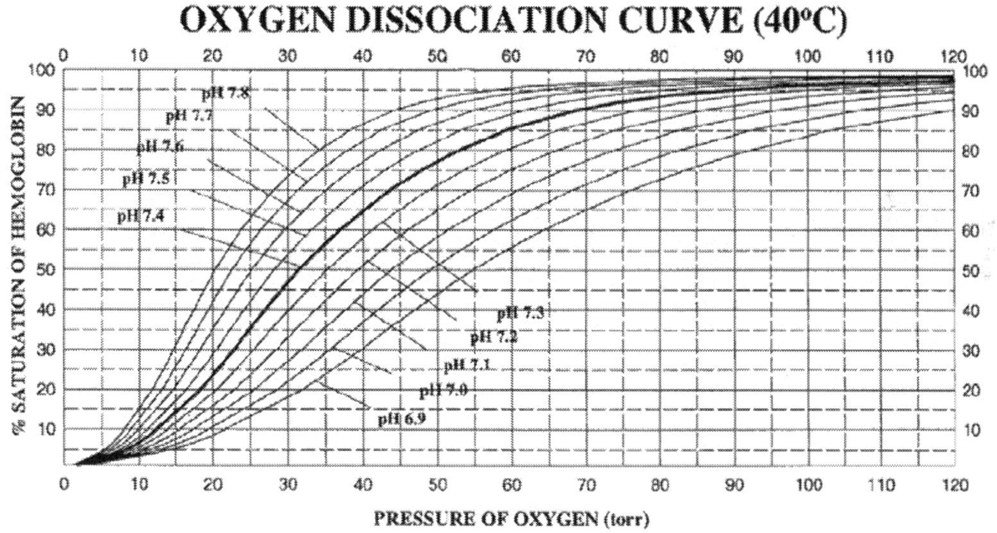

Figure 4: Effect of pH on the hemoglobin's oxygen-dissociation curve at 40°C

APPENDIX 4

Calculations

Below are examples of methods used to calculate right-to-left blood shunt fraction, alveolar dead space fraction, partial pressure of O_2 in mixed venous blood, and base excess (BE).

A. RIGHT-TO-LEFT BLOOD SHUNT FRACTION

1. Physiological shunt fraction ($\dot{Q}Ps/\dot{Q}$) and $(Ai\text{-}a)PO_2$ calculations (Eqs. 1-6) for a subject breathing room air and having the following values:

PaO_2 = 80 mmHg, $PaCO_2$ = 40 mmHg, R = 0.8, pHa = 7.4, Hb = 15 g/100 ml blood, Body Temperature (T) = 37°C, O_2 extraction = 5 vol%, Barometric Pressure (BP) = 747 mmHg.

$$PAiO_2 = (747 - 47)0.2094 - \frac{1-0.2094(1-0.8)}{0.8}40 = 98.6 \text{ mmHg} \ldots \quad (1)$$

$\%SAiO_2 \approx 97.5\%$ (at $PAiO_2$ = 98.6, pHa = 7.4 and T = 37°C)

$$CAiO_2 = 98.6 \times 0.0031 + (15 \times 1.34)0.975 = 19.9 \text{ vol\%} \ldots \quad (2)$$

$\%SaO_2 \approx 96\%$ (at PaO_2 = 80, pHa = 7.4 and T = 37°C)

$$CaO_2 = 80 \times 0.0031 + (15 \times 1.34)0.96 = 19.5 \text{ vol\%} \ldots \quad (3)$$

Since extraction is 5 vol%

$$C\bar{v}O_2 = CaO_2 - 5 = 14.5 \text{ vol\%} \ldots \quad (4)$$

$$\frac{\dot{Q}Ps}{\dot{Q}} = \frac{19.9-19.5}{19.9-14.5} = 7.4\% \ldots \quad (5)$$

$$(Ai\text{-}a)PO_2 = 98.6 - 80 = 18.6 \text{ mmHg} \ldots \quad (6)$$

2. Conductive shunt fraction ($\dot{Q}Cs/\dot{Q}$) is calculated as above, with blood samples taken while the subject breathes 100% FIO_2

3. Shunt caused by $\dot{V}/\dot{Q}$ maldistribution and/or diffusion impairment ($\dot{Q}Ms/\dot{Q}$), is calculated as follows (Eq. 7):

$$\frac{\dot{Q}Ms}{\dot{Q}} = \frac{\dot{Q}Ps}{\dot{Q}} - \frac{\dot{Q}Cs}{\dot{Q}} \ldots \quad (7)$$

B. ALVEOLAR DEAD SPACE FRACTION

There are two ways to calculate $\dot{V}Ad/\dot{V}\bar{A}$.

1. Both $PaCO_2$ and $P\bar{A}CO_2$ are available (Eq. 8).

Assume the following values: $PaCO_2$= 40 mmHg and $P\bar{A}CO_2$ = 30 mmHg.

$$\frac{\dot{V}Ad}{\dot{V}\bar{A}} = \frac{PaCO_2 - P\bar{A}CO_2}{PaCO_2} = \frac{40-30}{40} = 25\% \ldots \quad (8)$$

2. $P\bar{A}CO_2$ is not available (Eqs. 9-15)

The fraction of alveolar dead space ventilation can still be calculated as long as we know the values of VCd, VT, f, $\dot{V}O_2$, R and $PaCO_2$.

Assume: VCd = 150 ml (BTPS), VT = 670 ml (BTPS), f = 11, $\dot{V}O_2$= 250 ml/min (STPD), R = 0.8, $PaCO_2$ = 40 mmHg, BT = 37°C.

$$\dot{V}E = VT \times f = 0.67 \times 11 = 7.37 \text{ l/min (BTPS)} \ldots \quad (9)$$

$$\dot{V}Cd = VCd \times f = 0.15 \times 11 = 1.65 \text{ l/min (BTPS)} \ldots \quad (10)$$

$$\dot{V}\bar{A} = \dot{V}E - \dot{V}Cd = 7.37 - 1.65 = 5.72 \text{ l/min (BTPS)} \ldots \quad (11)$$

$$\dot{V}CO_2 = \dot{V}O_2 \times R = 0.25 \times 0.8 = 0.2 \text{ l/min (STPD)} \ldots \quad (12)$$

$$\dot{V}Ai = \frac{863 \times \dot{V}CO_2}{PaCO_2} = \frac{863 \times 0.2}{40} = 4.32 \text{ l/ min(STPD)} \ldots \quad (13)$$

$$\dot{V}Ad = \dot{V}\bar{A} - \dot{V}Ai = 5.72 - 4.32 = 1.4 \text{ l/min (BTPS)} \ldots \quad (14)$$

$$\frac{\dot{V}Ad}{\dot{V}\bar{A}} = \frac{1.4}{5.72} = 24.5\% \ldots \quad (15)$$

C. MIXED VENOUS PO_2 ($P\bar{v}O_2$), INDICATIVE OF AVERAGE TISSUE OXYGENATION

To estimate $P\bar{v}O_2$ one needs first to calculate $\%S\bar{v}O_2$ (Eqs. 16-22). A way to do so is by calculating the fraction $C\bar{v}O_2/O_2$-capacity.

The following values are needed: PaO_2, $\dot{V}O_2$, $\dot{Q}$, Hb, Body Temperature (T), pHa and $pH\bar{v}$.

Assume: $PaO_2 = 98$ mmHg, $\dot{V}O_2 = 250$ ml/min (STPD), $\dot{Q} = 5$ l/min, Hb = 15 g/100 ml blood, T = 37°C, pHa = 7.4, $pH\bar{v} = 7.35$.

$SaO_2 \approx 98\%$ (at $PaO_2 = 98$, pHa = 7.4 and T = 37°C)

$$CaO_2 = 98 \times 0.0031 + (15 \times 1.34)0.98 = 20 \text{ vol\%} \ldots \qquad (16)$$

$$\frac{\dot{V}O_2}{\dot{Q}} = (CaO_2 - C\bar{v}O_2) \ \ldots \qquad (17)$$

$$\frac{0.25}{5} = (0.2 - C\bar{v}O_2) \ \ldots \qquad (18)$$

$$C\bar{v}O_2 = 0.2 - \frac{0.25}{5} = 15 \text{ vol\%} \ \ldots \qquad (19)$$

$$\%S\bar{v}O_2 = \frac{C\bar{v}O_2}{O_2 \text{ capacity}} \ \ldots \qquad (20)$$

$$\%S\bar{v}O_2 = \frac{15}{1.34 \times 15} = 74.6\% \ \ldots \qquad (21)$$

Corrected for Bohr shift due to $pH\bar{v} = 7.35$

$$P\bar{v}O_2 = \sim 42 \text{ mmHg} \ldots \qquad (22)$$

Note: this calculation introduces a small error, because $C\bar{v}O_2$ is the sum of dissolved O_2 and Hb-associated O_2, whereas O_2-capacity is just Hb-associated O_2. However, due to the low PO_2 of venous blood, the dissolved O_2 is quite low (dissolved O_2 cannot be calculated because we don't know $P\bar{v}O_2$). For a more precise calculation see below (**D. Note:**)

D. HOW TO ESTIMATE PaO_2 KNOWING THE VALUES OF RIGHT-TO-LEFT BLOOD SHUNT FRACTION AND O_2-EXTRACTION (Eqs. 23-32)

Assume: PB = 760 mmHg, Hb = 15 g/100 ml blood, FiO_2 = 20.94%, R = 0.8, $PaCO_2$ = 40 mmHg, pHa = 7.4, $\dot{Q}Ps/\dot{Q}$ = 20%, and $(Ca - C\bar{v})O_2$ = 5 vol%.

$$PAiO_2 = (760 - 47)0.2094 - \frac{1-0.2094(1-0.8)}{0.8}40 = 101.4 \text{ mmHg} \ldots \quad (23)$$

$$\%SAiO_2 \approx 98\%$$

$$CAiO_2 = 101.4 \times 0.0031 + (15 \times 1.34)0.98 = 20 \ldots \quad (24)$$

$$\frac{\dot{Q}Ps}{\dot{Q}} = 0.2 = \frac{20-CaO_2}{20-(CaO_2-5)} \ldots \quad (25)$$

$$CaO_2 = 18.75 \text{ vol\%} \ldots \quad (26)$$

$$O_2 \text{ capacity} = 15 \times 1.34 = 20.1 \text{ vol\%} \ldots \quad (27)$$

$$\%SaO_2 \approx \frac{CaO_2}{O_2\text{capacity}} \approx \frac{18.75}{20 \times 1.34} \approx 93.3\% \ldots \quad (28)$$

$$PaO_2 \approx 66 \text{ mmHg} \ldots \quad (29)$$

<u>**Note**</u>: this calculation introduces a small error because CaO_2 is the sum of dissolved O_2 and Hb-associated O_2, whereas O_2-capacity is just Hb-associated O_2. To obtain a more precise value of PaO_2, one can estimate the dissolved O_2 at $PaO_2 \approx 66$ mmHg, subtract its value from CaO_2 and recalculate the $\%SaO_2$, as follows:

$$\text{Dissolved } O_2 = 66 \times 0.0031 = 0.205 \text{ vol\%} \ldots \quad (30)$$

$$\%SaO_2 \approx \frac{18.75-0.205}{20 \times 1.34} \approx 92.3\% \ldots \quad (31)$$

$$PaO_2 \approx 64 \text{ mmHg} \ldots \quad (32)$$

E. BASE EXCESS (BE)

To estimate the Base Excess (BE, Eqs. 33-40) one needs to know the values of $PaCO_2$, pHa and Hb.

Assume: $PaCO_2$ = 36 mmHg, pHa = 7.3 and Hb = 14 g/100 ml blood.

By means of the Henderson-Hasselbalch equation (Eq. 33) we calculate the **"actual"** bicarbonate concentration: $[HCO_3^-]_{actual}$

$$pH = 6.1 + \log\frac{[HCO_3^-]}{\alpha \times PaCO_2} \ldots \quad (33)$$

$$\log[HCO_3^-]_{actual} = 7.3 - 6.1 + \log(36 \times 0.0301) \ldots \quad (34)$$

$$[HCO_3^-]_{actual} = 17.2 \text{ mEq/l plasma} \ldots \quad (35)$$

By means of the buffer capacity (BC) equations (Eqs. 36 and 37), we calculate what would be the value of the **"predicted"** bicarbonate concentration ($[HCO_3^-]_{predicted}$, Eqs. 37 and 38) if pHa = 7.3 had been reached as a result of a pure, uncompensated, respiratory condition.

$$BC = \frac{8.2 + (1.56 \times 15)}{3} = 10.5 \ldots \quad (36)$$

$$-10.5 = \frac{24 - [HCO_3^-]_{predicted}}{7.4 - 7.3} \ldots \quad (37)$$

$$[HCO_3^-]_{Predicted} = 25.05 \text{ mEq/l (plasma)} \ldots \quad (38)$$

The base excess (BE, Eqs. 39 and 40) is the difference between actual and predicted $[HCO_3^-]$

$$BE = [HCO_3^-]_{Actual} - [HCO_3^-]_{Predicted} \ldots \quad (39)$$

$$BE = 17.2 - 25.05 = -7.85 \text{ mEq/l (plasma)} \ldots \quad (40)$$

Further Reading

HISTORY OF RESPIRATION

Kiley JP. Advancing respiratory research. Chest 2011;140:497-501.

Massaro D. The 20th century in respiratory physiology: one view. Ann. Rev. Physiol. 2000;62:951-960.

Mitzner W. Mechanics of the lungs in the 20th century. American Physiological Society, Comprehensive Physiology, 2011;1:2009-2027.

Otis AB, Rahn H. Development of concepts in Rochester, New York, in the 1940s. In: West JB ed. Pulmonary gas exchange. Vol. 1. Ventilation, blood Flow, and diffusion. New York: Academic Press;1980, Chapter 2, pp. 33-66.

Perkins JF Jr. Historical development of respiratory physiology. In: Fenn WO, Herman Rahn H. eds. Handbook of Physiology, Section 3: Respiration, Vol. 1. Washington, DC: American Physiological Society; 1964, Chapter 1, pp. 1-62.

Riley RL. Development of the three-compartment model for dealing with uneven distribution. In: West JB ed. Pulmonary Gas Exchange. Vol. 1. Ventilation, Blood Flow, and Diffusion. New York: Academic Press; 1980, Chapter 3, pp. 67-85.

West JB. Historical development. In: West JB ed. Pulmonary Gas Exchange. Vol. 1. Ventilation, Blood Flow, and Diffusion. New York: Academic Press; 1980, Chapter 1, pp. 1-32.

West JB. A century of pulmonary gas exchange. Am J Respir Crit Care Med. 2004;169:897-902.

RESPIRATORY PHYSIOLOGY - GENERAL

Cloutier MM. Respiratory Physiology. The Mosby Physiology Monograph Series. London: Mosby; 2006.

Comroe JH. Physiology of Respiration: An Introduction. 2nd ed. Chicago: Year Book Medical Publisher Inc.; 1979.

Cotes, JE, Chinn DJ, Miller MR. Lung Function: physiology, measurement and application in medicine (6th Ed.). Hoboken, NJ: Wiley-Blackwell; 2006.

Hlastala MP, Berger AJ. Physiology of respiration. 2nd ed. New York: Oxford University Press; 2001.

Levitzky MG. Pulmonary physiology (Lange Physiology Series). 7th ed. New York: McGraw-Hill Medical; 2007.

Lumb AB. Nunn's Applied respiratory physiology. New York: Churchill Livingstone; 2010

Mines AH. Respiratory physiology. 3rd ed. New York: Raven Press; 1993.

Riley, R.L. and Cournand, A. "Ideal" alveolar air and the analysis of ventilation-perfusion relationships in the lungs. J Appl Physiol. 1949;1:825–847.

Riley RL, Cournand A, Donald KW. Analysis of factors affecting the partial pressures of oxygen and carbon dioxide in gas and blood of lung: methods. J Appl Physiol. 1951;4:102-120.

Schwartzenstein R, Michael J, Parker MJ. Respiratory physiology: A clinical approach. The Integrated Physiology Series. Philadelphia: Lippincott Williams & Wilkins; 2005.

Slonim NB, Hamilton LH. Respiratory Physiology 5th ed. St. Louis: The C.V. Mosby Company; 1987.

Wagner PD, Saltzman HA, West JB. Measurement of continuous distributions of ventilation-perfusion ratios: theory. J Appl Physiol.1974;36:533–537.

Weibel ER. The Pathway for oxygen – structure and function in the mammalian respiratory System. Cambridge, MA: Harvard University Press; 1984.

West, JB, Dollery CT, Naimark A. Distribution of blood flow in isolated lung: relation to vascular and alveolar pressures. J Appl Physiol. 1964;19:713-724.

West JB. ed. Pulmonary Gas Exchange - Ventilation, Blood Flow, and Diffusion. New York: Academic Press; 1980.

West JB. Ventilation/blood flow and gas exchange. 4rd ed. Oxford: Blackwell Scientific Publications; 1985.

West JB. Respiratory physiology: people and ideas. People and Ideas Series. New York: Oxford University Press; 1996.

West JB. Respiratory physiology: the essentials. 9th ed. Philadelphia: Lippincott Williams & Wilkins; 2011.

ACID-BASE BALANCE

Faibel S, Topf J. The fluid, electrolyte, and acid-base companion. Alert & Oriented Publishing Company; 1999.

Halperin, M.L. and Goldstein, M.B. Fluid, Electrolyte and Acid-Base Physiology: A Problem-Based Approach. Philadelphia: Saunders-Elsevier; 1998.

Preston RA. Acid-base, fluids, and electrolytes made ridiculously simple. 2nd ed. Med Master Inc.; 2010.

RESPIRATORY PATHOPHYSIOLOGY

Ali J, Summer W, Levitzky M. Pulmonary pathophysiology. Lange Physiology Series. New York: McGraw-Hill; 2004.

Juzar A, Summer WR, Lewitzky MG. Pulmonary pathophysiology: a clinical approach. 3rd ed.; A Lange Medical Book. New York: McGraw-Hill Medical; 2009.

West JB. Pulmonary pathophysiology: the essentials. 8th ed. Philadelphia: Lippincott Williams & Wilkins; 2012.

RESPIRATORY MEDICINE

Albert RK, Spiro SG, Jett JR. Comprehensive Respiratory Medicine. London: Mosby; 1999.

Bordow RA, Ries AL, Morris TA. eds. Manual of Clinical Problems in Pulmonary Medicine. 6th ed. Philadelphia: Lippincott Williams & Wilkins; 2005.

Kryger MH. ed. Introduction to respiratory medicine. 2nd ed. New York: Churchill Livingstone; 1990.

Spiro SG, Silvestri GA, Agusti A. Clinical respiratory medicine: expert consult - online and print. 4th ed. Philadelphia: W.B. Saunders Company; 2012.

Weinberger SE, Cockrill BA. Principles of pulmonary medicine. 5th ed. Philadelphia: W.B. Saunders Company; 2008.

RESPIRATION AT HIGH ALTITUDE

Reeves JT, Leon-Velarde F. Chronic mountain sickness: recent studies of the relationship between hemoglobin concentration and oxygen transport. High Alt. Med. Biol. 2004;5:147-155.

Zubieta-Castillo G Sr, Zubieta-Castillo, GR Jr, Zubieta-Calleja L. Chronic mountain sickness: the reaction of physical disorders to chronic hypoxia. J Physiol Pharmacol. 2006;57 (Supp. 4):431-442.

Bärtsch, P. and Gibbs, J.S.R, Effect of altitude on the heart and the lungs. Circulation 116:2191-2202, 2007

Sutton, J.R. *et al.*, Operation Everest II: oxygen transport during exercise at extreme simulated altitude. J. Appl. Physiol. 64:1309-1321, 1988

Index

A

Acclimatization to high altitude 228
  blood changes 229
  erythropoietin synthesis stimulation 229
Acetazolamide
  used for treating alkalosis at high altitude 230
Acetylene absorption
  used for monitoring pulmonary capillary flow 31
Acid-base balance
  adding an acid load at constant PCO_2 128
  adding an acid load to a closed system 127
  adding an acid load while allowing PCO_2 to change 128
  at high altitude 225
  blood buffering capacity (BC) 132
  blood-buffer line 131
  clinical cases
    flail chest 148
    morphine overdose 145
    panic attacks 148
    pyloric stenosis 146
  clinical methods for evaluation of
    the Singer-Hasting method 140
    the standard bicarbonate/base excess method 140
  CO_2/HCO_3^- - buffering 126
  conceptual approach for disorders of
    step 1, Blink 142
    step 2, compensation formula 143
    step 3, anion gap 144
  during exercise 221
  during exercise at high altitude 228
  effect of hemoglobin on the *in vitro* blood-buffer line 132
  Henderson-Hasselbalch equation 124, 126

Camillo Peracchia and Nasr H. Anaizi

ionization and dissociation constants 124
normal values 408
pH buffering 125
slykes
units of buffering capacity (mEq/l per pH unit) 132
Acid-base disorders
evaluation 136–40
metabolic 134–36
respiratory 133–34
Acidemia
sensitivity of carotid bodies to 211
Acute mountain sickness (AMS)
increased cerebral blood flow in 229
role of hypoxemia and alkalosis in 229
symptoms of 229
Adaptation
to high altitude 230
Adenocarcinoma
lung cancer
less frequent in non-smokers 264
Adenoid hypertrophy
role of in sleep apnea 213
Adenosine-5'-triphosphate (ATP)
role of in medullary chemosensitive response 211
Air pollutants
effect on cilia function 243
Airways
alveolar ducts 37
histology 44
anatomy 36–37
cilia structure 42
collaps tendency in expiration 73
dilatation during exercise 218
dynamics during breathing cycle 72–76

gas flow
laminar *versus* turulent 68
resistance 70
histology 41–44
juxta-capillary receptors (J-receptors) 46, 244, 252, 253
obstructive diseases of
asthma 241
bronchiolitis 238
chronic bronchitis 235
emphysema 233
extrathoracic obstruction 265
mixed emphysema and chronic bronchitis 237
respiratory bronchioles
histology 44
viral infections as asthma triggers 241
Alexandria
burning of the library 5
Alpha1-antitrypsin
deficiency
role in COPD 31
Alveolar
dead space
fraction calculation *See* Calculations
dead space fraction equation 180
gas equation 93, 170, 410
derivation 397
ideal compartment 168
ideal gas 92
ideal ventilation
relationship to $PaCO_2$ and metabolic rate (CO_2 production) 97, 411
ideal *versus* arterial PO_2 92
sacs
histology 44
Alveolar-capillary-block syndrome

first described by Austrian, R. *et al.* 22
Alveoli
anatomy 37
blood-gas barrier 46
cathelicidins 32
cell types 1 and 2 45
defensins 32
evidence for a continuous cellular layer in alveoli
reported by N. Low and confirmed by C.C. Macklin 24
evidence for liquid layer coating the alveolar surface
provided by C.C. Macklin and confirmed by E.R. Weibel and J.Gil 24
granular pneumocytes, (cells type 2) 57
histology 44–46
Kohn's pores 37
role in spreading infection to contiguous alveolar sacs in bacterial pneumonia253
mesothelial cells 46
surfactant
cathelicidins 57
collectins 57
defensins 57
role in maintaining alveolar stability 58
SPs proteins 32, 57
Amine Precursor Uptake Decarboxylation cells (APUD), *See* Feyrter's cells
Amyotropic Lateral Sclerosis (ALS)
consequences to respiratory mechanics of 258
Anaerobic threshold 212
Andes dwellers
adaptation to high altitude of 231
Aneurysm
abdominal
clinical case 335
Anion gap *See* Acid-base balance: conceptual approach for disorders of
Ankylosing spondylitis
consequences to respiratory mechanics of 260

effect on chest wall compliance 61
Aortic bodies
chemoreceptors 205
sensitivity to hypoxia 210
Apneustic center *See* Control of breathing:neural, *See* Control of breathing:chemical
named by T. Lumsden 202
Arachnoid plexus *See* Control of breathing:chemical
ARDS
Adult Respiratory Distress Syndrome See Respiratory failure
Arterial
$PaCO_2$
relationship to alveolar ideal ventilation and metabolic rate (CO_2 production) 97
pulmonary pressure during exercise 220
Aspergillosis infection
bronchiectasis as consequence of 237
Aspirin
asthma trigger 241
Asthma
atopy as cause of 241
beta-2-agonists
effective in reducing maldistribution shunt-like effect 241
expiratory work in 76
in patient with patent foramen ovale
case study 288
pathology and functional consequences of 241
triggers of acute attacks 241
Atopy
hereditary condition coausing incresed IgE, predisposing for asthma 241
ATP *See* Adenosine-5'-triphosphate (ATP)
ATPS
state of gases at ambient conditions 83, 392
Autoimmune deficiency syndrome
rare cause of emphysema 234
Azygos veins 40

B

Base Excess (BE)
  calculation *See* Calculations
Bernoulli's principle 74
Beta blockers
  asthma triggers 241
Beta-2-agonists *See* asthma
Blink *See* Acid-base balance: conceptual approach for disorders of
Blood Brain Barrier (BBB) 206
Blood pressure
  pulmonary *versus* systemic 150
Blood-gas barrier *See* Alveoli
Bohr effect
  acidosis causes right shift of O_2 dissociation curve 114
Bohr's method for calculating dead space 88
Bombesin *See* Feyrter's cells
Bötzinger complex *See* Control of breathing:neural
Boyle-Marriotte' law *See* Gas:laws:Boyle-Mariotte's law
Brain
  Blood Brain Barrier (BBB) 206
  Interstitial Fluid (ISF) *See* Control of breathing:chemical
Breathing
  work of 76
Bronchi
  anatomy 36
  histology 42
Bronchiectasis
  in Kartagener's syndrome 237, 242
  pathology and functional consequences of 237
  resulting from
    fungal infection (aspergillosis) 237
    measles 237
    pertussis 237
Bronchioles

anatomy 37
bronchiolitis-induced obstruction of 238
canals of Lambert 37
Clara cells 44
histology 44
Bronchiolitis
Bronchiolitis Obliterans Organizing Pneumonia (BOOP) 238
caused by Respiratory Syncytial Virus (RSV) in infants 238
complication of Hematopoietic Stem Cell Transplantation (HSCT) 238
follicular
complication of rheumatoid arthritis or Sjögren's disease 238
Obliterative Bronchiolitis (OB) 238
pathology and functional consequences of 238
Bronchoconstriction
hypocapnic cause of 185
Broncho-pulmonary anastomoses
conductive (anatomical) shunt caused by 178
BTPS
state of gases at body conditions 83, 392
Buffer capacity 126, 132
equation 411

C

Calcitonin *See* Feyrter's cells
Calculations
mixed venous PO_2 417
shunt fraction 415
Canals of Lambert *See* Bronchioles
Capacities *See* Lung:volumes
Carbon dioxide
carbamino (hemoglobin-bound CO_2) 116
$PaCO_2$
relationship to alveolar ideal ventilation and metabolic rate (CO_2 production) 97
production 85
production equations 394, 410

retention with oxygen therapy 193
role in regulating O_2 binding to hemoglobin 114
transport 116–20
Carbon monoxide
lung diffusion capacity (DLCO) 105
Carbonic acid 8
Carbonic anhydrase
acetazolamide, inhibitor of 230
catalytic activity in CO_2 hydration mechanism 117
Carcinoma
small-cell type *See* Feyrter's cells
Cardiac failure
in COPD patient with mitral valve regurgitation 280–88
Carotid bodies
chemoreceptors 205
sensitivity of hypoxia 209
sensitivity to acidemia, hyperkalemia and hypercapnia 211
Cathelicidins 32, *See* Alveoli:surfactant
Cervical Magnetic Stimulation (CMS)
used for stimulating diaphragm contraction 32
Charles' law *See* Gas:laws:Charles' law
Chemoreceptors *See* Control of breathing:chemical
Chest wall
compliance 60
basis of 61
normal value of 66
Cheyne-Stokes breathing 267
Chronic bronchitis
functional consequences of 235
Chronic Obstructive Pulmonary Disease See COPD
Cigarette smoke
effect on cilia function 243
impaired macrophage function by 243
role in COPD *via* inhibition of anti-proteases 31

Cilia
impaired function of
by cigarette smoke and pollutants 243
by high FIO_2 breathing 243
by viral infections 243
in Kartagener's syndrome 242
malfunction in bronchiectasis 237
Circulation
normal values 408
pulmonary
anatomy 38
at high altitude 224
during exercise 220
vascular resistance 151–54
pulmonary *versus* systemic blood pressure values 150
systemic
at high altitude 225
during exercise 221
Clara cells *See* Bronchioles
Collagen diseases
pulmonary fibrosis caused by 244
Collectins *See* Alveoli:surfactant
Compensation formula *See* Acid-base balance: conceptual approach for disorders of
Compliance 53
Computed technology (CT)
used for monitoring pulmonary circulation 31
Control of breathing
anaerobic threshold 212
central controller 198
central sleep apnea (CSA) 213
role of Ondine's curse in 214
chemical 205–11
central chemoreceptors 205
peripheral chemoreceptors 205

disorders of
apneustic breathing 267
ataxic breathing 267
Cheyne-Stokes breathing 267
cluster breathing (Biot's respiration) 268
in neurological diseases 266
Kussmaul's respiration 268
secondary to lung diseases 268
Sleep Apnea-Hypopnea Syndrome (SAHS) 269
during exercise 211–12
during sleep 212–14
effectors 198
neural 198–205
neurogenic mechanism activated at onset of exercise 212
neuro-receptors
histology 46
role of oxygen first demonstrated by E.F.W Pflüger 13
sensors 198
Sleep Apnea Hypopnea Syndrome (SAHS) 213
stages of sleep 212
COPD 41
bronchiectasis 237
case study 280
complicated by bacterial pneumonia and pneumothorax
problem based learning (PBL) case 373–90
complicated by ruptured coronary artery
case study 313–20
complicated by tension pneumothorax
case study 297
mixed emphysema and chronic bronchitis
functional consequences of 237
pathology and functional consequences of 233–37
pure chronic bronchitis (COPD type B)
functional consequences of 235

pure emphysema (COPD type A)
functional consequences of 233
respiratory failure following operation for abdominal aneurysm
case study 335
role of cigarette smoke 31
role of α1-antitrypsin deficiency 31
Coronary artery
ruptured during angioplasty in COPD patient
case study 313
Cutis laxa
rare cause of emphysema 233
Cystic fibrosis
pathology and functional consequences of 239
staphylococcus and pseudomonas infections in 240
Cystic Fibrosis Transport Regulator (CFTR)
genetic defect of, in cystic fibrosis 239

D

Dalton's law *See* Gas:laws
Davenport diagram 129, 133
Dead space
alveolar 180–82
definition 91
equation 180
quantification 180
conductive (anatomical) 80
calculated by Bohr's method 88
derivation of equation 394
quantification methods 87
equations for measuring wasted ventilations in conductive, physiological and alveolar dead space compartments 410
Fowler's method for measuring conductive dead space 87
physiological
derivation of equation 394
quantification 89

quantification methods 89
Defensins *See* Alveoli:surfactant
Diaphragm *See* Respiratory muscles
Diaphragmatic hernia
developed during labor
test case 363
Diffuse lung diseases *See* Fibrosis
Diffusion
Fick's law of 101
gas through membranes 8, 101–8
impairment at high altitude 223
measured by monoxide diffusion capacity (DLCO) 105
Diffusion impairment
during exercise at high altitude 226
hypoxemia caused by 190
venous admixture caused by 179
Dipalmitoyl lecithin (DPL) *See* Lung:surfactant
Diphosphoglycerate (2,3-DPG) 114–16
binding to hemoglobin of 110
increase at high altitude 229
role in regulating O_2 binding to hemoglobin 114
role of discovered by Chautin *et al.* 15
Drug users (intravenous)
rare cases of emphysema in 234
Ductus arteriosus
patent
cause of conductive (anatomical) shunt 179, 252
Dynein *See* Airways:cilia structure

E

Ehlers-Danos type IX syndrome
type of cutis laxa
rare cause of emphysema 234
Elastance 53
Emphysema

expiratory work in 76
functional consequences of 233
mechanism of airway collapse in expiration 73
types of 234
Erythropoiesis
hypoxia-stimulated at high altitude 229
Erythropoietin
synthesis stimulation at high altitude 229
Esophageal compression
by lung cancer invasion of mediastinum 265
Everest mount
barometric pressure 215
Exercise
(Ai-a)PO_2 gradient 220
acid-base balance 221
airway dilatation during 218
asthma trigger 241
effect on respiratory physiology at high altitude 226–28
effect on respiratory physiology at sea level 216–22
effect on ventilation-perfusion ratio 156
hyperpnea 218
metabolic changes 219
muscle metaboreceptors 218
neurogenic mechanism at onset of 212
neurohumoral theory 218
nocireceptors stimulation 218
pulmonary circulation 220
stimulatory impulses from brain to respiratory centers at onset of 212
systemic circulation 221
tissue oxygenation 220
ventilation-perfusion distribution 219
Expiration 51
accessory muscles 52
change on gas composition during 83

gas exchange 83
Expiratory flow limitation 73
Pride-Permutt's model 28
Eye damage
retrolental fibroplasia in infants exposed to high FIO_2 195

F

Fenn-Rahn diagram *See* O_2-CO_2 diagram
Feyrter's cells 42
neuroendocrine function of 42
small-cell carcinoma 43
Fibrosis
complicated by pneumonia
case study 271–80
pathology and functional consequences of 243
Fick equation
carbon dioxide production measured by 410
oxygen consumption measured by 410
Fick's law
diffusion across a barrier governed by 101
Flail chest
clinical case *See* Acid-base balance
consequences to respiratory mechanics of 260
Flow limitation *See* Expiratory flow limitation
Foramen ovale
opened by compression of right atrium 313
patent in asthmatic patient
case study 288
Forced Oscillation Technique (FOT) 30
Fowler's method for measuring conductive dead space volume 87

G

GABA receptors
role of during sleep 213
Gas

body stores *See* Gas exchange:gas stores
changes during expiration 83
changes during inspiration 81
different states of *See* ATPS:BTPS:STPD
diffusion through membranes 101–8
flow *See* Airways
fractional concentration 82
laws 412
Boyle-Mariotte's law 391
Charles' law 391
Dalton's law 412
ideal gas law 391
partial pressure 82
word invented by J.B. van Helmont 8
Gas exchange
acute hyperventilation and hypoventilation
effect on exchange ratio 94
alveolar dead space 92
alveolar ideal gas 92
carbon dioxide production 85
conductive (anatomical) dead space 85
quantification methods 87
effect of gravity on 164
expiration 83
gas stores 94
O_2-CO_2 diagram (Fenn-Rahn diagram) 94
oxygen consumption 83
equation 85
physiological dead space
quantification 89
right-to-left shunt (venous admixture) 91
Gas Silvestre
carbonic acid 8
Gay-Lussac's law *See* Gas:laws:Charles' law

Genioglossus muscle
  defective function of, in sleep apnea hypopnea syndrome 265, 269
Glycosaminoglycans *See* Bronchioles:Clara cells
Graham's law 102
Gravity
  effect on regional gas exchange 164
Guillain-Barré syndrome
  consequences to respiratory mechanics of 258

H

Haldane effect 119–20
HAPE *See* High altitude:acute pulmonary edema
Haplotypes
  selected for adaptation to hypoxia in Tibetans 231
Heart
  cardiac failure
    clinical case 280
  coronary artery
    ruptured during angioplasty in COPD patient
      case study 313
  patent foramen ovale in asthmatic patient
    case study 288
  pericardial effusion caused by lung cancer 265
  septal defects
    clinical case 316
    shunt caused by 179, 252
Hemoglobin
  carbamino CO_2 116
  effect on the *in vitro* blood-buffer line of 132
  heme group 109
  oxygen buffer properties of 162
  positive cooperativity of heme-heme interaction 111
  role in O_2 transport 109
  structure and function 109–16
Henderson-Hasselbalch equation 19, 124, 126, 411

Henry's law
  concentration of dissolved gas determined by 109
High altitude
  (Ai-a)PO_2 gradient 224
  acclimatization to 228–29
  acute and chronic mountain sickness 229–30
  acute mountain sickness 229
  acute pulmonary edema (HAPE) 230
  adaptation to 230
    haplotypes of Tibetans 231
    in dwellers of the Andes 231
    in Himalayans 231
  at rest
    acid-base balance 225
    diffusion impairment 223
    effect on metabolic rate of 222
    effect on ventilation 222
    pulmonary circulation 224
    systemic circulation 225
    tissue oxygenation 224
    ventilation-perfusion distribution 224
  atmospheric changes from sea level 215–16
  chronic mountain sickness 230
    Monge's disease 230
    polycytemia 230
  effect on respiratory physiology 222–25
  exercise
    acid-base balance 228
    gas exchange 226
    pulmonary circulation 227
    systemic circulation 227
    tissue oxygenation 227
    ventilation-perfusion distribution 226
Himalayans

adaptation to high altitude of 231
History of respiration
17th century 7–9
18th century 9–11
19th century 12–15
20th century 15–29
before common era 3–4
Chinese understanding of breathing 4
Ebers papyrus 4
Greco-Roman times 4–5
middle ages 6
mistaken belief that arteries carry air 4
recent development 29–33
renaissance 6–7
the three golden decades of the 20th century - 1940-1970 20–27
Horner's syndrome
Pancoast tumors (apical), cause of 265
Hyaline membrane*See* Respiratory failure:Infant Respiratory Distress Syndrome (IRDS)
Hypercapnia
caused by oxygen therapy 193
respiratory response to 206, 208
sensitivity of carotid bodies to 211
Hypercapnic Hypoxic Respiratory Failure (HHRF) 191
Hyperkalemia
sensitivity of carotid bodies to 211
Hyperpnea 98
Hyperventilation
acute
effect on exchange ratio (R) 94
neurogenic 266
Hypocapnic bronchoconstriction 185
Hypocomplementemic Urticarial Vasculitis Syndrome (HUVS)
rare cause of emphysema 234
Hypothalamus

supra-chiasmatic nuclei
role of in sleep 212
Hypoventilation
acute
effect on exchange ratio (R) 94
hypoxemia caused by 187, 189
neurogenic 266
Hypoxemia 187–92
causes of 187
diffusion impairment as cause of 187, 190
Hypercapnic Hypoxic Respiratory Failure (HHRF) 191
hypoventilation as cause of 189
Hypoxic Respiratory Failure (HRF) 191
respiratory response to 209
shunts as cause of 187
ventilation-perfusion maldistribution as cause of 187
Hypoxia
in muscles during exercise 219
Hypoxic breathing
hypoxemia caused by 190
Hypoxic Respiratory Failure (HRF) 191
Hypoxic vasoconstriction 185

I

Ideal
alveolar ventilation
relationship to $PaCO_2$ and metabolic rate (CO_2 production) 97
Ideal alveolar compartment 168
Ideal gas law *See* Gas:laws:ideal gas law
Idiopathic Pulmonary Fibrosis (IPF) *See* Fibrosis
Inert-gas-elimination technique
developed by J.B. West 186
Inhalant-related diseases
pulmonary fibrosis caused by 243
Innominate vein *See* Lung:lymphatic circulation

Inspiration 50
accessory muscles 52
gas exchange 80
mechanism of 51
Inspired gas
changes from ambient to alveolar compartment 81

J

J-receptors 46, 244, 252, 253

K

Kartagener's syndrome
bronchiectasis, sinusitis and situs in*versus* in 237, 242
Klebsiella pneumoniae
agent of bacterial pneumonia 253
Kohn's pores *See* Alveoli
Kulchitsky's cells (K-cells) *See* Feyrter's cells
Kyphoscoliosis
consequences to respiratory mechanics of 259
effect on chest wall compliance 61

L

La Rinconada
Peruvian town 216
Laplace, P.S.
law of 56
Large cell carcinoma
lung cancer
less frequent in non-smokers 264
Larynx
histology 42
Leukocytes, polymorphonuclear
depressed function of
by chemotherapy 243
in leukemia 243
role in pathogenesis of bacterial pneumonia 253

Lung
  anatomy 35
  cancer
    functional consequences of 264
  collapsed in cancer patient
    case study 327–35
  compliance 53
    effect of emphysema and fibrosis on 54
    effect of surface tension and surfactant on 55
    normal value of 66
    structural basis of 55
  elastance 53
  functional equivalent of real lung 166–68
  infectious diseases of 253–55
  innervation 40
    non-adrenergic, non-cholinergic (NANC) fibers 41
  interdependence theory of lung parenchima 24
  lymphatic circulation 40
  perfusion distribution
    studied in isolated lungs 156
  surfactant 56
    administered following drowning
      test case 354
  three-compartment-model or real lung 168–71
  trabeculae 35
  volumes
    changes with age 50
    conversion 391
    effect of emphysema and fibrosis on 50
    Expiratory Reserve Volume (ERV) 48
    Functional Residual Capacity (FRC) 47
    Inspiratory Capacity (IC) 48
    Inspiratory Reserve Volume (IRV) 48
    measured by plethysmography 49

measured by spirometry 48
measured by the inert gas dilution method 48
normal values 406
Residual Volume (RV) 48
Tidal Volume (VT) 47, 80
Total Lung Capacity (TLC) 48
Vital Capacity (VC) 48
Lung + chest wall
compliance
normal value of 66
Lung-on-a-Chip Microdevice 31
Lymphatic circulation *See* Lung

M

Macrophages
impaired function of
by cigarette smoke 243
role in pathogenesis of bacterial pneumonia 253
Magnetic method
used for stimulating respiratory muscles 31
Magnetic Resonance Imaging (MRI)
used for monitoring pulmonary circulation 31
Marfan syndrome
rare cause of emphysema 234
Measles
bronchiectasis as consequence of 237
Mechanics *See* Respiratory mechanics
Mediastinal diseases
mediastinal masses 264
pathology and functional consequences of 263–64
pneumomediastinum 263
Menstrual and pre-menstrual periods
asthma triggers 241
Mesothelial cells *See* Alveoli
Metabolic rate

effect of high altitude on 222
Metabolism
normal values 409
Metaboreceptors 218
Microscope, compound
invented by Dutch spectacle makers 7
Mitral valve regurgitation
cardiac failure in COPD patient
case study 280
Mitral valve stenosis
effect on lung's perfusion-distribution 156
Monod's model of allosteric-enzymes' behavior 110
Morphine overdose
clinical case *See* Acid-base balance
Mountain
acute sickness 229
chronic sickness (Monge's disease) 230
Muscular dystrophy
consequences to respiratory mechanics of 258
Myastenia gravis
consequences to respiratory mechanics of 258
Mycobacterium tuberculosis
agent of tuberculosis 255
Mycoplasma pneumoniae
agent of atypical pneumonia 253
Myoglobin
increased content at high altitude 229

N

Negative Expiratory Pressure (NEP) method 30
Neurohumoral theory *See* Exercise
Nociceptors
stimulated during exercise 218
Normal values *See* Values
Nose

histology 41
paranasal sinuses
histology 41

O

O_2-CO_2 diagram 94
Obesity
catabolic and anabolic signaling molecules 261
role in sleep apnea 213
Ondine's curse
neurogenic hypoventilation
impaired automatic control of breathing 266
role of in central sleep apnea (CSA) 214
Oxygen
(Ai-a)PO_2 gradient 92
effect of hyperoxemic and hypoxemic conditions on 175
(Ai-a)PO_2 gradient at high altitude 224
Bohr-integration-method for estimating mean PO_2 in alveolar capillary blood 15
change in pressure with altitude 215
consumption 83
consumption equation 393, 409
content equation 411
diffusion *versus* secretion controversy 16
dissociation curves 412
pH- and temperature-induced shift 412
dissolved O_2 determined by Henry's law 109
estimation of PaO_2 knowing shunt fraction and O_2-extraction *See* Calculations
extraction
measured by Fick equation 410
fraction in air first determined by Joseph Priestley 10
hypoxemia caused by hypoxic breathing (low PIO_2) 190
impaired cilia function by high FIO_2 breathing 243
independent discovery of by J. Priestley and C. W. Scheele 10
kiss of death of secretion hypothesis 16
lung diffusion capacity of 105

mechanism of binding to hemoglobin 109
mixed venous PO_2 calculation *See* Calculations
O_2-CO_2 diagram 94
role in control of breathing first demonstrated by E.F.W Pflüger 13
therapy 190–94
hyperbaric 194
toxicity 194–95
retrolental fibroplasia 195
transport 108–16

P

Pancoast tumors
superior sulcus tumors (apical lung cancers) 265
PBL *See* Problem Based Learning (PBL)
PEEP 193, 256, 257
effect on pulmonary vascular resistance of 153
prevention of alveolar collapse by PEEP ventilation 193
Pertussis
bronchiectasis as consequence of 237
pH
buffering 125–29
role in regulating O_2 binding to hemoglobin 114
Phlogiston
combustion theory 9
Phrenic nerve
stimulation by Cervical Magnetic Stimulation (CMS) 32
Plethysmography 49
Pleura
anatomy 35
histology 46
parietal
innervation by branches of phrenic and intercostal nerves 41
pleural space 35
visceral
innervation by branches of vagus nerve 41

Pleural effusion
caused by lung cancer 265
exudate formation in tuberculosis 255
pathology and functional consequences of 247
trasudate *versus* exudate 247
Pneumatic trough 10
instrument for collecting gases 8
Pneumococcus *See* Streptococcus pneumoniae
Pneumomediastinum
functional consequences of 263
Pneumonia
atypical 253
bacterial 253
Bronchiolitis Obliterans Organizing Pneumonia (BOOP) 238
caused by cancer related bronchial occlusion 265
caused by fungal or viral infection 253
caused by Mycoplasma pneumoniae 253
complicated by ARDS
case study 306–13
functional consequences of 253
in fibrosis patient
case study 271–80
lobar 253
Pneumotaxic center 19, *See* Control of breathing:neural
Pneumothorax 67
causes of 245
in cancer patient
case study 327
pathology and functional consequences of 245
tension type 67
functional consequences of 245
in COPD patient
case study 297–306
Poiseuille's law 70

Poliomyelitis
  consequences to respiratory mechanics of 258
Pollutants
  asthma triggers 241
Polymyositis
  consequences to respiratory mechanics of 258
Positive End Expiratory Pressure (PEEP) *See* PEEP
Problem Based Learning (PBL)
  COPD complicated by pneumonia and pneumothorax 373
Pulmonary
  arterial pressure during exercise 220
  artery
    branches 39
    pressure 150
  circulation
    anatomy 38–40
    at high altitude 224
    effect of gravity 155–56
    modern non-invasive monitoring techniques 31
  circulation during exercise at high altitude 227
  edema
    at high altitude (HAPE) 230
    functional consequences of 248
  embolism
    functional consequences of 250
    in diabetic patient following surgery
      case study 342–52
  function tests *See* Respiratory:function tests
  hypertension
    causes of 251
    pathology and functional consequences of 251
  hypocapnic bronchoconstriction 185
  hypoxic vasoconstriction 185
  vascular resistance

role of alveolar pressure in 153
role of blood flow in 154
role of lung volume in 151
wedge pressure 221
Pulmonary Capillary Wedge Pressure (PCWP) 154

Q

Quadriplegia
consequences to respiratory mechanics of 258

R

R lines *See* Respiratory exchange ratio (R)
Radiation
pulmonary fibrosis caused by 244
Respiratory centers *See* Control of breathing:neural
Respiratory exchange ratio (R) 84
blood R lines 162
effect of acute hyperventilation and hypoventilation, on 94
gas R lines 162
shape of HBO_2 dissociation curve and regional R values 160
Respiratory failure
Adult Respiratory Distress Syndrome (ARDS)
functional consequences of 256
following drowning
test case 354
hyaline membrane
in ARDS 256
in IRDS 257
in asthmatic patient with patent foramen ovale 288–97
in COPD patient operated for abdominal aneurysm
case study 335–42
lack of surfactant as cause of ARDS/IRDS 58
pneumonia complicated by ARDS 306
role of epithelial cells types 1 and 2 in ARDS 256
Respiratory mechanics

accessory muscles
expiration 52
inspiration 52
disorders of
in chest wall diseases 259, 260
in neuromuscular diseases 258
in obesity 262
dynamic properties 68–76
elastance 65
expiration 51
inspiration 50
most common function tests 77–78
normal values 407
pathology and functional consequences of disorders of 257–63
pneumothorax 67
static properties 52–67
surface tension and surfactant 54–59
work of breathing 76–77
Respiratory muscles
accessory expiratory 52
accessory inspiratory 38, 52
genioglossus muscle 265, 269
anatomy 38
diaphragm 38
magnetic stimulation of 32
ruptured during labor
case study 363
expiratory 38, 51
inspiratory 51
inter-costal 38
Respiratory Quotient (RQ) 84, 97
Respiratory Syncytial Virus (RSV)
bronchiolitis caused by 238
Restrictive diseases

functional consequences of 243–45
Retrolental fibroplasia
in infants exposed to high FIO_2 195
Reynold's number 69

S

SAHS *See* Sleep Apnea Hypopnea Syndrome (SAHS)"
Sarcoidosis
pulmonary fibrosis caused by 244
Septal defects *See* Heart
Serotonin (5-hydroxytryptamine) *See* Feyrter's cells
Shunt
$(Ai\text{-}a)PO_2$ gradient and magnitude of 175
alveolar 91
conductive (anatomical) 89
anastomoses between bronchial and pulmonary veins 40
caused by opening of foramen ovale 297
caused by venae minimae and broncho-pulmonary anastomoses 178
equation 412
fraction calculation of *See* Calculations
hypoxemia caused by 187
maldistribution-diffusion component of 175
eliminated by 100% O_2 breathing 175
physiological 89
physiological shunt fraction 171–75
types 178–80
Sleep *See* Control of breathing
Sleep Apnea Hypopnea Syndrome (SAHS) 28, 29, 214
control of breathing in 213–14
role of genioglossus muscle and tongue in 265, 269
Slykes
units of buffering capacity (mEq/l per pH unit) 132
Spirometer
gas volumes measured by 48
Squamous cell carcinoma

smoke-related lung cancer 264
Staphylococcus aureus
agent of bacterial pneumonia 253
Starling equation
fluid diffusion governed by 248
Steady state
change with acute hyper- or hypo-ventilation 95
STPD
state of gases at standard conditions 83, 392
Streptococcus pneumoniae (pneumococcus)
lobar pneumonia caused by 253
Superior Sulcus Tumors *See* Pancoast tumors
Surface tension 55
effect on lung compliance 55
Surfactant *See* Lung:surfactant
Surfactant containing proteins (SPs) *See* Alveoli:surfactant
Sympathetic nerves
lung innervation by 41

T

Temperature
role in regulating O_2 binding to hemoglobin 114
Thebesius veins
venae minimae 178
Three-compartment-model 168–71
functional equivalent of the real lung 91
Tibetans
adaptation to high altitude of 231
Tissue hypoxia
during exercise 219
Tissue oxygenation
at high altitude 224
during exercise at high altitude 227
Tonsil hypertrophy
role of in sleep apnea 213

Trachea
anatomy 36
histology 42
vascularized by branches of inferior thyroid artery 40
Trans Pulmonary Pressure (TPP) 63
Tuberculosis
cavities and fibrosis caused by 255
functional consequences of 255
granuloma formation in 255
pleural exudate effusion in 255

U

Unilateral/bilateral anterolateral stimulation 32

V

Vagus
lung innervation by 41
Valsalva maneuver 63
Veins
azigos 40
Vena cava (superior)
compression by mediastinal masses 264
Venae minimae (Thebesian veins)
conductive (anatomical) shunt caused by 178
Venous admixture *See* Shunt
Venous return
impaired
by mediastinal masses 264
by pneumomediastinum 263
Ventilation
effect of gravity on 157–59
effect of high altitude on 222
ideal 180
ideal *versus* effective 182–85
normal values 407

Ventilation-perfusion
improved distribution during exercise 219
inert-gas method for quantifying distribution, of 186
maldistribution
compensatory mechanisms 185–86
effect of gravity on 159–62
partial compensation by hypoxic vasoconstriction and hypocapnic bronchoconstriction 185
quantification 175–78
role in hypoxemia
determined by Rahn, Riley *et al*., and Otis *et al.* 22
ratio line 160
Venturi effect 74
Volume conversion equation 412

W

Water
composition
co-discovered by Lavoisier, A. Cavendish, H., Monge, G. and Watt, J. 10
vapor pressure values at different temperatures 406
Wedge pressure 221
Work of breathing 76

X

Xenon (^{133}Xe)
used to study lung perfusion-distribution 155

used to study lung ventilation-distribution *15*

Made in United States
Orlando, FL
04 November 2026

90200478R00270